AO Masters' Cases

Bernhard G. Weber

Minimax Fracture Fixation

AO Masters' Cases

Bernhard G. Weber

Minimax Fracture Fixation

with an introduction by René K. Marti

788 illustrations

Thieme

Design & typesetting: Sandro Isler, nougat, CH-4056 Basel
Illustrations: Sandro Isler, Zoe Koh, nougat, CH-4056 Basel
Scans: AO Media Service, CH-7270 Davos Platz

Library of Congress Cataloging-in-Publication Data is available from the publisher.

Legal restrictions

Great care has been taken to maintain the accuracy of the information contained in this publication. However, neither AO and/or Thieme, nor the editors and/or the authors can be held responsible for errors or any consequences arising from the use of the information contained in this publication. Contributions published under the name of individual authors are statements and opinions solely of said authors and not of AO Publishing or the AO Group.

Some of the product names, instruments, treatments, logos, designs, etc. referred to in this publication are also protected by patents and trademarks or by other intellectual property protection laws (eg, "AO", "ASIF", "AO/ASIF", "TRIANGLE/GLOBE Logo" are registered trademarks) even though specific reference to this fact is not always made in the text. Therefore, the appearance of a name, instrument, etc. without designation as proprietary is not to be construed as a representation by the publisher that it is in the public domain.

Hazards

The products, procedures, and therapies described in this work are only to be applied by certified and trained medical professionals in environments specially designed for such procedures. No suggested test or procedure should be carried out unless, in the user's professional judgment, its risk is justified. Whoever applies products, procedures, and therapies shown or described in this work will do this at his/her own risk. Because of rapid advances in the medical sciences, AO recommends that independent verification of diagnosis, therapies, drugs, dosages, and operation methods should be made before any action is taken.

Although all advertising material is expected to conform to ethical (medical) standards, inclusion in this publication does not constitute a guarantee or endorsement by the publisher regarding quality or value of such product or of the claims made of it by its manufacturer.

Distribution by Georg Thieme Verlag, Rüdigerstrasse 14, D-70469 Stuttgart, Germany and
Thieme New York, 333 Seventh Avenue, New York, NY 10001, USA

Printed in Germany

ISBN 3-13-139271-1
ISBN 1-58890-269-2

Introduction

René K. Marti

Summary

Despite his sometimes provoking ideas, Hardi Weber created many friends throughout his long-lasting career. The residents, visitors, and fellows who worked and stayed in contact with him became able to follow his constant evolution, take it over, and use it as a basis for further innovations. The duration of this process is why it took some time for his marginally modified ideas on the AO basic principles to be accepted and for him to be rediscovered worldwide as guest speaker on AO courses and committees.

His full training in orthopedic and trauma surgery resulted in his finding any general surgeons' consideration of fracture treatment as a side-occupation unacceptable, which led to some degree of confrontation. We are now well on the way to realizing his ideas; times have changed, former general trauma surgeons concentrate on lesions of the locomotor system, and in the near future orthopedic and trauma surgery will be one specialty, as in Hardi Weber's vision.

For Weber, the basis of orthopedic trauma surgery was biomechanical and biological knowledge in combination with technical skill and clinical instinct, which allowed for planned improvisation. Even if minimal invasive plate osteosynthesis (MIPO) was a logical further development of his MINIMAX techniques, he was afraid that 'cookbook surgery' would lead to incorrect indications and applications of the new implants. Relying on optimal asepsis, he clearly preferred open and not what he termed 'defensive' surgery in most situations.

In his opinion, basic implants can be adapted to the bone. He referred to the huge number of new anatomical plates as a "Beschlägeladen", which in German means more than just a hardware store.

On the other hand, he also realized that the new developments facilitate our work and that the training program of our young colleagues is no longer the same. They are used to indirect methods and some only know the anatomy from inside (endoscopy) or through the image intensifier. The non-reversible trend to superspecialization stimulates surgeons and manufacturers to create new implants, adapted to the anatomy.

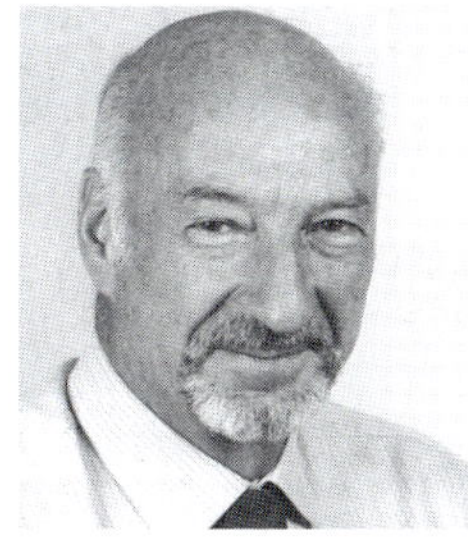

Bernhard Georg Weber (Hardi)
1927–2002

Dear Hardi,

Up until the day before your unexpected death, you were busy writing a book on your favorite trauma surgery topics. For me, it is both a great honor and pleasure to write the introduction, and the AO Foundation is delighted to recognize your merits by publishing your original ideas based on your extensive experience under the title: AO Masters' Cases—Minimax Fracture Fixation.

René Marti
Former co-worker
President of the AO Foundation 2002–2004

Especially for the many, really skilled orthopedic surgeons in the so-called developing countries, it is of great importance to read and see that good results do not only depend on implants and high-tech facilities.

Unfortunately, Hardi Weber's still relevant books dealing with the classification of malleolar fractures, pseudarthroses, fractures in children, special osteosyntheses, and external fixators are now out of print. Fortunately, however, in his last book he presents a summary of his most important contributions, with illustrations from his huge slide collection. It will certainly stimulate all of us to really reconsider asepsis, to analyze fracture patterns and their possible complications, and finally their optimal, but individualized treatment possibilities. Many surgeons worldwide, including myself, will confirm that Weber's technical and more philosophical contributions have influenced and will continue to influence our own view of orthopedic surgery.

Finally—certainly also in the name of Hardi Weber—I would like to thank AO International and especially AO Publishing for recognizing the importance of Hardi Weber's message and publishing the book in an extremely short time after his unexpected death.

Asepsis

When Prof Dr B.G. Weber took over the Orthopedic Department at the County Hospital in St. Gallen in 1967, the reported infection rates in trauma surgery and total joint replacement were too high. That was the period when the use of prophylactic antibiotics and antibiotic-loaded cement was advocated.

It was during my residency in St. Gallen that Weber, inspired by John Charnley, introduced the vertical laminar flow 'greenhouse' to diminish airborne contamination. At the same time, classical aseptic principles were perfected to avoid infection rising through skin incisions. The effectiveness of those anti-infection measures has been proven with multiple scientific studies, with and without antibiotic prophylaxis. The message is clear: Relying on antibiotics is not the way forward. We still primarily require a coordinated performance from the whole team to achieve the goal of integrated aseptic surgery, starting with the classical aseptic principles and with additional clean air. Young surgeons have a tendency to rely on antibiotics, but more ritual and more discipline seem to be necessary. We are clearly missing the 'dragon-like' chief nurse that forced us, the older generation, to respect optimal asepsis. Unfortunately, they are no longer so prominent and have been degenerated to office managers.

MINIMAX principle

By intuition and as a result of meticulous documentation, the St. Gallen Orthopedic Department, with Hardi Weber as a leader, already continuously adapted the classical, may be maximal invasive, AO principles in the 1960s. Careful anatomical joint reduction, more attention to the soft tissues and just stable but not per se rigid internal fixation was a logical, experience-based consequence. MINIMAX, maximum effect with a minimum of material and effort, still respecting basic biomechanical principles, was Weber's slogan, comparing the effectiveness with the well known portable fire extinguisher.

It has taken quite a period for this message to be adopted by those other than St. Gallen trainees. New slogans like atraumatic and biological osteosynthesis ending with minimal percutaneous internal fixation have been created.

The MINIMAX principle can be considered to fall between rigid maximal fixation and minimal invasive percutaneous procedures.

Weber poses some questions concerning new implants and clearly shows that a skilled surgeon can apply the main goals of the AO philosophy with a minimum of standard implants or external fixators—as long as basic biomechanical principles are respected.

Lower leg fractures

In 1966, Hardi Weber published his still valid classification of ankle fractures and their specific ligament lesions. The combination, lower leg and ankle fractures, was almost unknown at that time. After meticulous analysis of his huge slide collection, Weber compares the lower leg with the forearm and concludes that lower leg fractures are not just a broken tibia. The fibula, including syndesmotic ligaments and the membrana interossea (SLIM), need our attention to avoid malunion of the ankle joint. To aid expectation of the unexpected, Weber presents an extensively documented and illustrated new classification of lower leg fractures that respects potential ankle fractures, or in other words, he presents an additional classification of ankle fractures.

His therapeutic suggestions are clear, based on personal experience, and it is our task to prove that modern techniques like minimal invasive procedures, percutaneous plate insertions, or unreamed nails produce similar or better results. In his opinion, many fracture types still need open surgery because of the benefit of greater technical precision than can be achieved with defensive minimal invasive procedures.

Open fracture of the lower leg

For the treatment of open fractures, Weber advocates a clear, still valid prevention of contamination and a refined MINIMAX fixation technique that respects the bone and soft-tissue damage. Original standard implants can be used in different ways, the challenge being the skillful application of screws, plates, nails, external fixators, and soft-tissue management. Additional tissue violation must be avoided. Fixation techniques vary from case to case; multiple case presentations have shown nonstandard plating may be less traumatic than intramedullary nailing. He demonstrates that both temporary and permanent external fixation using the original threaded rod is a minimal invasive stable fixation that can be achieved with a few elements. The minimal open local internal fixation protected with an external fixator will provoke new useful discussions, as is the case for skin-lesion management.

Ankle joint

In this chapter, Weber returns to his favorite joint, the ankle and its neighborhood. He describes extremely useful hints and tricks in primary fracture treatment and secondary reconstructions, including author-specific techniques of supramalleolar osteotomy and joint fusions. The roots of the now popular mini-invasive simple Achilles tendon suture followed by functional aftercare are in St. Gallen, as are those of anatomical reconstruction of the lateral ligament complex.

Nonunions

Uncritical applications of the early AO principles of internal fixation clearly produced new types of nonunions. After conservative treatment, bony hypertrophy was the classic manifestation of a nonunion; vascular disturbance, especially following infection, led to atrophic real pseudarthrosis. St. Gallen was an international center for treating failed internal fixations. Weber's contributions to biological analysis, classification, and finally the biomechanically optimal surgical treatment have not changed essentially in 30 years (Weber BG, Čech O, Pseudarthrosen, 1973). Only expressions such as hypertrophic, normotrophic, and atrophic nonunions have been replaced by two types, biologically active and biologically inactive.

In the treatment of septic-defect nonunions, major changes have occurred, based on Ilizarov's contributions. Nevertheless, Weber's classical approach using an external fixator for stabilization and autogenous bone graft for biological stimulation are still used in the majority of the cases.

Autogenous bone transplantation

Even autogenous bone grafts, the best available material to restore bone defects, needs well vascularized and mechanically stable surroundings to avoid resorption. Weber demonstrates in multiple examples indication, behavior, integration, and transformation of transplanted autogenous bone grafts and mentions how to avoid potential morbidity at the different harvest sites. There are many examples of biological, MINIMAX—spine fusion—techniques with excellent results, worthy of consideration by spinal surgeons. Some other examples, such as lengthening procedures, may need to be seen in another light, namely diaphyseal callus distraction, using the same devices—Wagner lengthening device or Synthes external fixators.

Hardi Weber clearly demonstrates that autogenous bone grafting is an art that needs careful preoperative evaluation and an adapted postoperative treatment. In which case, even open cancellous bone grafts have still their indications. The results of this type of surgery depend on small details that are discussed here and are based on a very well described, extensive, personal experience.

Foreword

This book was written because of the repeated encouragement of former residents of mine at the Orthopedic Department of the County Hospital, St. Gallen, Switzerland (heads: M.E. Müller, 1960–1967, B.G. Weber 1967–1986, F. Magerl 1986–1994).

It is a historical document covering 1960–1994. Our Department developed its own identity regarding cold orthopedics and trauma surgery, which has become imprinted on all of us as surgeons.

In St. Gallen, we were assigned all sorts of disorders of the locomotor system to treat, trauma included, as is the norm in the Anglo-Saxon world, as well as in France, Italy, Holland, Belgium, and Scandinavia. In contrast, in Germany, Austria and also partially in Switzerland, trauma in general and fracture care specifically are claimed by general surgeons and mainly by so-called trauma-surgeons such as their former teachers L. Böhler and H. Bürkle-Delacamp. With this background, it is no wonder that the 'St. Gallen School', under the leadership of orthopedic surgeons, who had also qualified in general surgery, produced a certain degree of conflict with the Swiss AO members, who were general surgeons. General and trauma surgeons view problems differently to orthopedic surgeons.

The St. Gallen orthopedic fracture care unit, our local style according to Schlich, is laid out in this book. Such a document may encourage young orthopedic surgeons to stay interested in trauma surgery.

The history of the early AO Switzerland and the early AO International has been described by R. Schneider (1969, 1983), U. Heim (2001), and most comprehensively by Th. Schlich (2002). From the foundation of the AO in 1958 till now, the original AO principles have been gradually modified—some would say softened up—by continuous small revolutions. Originally, anatomical open reduction and (stable rigid) internal fixation (ORIF) provided functional postoperative treatment with the aim of avoiding all degrees of 'fracture disease'. These basic AO principles, with their target of 'Back to Normal' are despised today in favor of 'biologically minimal invasive' fixations.

Reduction is sufficient when alignment of shaft fragments and 'virtual' repositioning of articular fractures is achieved with the support of imaging and navigation. New, newer and newest implants are offered and recommended by the producers. Willing contemporary accident surgeons are organizing meetings and instructional courses with the aim of making us believe that their new philosophies and the modern 'implants' involved are indispensable.

"Il faut assurément des années de chirurgie orthopédique pour établir des techniques, préciser des indications et apprécier des résultats. Il faut surtout une bien plus longue expérience chirurgicale pour oser innover."

"Beyond all doubt, years and years of orthopedic surgery are needed to establish techniques, to define indications, and to judge results. Above all, an even much longer surgical experience is mandatory to dare innovations."

Pol Le Coeur, 1938

In 2000, Terry Canale and Augustus Sarmiento discussed various changes in the American orthopedic community. They recommended a return to more caring for the patients, more compassion for the profession, and criticized new technologies. Canale and Sarmiento's reflections accord with my 45-year experience in orthopedic and trauma surgery in Europe. "...Orthopedics is no longer a well-defined body of knowledge, acquired through a long and sophisticated period of training, but a series of surgical operations which anyone with a modicum of manual skill should be able to perform..." says A. Sarmiento. In other words: Today's surgeons, treating trauma, should find their way back from being jobbers to professionals. The 'normal' training has become shorter and shorter, as have the presence hours in the hospital, reducing from approximately 80–50 h a week with the result that together with the increasing number of interns and residents, quantity and quality of training is 'diluted', with a trend to homoepathic dosage. This deficit cannot be compensated for by attending workshops and meetings and by the use of e-technologies, navigation, and robotics.

Till 25 years ago, St. Gallen residents were trained for 10–15 years. To various degrees thereafter they enjoyed professional success and satisfaction. Many of them became teachers and continued to train their own pupils in the spirit Canale and Sarmiento tried to reactivate in the United States of America.

In this book, the orthopedic surgeons from St. Gallen will find patients and cases they operated on according to our local principles of fracture care. In retrospect, I thank them for their collaboration during their residency in St. Gallen. I thank them for the friendship that I enjoy and share with them at every occasion. We are also enjoying the late recognition of our St. Gallen AO concepts outside of Switzerland, mainly by our colleagues in the American AO, approximately 20 of whom came to us as visiting fellows.

With the following list—in alphabetical order—I express my deep respect for my last chief of surgery and for my former residents, and current residents and partners:

Jean-Pierre Ackermann, Peter Aebersold, Parvis Afchampour, Theodor Albrecht, Annemarie Anderhub, Miguel Aparicio, Felix Augstburger, Klaus Barth, Pal Benum, Pierre Berruex, Lukas Birrer, Andreas Bischof, Roman Bischofberger, Georg Blatter, Roland Blatter, Alexandre Boitzy, Hans-Ruedi Bollag, Peter Andreas Brändli, Christian F. Brunner, Hansbeat Burch, Peter Burkart, Felix Buschor, Marco Casanova, Oldrich Čech, Eric Courvoisier, Alfred Debrunner, Maurus Dörig, Dietrich Dressler, Marcel Duc, Jan Dvorak, Andreas Egli, Pieter Elzenga, Thomas Fiechter, Edi Fornaro, Hossein Forudastan, Ueli Freihofer, Franz Freuler, Ernesto Frick, Dieter Domenic Gmür, Tilman Goerttler, Walter Grädel, Silvio Grass, Dieter Grob, Mavrtin Gubler, Hans Güntert, Felix Hardegger, Günther Henke, Paul Holenstein, Heinrich Huber, Rainer Janssen, Remigi Joller, Peter Jörg, François Kaech-Dehm, Fritz Kägi, Urs Kappeler, Adi Klammer, Hanspeter Knüsel, Reinhard Kölbel, Werner König, George Kouwenhoven, Josef Kramer, Jörn Urs Kübler, Poulose Kulangara, Ulrich Kunath, Marcel Lauber, Paul Lauber, Karl L. Ledermann, Hans-Leopold Lehner, André Liberek, René Liechti, Jean-Jacques Loertscher, Friedrich Paul Magerl, René Konrad Marti, Georges Mayor, Peter Mehmann, Wolfgang Meier, Alfons Merki, Christoph Meuli, Hans-Rudolf Meyer, Fritz Minger, Gerold Müller, Giacomo P. Müller, Hanny Müller, Maurice E. Müller, Andrea Mumenthaler, Harald Nittner, Jörg Oberhammer, Otto Oest, Eduardo Patow, Daniel Pelet, Ernst Raaymakers, Valentin Rehli, Alfred Reichen, Marco Rimoldi, Lorentz Rolfsen, Manfred Ruckelshausen, Georg Bernhard Ruflin, Axel Rüter, Ulrich Saxer, Urs Albert Schneider, Gottfried Segmüller, Gontran Sennwald, Hans-Peter Sieber, August Spiess, Fritz-Beat Sprenger, Ruedi Spring, Regula Steiger, Hans Steinhauer, Ueli Stucki, Karl Gerhart Stühmer, Frithjof Süssenbach, Reto P. Tissi, Adrian Urfer, Harold Vasey, Bruno Walser, John Ward, Peter Wettstein, Luc Weydert, Ulrich Wiedmer, Benedikt Winkler, Georges Wohlgensinger, Robert Wohlwend, Christoph Wolfensberger, Otto Wörsdörfer, André Wyss, Michel-Bertrand Zadory, Herbert Zimmermann, Klaus Zöch, Jürg Heinrich Zweifel.

I also thank very much Silvia Noto, my secretary, Anneliese Spitz and Veronica Baur, photographic laboratory, County Hospital, St. Gallen for their great work in the production of this book.

Bernhard G. Weber
Fall 2002

Preface

„Et surtout il n'y a pas de culture sans liberté."

„And above all, there is no culture without liberty."

Eugène Ionesco, 1979

This book does not compete in any way with the AO Manuals. But those, who read this book must be familiar with the AO principles and the AO textbooks. Although this book is not a textbook, it does discuss selected fracture subjects, most of which—though not all—have already been outlined in former publications. It addresses specialists in orthopedic surgery, especially in trauma care, and not 'beginners'. The reader is confronted with solutions to problems that are in some way different from the AO gospel. Those readers who know our rules, elaborated in St. Gallen, will find themselves at home with their own experience. The other readers will find our interpretation of the 'official' AO challenge—back to normal. Not implants, but treatments with original implants are discussed.

The chapters have been arbitrarily chosen according to the importance we feel they deserve. The described problems and solutions are based on approximately 125,000 performed operations, half and half trauma and cold orthopedics from 25 years at the Orthopedic Department, County Hospital, St. Gallen, and on approximately 20,000 operations performed by myself. The described surgery is approved, that is to say evidence based. Statistics may be found in other of our publications. According to the Pisa Study, figures are now more easily read than the written word, so the large number of cases and figures may speak for themselves.

The x-ray series have been chosen from my collection of about 80,000 slides taken from 1960 till now. All x-ray figures were produced photographically without electronic manipulation, in other words: They are real. Most x-rays are dated, which allows us to recognize when the patients were treated and when they were followed-up. Important to note is that through all the years the original standard implants were used. The surgery in contrast was and is not always 'standard' according to the AO gospel of the time. Surgical experience compares with the findings in a bore-core of the Arctic ice-shield. This book is a selection of the bore-core findings of my 40 years' surgical activity.

The local St. Gallen AO style, as it was named by the historian Th. Schlich, is expressed here.

Bernhard G. Weber
Fall 2002

Table of contents

3 Lower leg fractures with and without involvement of the ankle joint

4 Open fractures of the lower leg

5 Trauma of the ankle joint and of its neighborhood

6 Biodynamics, classification, and treatment of nonunions

7 Autogenous bone transplantation

1 Asepsis and the risk of infection
From conventional asepsis to sterile enclosure

1 Introduction

Pasteur (1822–1895) and Koch (1843–1910) discovered microorganisms as a source of fermentation, decay and infection. Based on this knowledge, the prevention of postoperative infection became possible for the first time.

In the 1867 publication 'On the antiseptic principle in the practice of Surgery', Joseph Lister [1] describes **antisepsis** by atomized carbolic acid in the operating room and by carbolic acid wound dressings. He assumed and proved that **wound contamination and infection** were **airborne**. Lethality after amputations dropped from 43–15% under his antiseptic principle.

Semmelweis (1818–1865) perceived puerperal fever **as contamination and infection** through the **dirty hands** of the obstetrician and the midwife. His meticulous **disinfection of the hands** with calcium chloride reduced the lethality after delivery impressively—**asepsis** was born.

From the end of the 19th century, Lister's antisepsis was step-by-step replaced by the development of **classical asepsis**. Direct contamination of the wound with surgical material, hands, and instruments was prevented. **Sterilization of surgical material**, disinfection of the hands of the surgical team, mouth-nose masks, sterile gloves, sterile draping, disinfection of the patient's skin and finally skin coverage with iodine impregnated adhesive plastic drapes became routine.

With the perfection of classical asepsis, infections following aseptic surgery and childbirth became rarer, but they continued to be frightening events, the horror of surgery.

Flemming discovered penicillin in 1928 and Domagk discovered sulfonamid prontosil in 1935. Successful antibiotic treatment of infected wounds, of pneumonia and other conditions became available. Gradually, these and new antibiotics since the late 1940s have been used prophylactically, becoming routine for many surgical procedures nowadays.

Since **prophylactic antibiotics** have been administrated and since operating rooms have been equipped with modern airconditioning systems, airborne contamination no longer seems to be a major problem, at least at first sight.

Blood loss control, ever better tolerated anesthesias, and prophylactic antibiotics have permitted amazing progress in surgery [2]. Mankind is continuously informed by the mass media about what contemporary surgery, standard and heroic, is able to offer. When watching such surgery on television, the operating rooms are usually crowded with people: the operating team, the anesthetic team, the supply team, navigational and robotic equipment, and television teams and observers. The air in the operating room must be loaded with particles and microbes released by everybody present. Without the advantage of prophylactic antibiotics, surgery would collapse under the inevitable airborne contamination.

The load of microbes in operating rooms is well known [3–10]. Therefore prophylactic administration of antibiotics [11, 12] is the concession by the surgeons to the fact that the open wound is inoculated during surgery and that potential infection must be prevented prophylactically. **'Prophylactic', however, is the wrong expression;** one should speak of **therapeutic antibiotics against contamination and infection**. More and more microbes are generating strains that resist antibiotics and they are growing to be a serious menace to mankind [13–16].

Not every branch of surgery suffers the same risk of infection of airborne contamination [17, 18]. Surgery on well vascularized soft tissues is less burdened by infections. The patient's own antimicrobial defense and the prophylactic antibiotics are the victors in the battle with wound contamination.

Implant surgery suffers from a higher infection risk [17–21]. Infection after implant surgery may end in disaster for the patient, in spite of antibiotic preventive and anti-infection treatment. Implants are foreign bodies without a blood supply and without self-defense. At the time of surgery and shortly after, they are surrounded by a contaminated dead space. Antibiotics may fail when the necessary local concentration level is not reached.

Surgically treated complex and open fractures have an infection rate several times higher than simple and closed fractures [1, 18]. Open fractures suffer from disruption of the blood supply to fragments, from damaged devitalized tissues and from dead spaces left behind, regardless the type of treatment. Surgically treated closed fractures, in contrast, enjoy much less blood supply deficit and less soft-tissue damage. The local resistance is undisturbed due to intact vascularity. Antibiotics can reach the site of contamination. Nevertheless, all operated on fractures are at risk of infection if they are not protected by prophylactic antibiotics.

When general surgeons do not perform implant surgery or open reduction and internal fixations of fractures, they are not as aware of the risk of infection [18]. It is interesting to note that **minimal invasive trauma surgery** was mainly initiated by so-called trauma and general surgeons. They seem to believe the risk of infection to be reduced when fractures are not opened generously, as has been recommended by the AO [22] since 1960.

The enthusiasm for minimal invasive fracture treatment, ie, 'keyhole-surgery', is not at all shared by orthopedic surgeons operating under **sterile enclosure conditions**. They do not have the problem of airborne contamination and take **advantage of open surgery** [18]. 'Precision surgery' is only possible with open reduction, open osteotomy, open arthroplasty. Such quality challenge calls for a supplement to classical asepsis and to prophylactic antibiotic administration. Airborne contamination either directly into the open wound or indirectly via instruments, implants and the surgeon's hands must be avoided [4, 23] in analogy to the pharmaceutical, food and electronic industries by **surgery in a clean-air environment**.

Increasing concern over viral transmission of HIV and hepatitis, enforces more and more precautions to minimize the risk for patients and for staff alike [24]. The same awareness should be raised regarding airborne contamination and infection.

2 How does airborne contamination and infection occur?

Each person is a permanent source of microbe release: With shed hair and skin cells, with droplets from the respiratory tract and via the anus, microbes are released into the clothes and from there into the ambient air. Moschner [25] counted 1 million microbes released from a person every minute and identified their leakage out of modern operating room gowning (Fig. 1-1).

The more people in an operating room [26] and the poorer its ventilation equipment, the higher the air content of particles and microbes [27–31]. In contrast: In the Arctic and in the high mountains, the air is bacteriologically clean. In this environment, man and animals as a source of microbes are absent or rare.

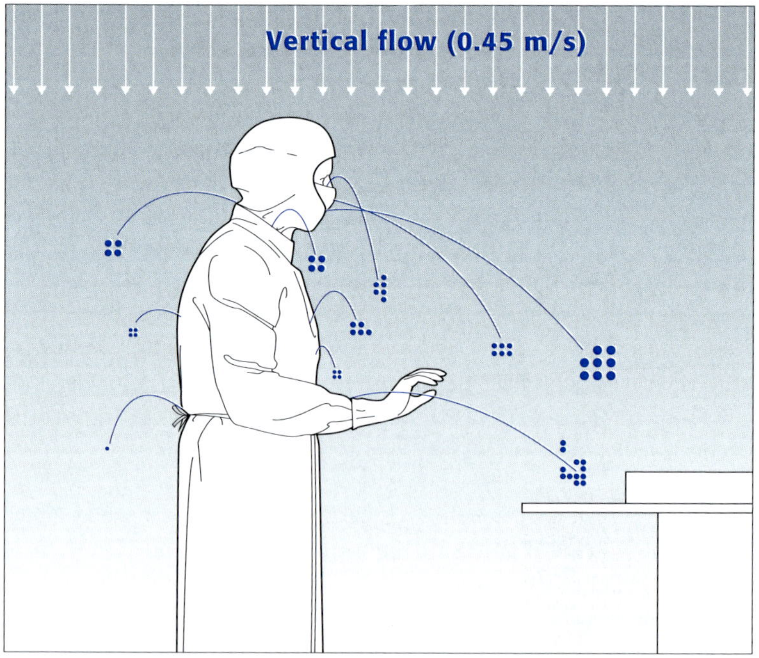

Fig. 1-1 Modern gowning and particle-germ release.
1 million particles or germs are generated per minute by one person. In spite of modern gowning, remarkable leakage occurs from the head and sleeves. (Figure redrawn with permission of Carsten Moschner.)

3 How to lower the number of microbes in operating rooms

In spite of prophylactic antibiotic treatment, the classical aseptic principles should be maintained [27, 32, 33]. In fact, the asepsis should be 'augmented' by the prevention of airborne contamination.

According to common sense, the best way to prevent the release of microbes would be the enclosure of every person in a microbe-proof gown with body-exhaust system (Fig. 1-2). This solution, however, is logistically impossible for everyone in the operating theatres.

The second best solution is to reduce the number of people as far as possible close to the open wound. This can be achieved by dividing the theater into two zones [29, 34–38]. Everyone that has nothing directly to do with the surgical procedure is banned from the open wound (Fig. 1-3).
The **very best way to prevent airborne contamination** is the **Whitcomb-Charnley system** [4–7, 10, 23, 36–38, 39–45]. The surgical team works in a sterile enclosure that is ventilated with sterile air. The team is meticulously gowned with microbe-proof clothing and gloves [43, 46–48]. The body-exhaust system continuously removes the contaminated respiration air and the air from inside the gown [9, 41, 42, 44, 45] (Fig. 1-4).

The vertical airflow prevents the potentially contaminated air circulating uncontrolled in the theater. Numerous tests with sterile smoke (sulphuric acid aerosol) visualize the difference between conventional and Whitcomb-Charnley air-control in the operating room (Fig. 1-5).

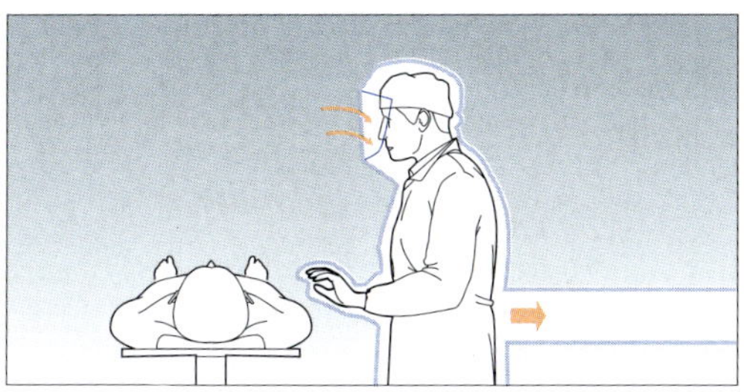

Fig. 1-2 Unrealistic proposal.
Body-exhaust system for all personnel working in the operating theaters.

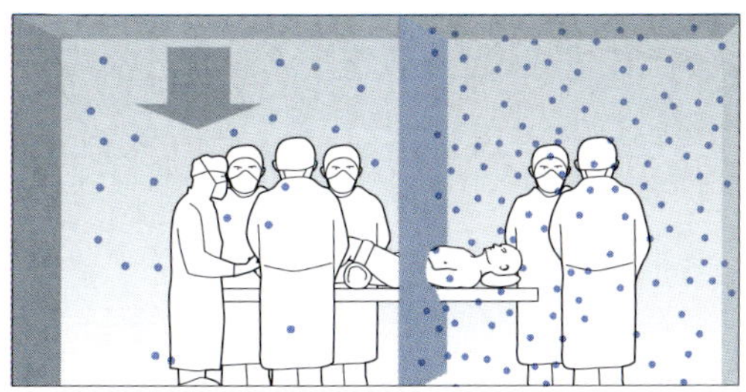

Fig. 1-3 Realistic proposal.
Separation of the area of surgery from the other areas in the operating theater by a separating wall. Fewer people produce less air contamination and fewer airborne bacteria (blue dots).

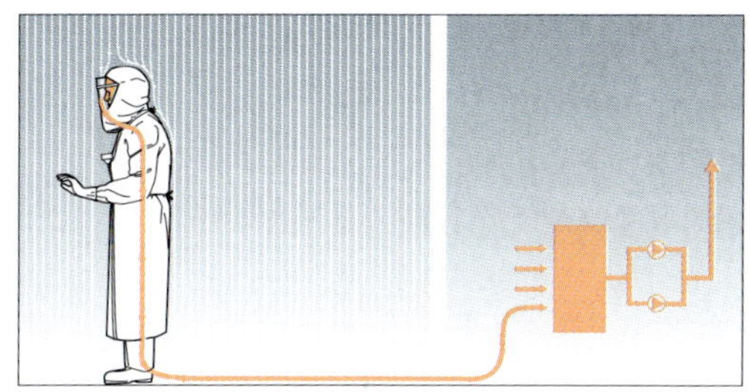

Fig. 1-4 Best proposal: Whitcomb-Charnley Principle. Body-exhaust suits. Vertical flow of sterile air in an enclosure, separated from the operating theater. Evacuation of respiration air and particles from inside: output 35 litres air per minute per person.

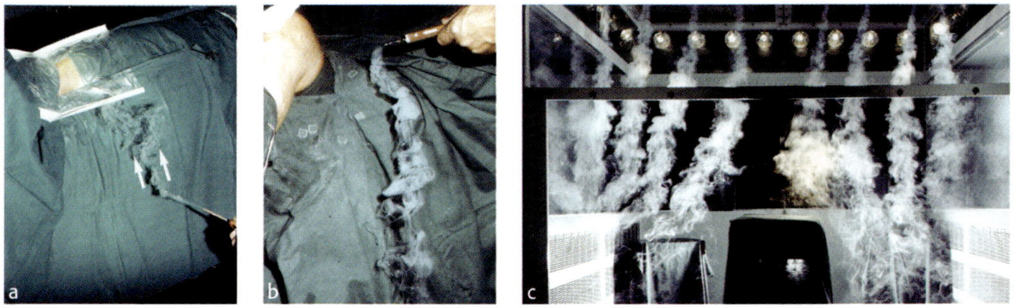

Fig. 1-5a–c Smoke tests.
a Modern, but conventional air conditioning: Contaminated air circulates uncontrolled and down-up in the thermal of the lamps.
b Sterile vertical flow: Air flows downward with a speed of 0.5 m/sec.
c Smoke test in the enclosure: Piston-like vertical airflow washes away all potential polluting particles and germs continuously.

4 Bacteriological investigations

Since 1970, most of our orthopedic surgery at our former and current institution has been performed under Whitcomb-Charnley conditions, typically joint replacement, internal fracture fixation, repair of ruptured Achilles tendon, and other surgery with infection risk.

In the 1970s, in collaboration with the Swiss University of Technology (ETH), Zürich, and with the Institute of Hygiene, we performed extensive bacteriological investigations [29, 34, 36, 39–42, 44, 45, 49]. The bacteriology in different theaters in the same operating theater suite was investigated. The same surgeons and the same staff worked under different conditions:

- In a sterile enclosure with a body-exhaust system.
- In a theater divided into two zones with a body-exhaust system.
- In two conventional theatres with conventional gowning.

Bacteriological samples were taken with Anderson and Sartorius samplers [35] (Fig. 1-6a–g) from the air in the theater, from the neighborhood of the open wound, from the instrument table, and from the front of the operating surgeon at the level of the chest and stomach. Swab tests were taken from the skin incision and from the depth of the wound. Patch tests were taken from the mouth-nose mask, from the gown front, from the forearms and the hands of the surgeon and the scrub nurse. Encouraged by our results, similar investigations have been performed at other institutions [50–52].

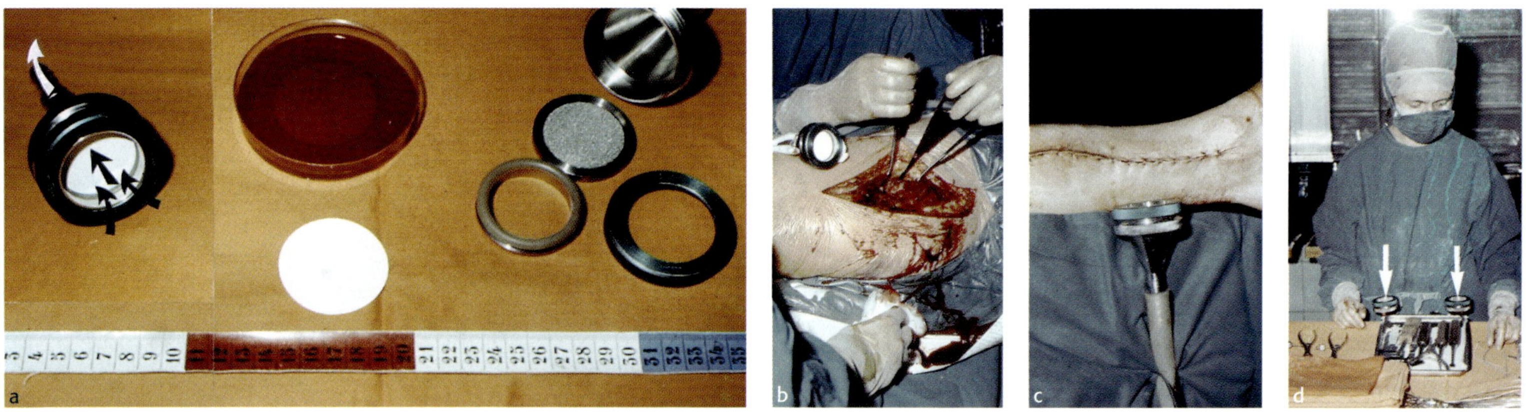

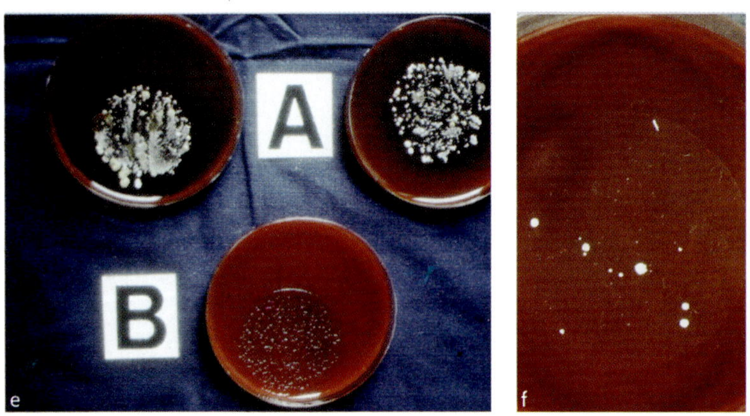

Fig. 1-6a–f Sartorious filter technique.

a The sterile equipment: mounted air collector to be fitted on a sterile hose and a pump aspirating air. Petri dish to accept the gelatine filter from the air collector. Dismantled air collector.

b Air germ collection close to the operating field. Hip replacement.

c Fracture fixation while air germ collecting.

d Germ collection from the instrument table.

e Bred petri dishes:

A From two modern but conventional theaters: masses of germ colonies.

B From the sterile enclosure: no germ growth.

f From the germ-stop wall theater: only a small number of airborne colonies. Staphylococcus albus and aureus are recorded.

4.1 Counting of airborne bacteria

Fig. 1-7 shows the outcome of airborne bacteria counting in different operating theaters from 8–12 o'clock during surgery:

OR 1 Sterile enclosure with body-exhaust system: almost zero load.

OR 2 Separating-wall theater with body-exhaust system: bacterial load below 100/m³ air, peak of 400/m³ at the time of the preparation for the second operation around 9 o'clock.

OR 3 Old-fashioned theater built 1960. Conventional gowning: bacterial load 200–550/m³ air.

OR 4 Modern theater built 1972, DIN-Norm 1946/4, conventional gowning: bacterial load 200–250/m³ air with two peaks at the time of the preparation for surgery after 8 and 10 o'clock.

In the separating-wall theater, bacteria were counted on both sides of the wall (Fig. 1-8): in the surgical section, the load was below 100/m³. The high peak occurred at the time of fluoroscopy, when the wall had to be opened to bring in the x-ray machine. On the other side of the wall, the bacterial load was always higher between 50–350 bacteria/m³.

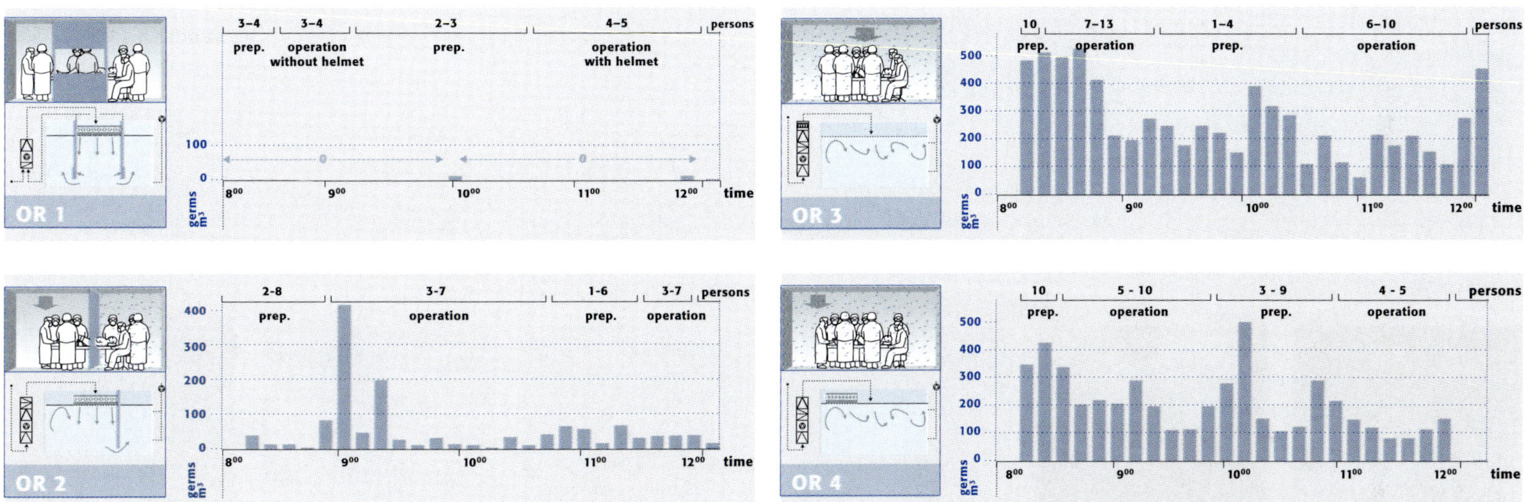

Fig. 1-7 Different germ pollution in different theaters. Air tests from 8–12 o'clock during surgery.
OR 1 Sterile enclosure.
OR 2 Germ-stop wall and conventional gowning.
OR 3 Conventional theater.
OR 4 Conventional modern theater.
The pollution load is impressive:
OR 1 Almost zero germs.
OR 2 Moderate pollution.
OR 3 Heavy load up to 500 germs/m³.
OR 4 Heavy load up to 400 germs/m³.
The highest levels occur during the patients' preparation—the sterile enclosure is outstanding in quality.

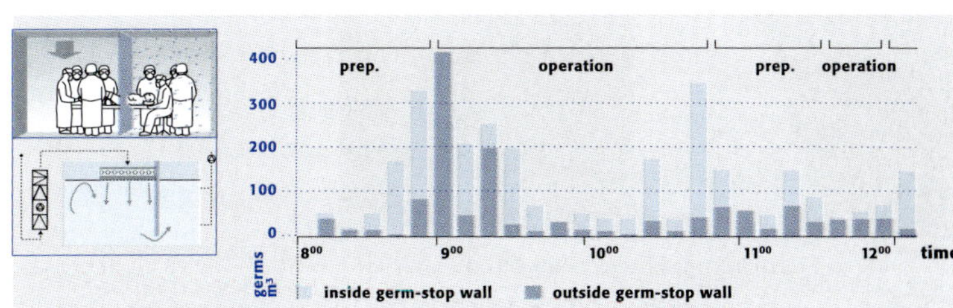

Fig. 1-8 Air pollution in the germ-stop wall theater and immediately outside. The pollution is evidently lower in the operating area (black columns) than in the 'outside' anesthesia area (gray columns). The highest peaks occur fortunately during the patients' preparation and not during surgery—which is nevertheless cold comfort.

4.2 Swab tests taken from the incision prior to skin closure (Fig. 1-7)

OR 1	20% positive tests under standard skin-preparation and adhesive plastic-sheet coverage [53] (before 1984). 0% positive tests when the skin-incision was also disinfected and covered with iodine/Betadine-soaked towels (since 1984).
OR 2	40% positive tests
OR 3	80% positive tests
OR 4	60% positive tests

This investigation reveals two sources of wound contamination:

- airborne,
- from the skin incision itself, releasing bacteria from hair follicles, sebaceous bulbs and sweat glands.

20% positive tests in the sterile enclosure are from the skin alone since the air is free of bacteria. Logically, the tests became negative when the skin incision was disinfected instantly and continuously with Betadine-soaked towels.

4.3 Swab tests deep from the wound and infection rate

Evaluation of 2,034 aseptic orthopedic operations in 1983:

OR 1	Swab+	6.5%	infection rate	0.45%
OR 2	Swab+	9.5%	infection rate	1.15%
OR 3	Swab+	9.8%	infection rate	2.80%
OR 4	Swab+	9.95%	infection rate	3.15%

75% of the positive swab tests in OR 1 are from patients who had previously had surgery in a conventional theater—they were bacteria carriers with a high risk of infection.

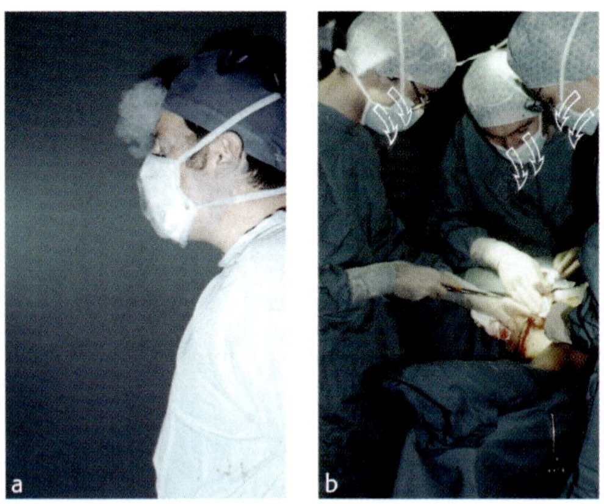

Fig. 1-9a–b Conventional head protection.

a Today's masks are inefficient. They do not retain germ-loaded respiration air (test with cigarette smoke).

b Unprotected skin is continuously 'losing' particles and germs (arrows).

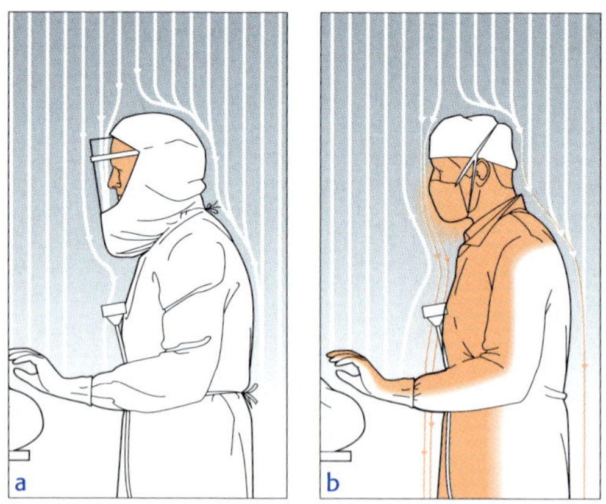

Fig. 1-10a–b Self-contamination in vertical airflow.

a Body-exhaust equipment prevents self-contamination. Patch tests negative.

b Conventional head protection allows self-contamination, the more contamination, the poorer the head protection is. Patch tests positive.

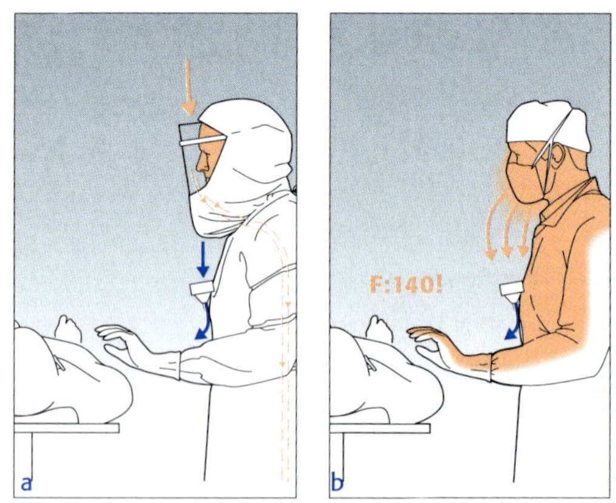

Fig. 1-11a–b Self-contamination in vertical airflow measured with the Sartorius technique.

a Body-exhaust equipment: 0.25 germs/m^3 air.

b Standard head protection: 35 germs/m^3, ie, factor 1:140 of cleanliness with scaphander compared with the mouth-nose mask.

4.4 Patch tests

Patch tests taken in the sterile enclosure with a body-exhaust system were almost all negative. In contrast, most patch tests were positive in the conventional theaters.

Of special interest was the question: "Is there a difference in the vertical flow of the enclosure if an exhaust-system scaphander or if conventional cap and mask are used?"

The answer:

- Patch tests under exhaust conditions were negative.
- Patch tests were, in contrast, regularly positive when the surgeons used standard head protection. The source of the bacteria was identified with patch testing from the surgeons' face and from the leakage of the mouth-mask (Fig. 1-9). The self-contamination runs downwards along the chest to the stomach and along the arms to the surgeons' hands (Fig. 1-10).
- Sartorius-sampling exhibited a bacterial load ratio of 1:140 (Fig. 1-11).

These results require meticulous gowning and head protection of the surgical team. Most importantly, low germ release depends on perfect sterile caping and masking (Fig. 1-12). However, total bacteria release is only eliminated when a body-exhaust system with head scaphander is used.

Horizontal flow is much less efficient. Our own experiments (Fig. 1-13) lack the 'laminar' wash-out effect of corresponding vertical flow.

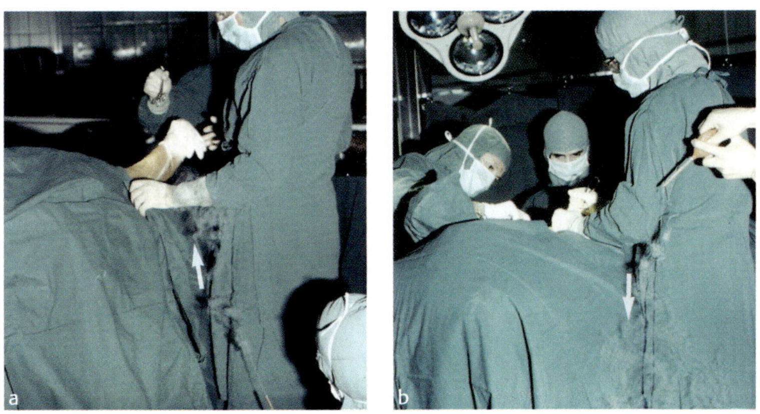

Fig. 1-12a–b Air pollution in different air conditions.
a In the conventional theater, the air circulates (smoke probe) upwards (arrows) in the thermal of the lamp above the operating field. Germ release mixes with the uncontrolled airflow and pollutes the whole ambient atmosphere.
b In vertical flow, particles orgerms are directed downwards to the open wound according to the smoke test (arrow).

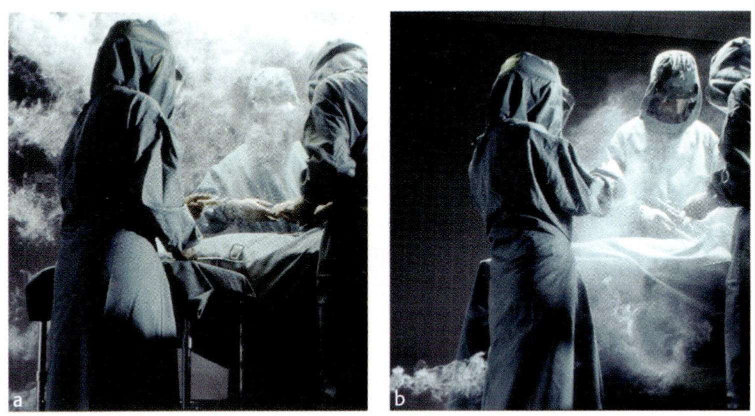

Fig. 1-13a–b Air turbulence in horizontal flow.
a In horizontal flow, objects (lamp, operation table, etc) and the team generate uncontrollable turbulence with a high risk of wound contamination.
b In addition, there is a tendency for flow deviation from the floor upwards to the wound.

5 Germ spectrum

- Airborne germs, collected with Anderson and Sartorius sampler:

Staphylococcus albus	70%
Staphylococcus aureus	20%
Streptococcus haemoliticus	5%
Other	5%

- Swab tests from the skin incision and deep from the wound:

Staphylococcus albus	80%
Staphylococcus aureus	14%
Enterococcus, E. coli	3%
Klebsiella	1%
Pseudomonas	1%
Streptococcus haemolyticus	1%

- Germs found in infections following primary and secondary total hip replacement and revisions:

Staphylococcus albus	56%
Staphylococcus aureus	19%
Streptococcus haemoliticus	12.5%
Enterococcus, E. coli	6%
Clostridium perfringes	6%

6 Sterile enclosure and antibiotics

The Nelson and the Lidwell **[54, 55]** reports (below) demonstrate that antibiotics are lowering the infection rate both in the conventional and in the enclosure theater. The question of which cases fall through the net of prevention remains unanswered, however.

Nelson report—total hip replacements (THR)

	w/o antibiotics	w/antibiotics	Total
Conventional operating room	1,880/109 5.8	6,791/90 1.3	8,671/199 2.3
Ultraclean operating room	2,754/17 **0.6**	2,754/17 **0.6**	5,484/35 **0.6**
Total	4,610/127	9,545/107	1,4155/234

Lidwell report—total hip and knee replacements*

	w/o antibiotics	w/antibiotics	Total
Conventional operating room	1,161/39 3.4	2,968/24 0.8	4,133/63 1.5
Ultraclean operating room	1,060/13 1.2	2,863/10 0.3	3,922/23 0.6
Total	2,221/52	5,831/34	8,055/86

* There was little difference in the (infection) rate between patients with replacement hips (6,781/69; 1.02%) and those with replacement knees (1,274/17; 1.33%).

Our own investigation from 1970–1981 for THR in the sterile enclosure showed the following results:

Primary THR	**1,367**	**0.36%**	infections ratio 1:10!
Secondary THR	**874**	**3.8%**	infections
Total	2,241	1.74%	infections

2,241 THRs were analyzed without or with antibiotics.

Total hip replacement 1970–1975 without antibiotic prophylaxis:

Primary THR	**0.6%**	infections
Secondary THR	**4.0%**	infections
Total	1.8%	infections

THR 1976–1981 with antibiotic prophylaxis:

Primary THR	**0.16%**	infections
Secondary THR	**5.20%**	infections
Total	1.49%	infections

The analysis shows that the infection rate is lowered with antibiotics only in primary, 'virgin' THR, but not in cases of secondary THR. In the secondary THR, the primary surgery had been performed in a conventional theater, either in our own operating theater or elsewhere. This suggests that these patients are carriers of antibiotic-resistant germs or suffer from locally reduced resistance or that antibiotics do not reach the necessary bactericidal concentration locally.

The 'Ackermann' report from 1983 discusses our resident P. Ackermann's study of swab tests and infection rates in our four different theaters with the following results from 1,774 operations:

	Sterile enclosure	Separation wall	Conventional old theater	Theater DIN 1946
No of operations	672	885	286	191
No of swab tests	44	84	28	19
Positive swab tests	6.5%	9.5%	9.8%	9.95%
No of infections	3	10	8	6
% infections to positive swab tests	6.8%	11.9%	28.6%	31.5%
% infections to no of operations	0.45%	1.15%	2.8%	3.15%

The positive swab tests ranged between 6% and 10% in the four theaters. The infections per positive swab test exhibited a ratio of 1:2:4:5. The infection rate related to the different theatres exhibited a ratio of 1:3:6:7. All 1,774 operations were primary aseptic ones, orthopedics and open fixations of closed fractures, done by the same surgeons and staff along the same technical criteria. The only relevant difference was a different air condition and different gowning. Body-exhaust equipment was always used in the enclosure, but was only used occasionally in the separation wall theater and never in the two conventional operating rooms.

In the enclosure, systemic antibiotics and antibiotic-loaded bone cement were used only for the secondary total hip replacements or in cases of revisions. Antibiotics, however, were routinely used in all other three theaters.

The infection rates favor the enclosure for preventing infections.

These results also justified the current surgical practice of using antibiotics prophylactically and antibiotic-loaded bone cement for THR when ultraclean air facilities are not available, otherwise, the infection rates would be higher.

7 Actual infection rate report 1999–2000

In 1999 and 2000 in our orthopedic institution at Rosenberg, St. Gallen and Heiden, 5,600 aseptic orthopedic operations were performed by ten surgeons in three theaters: two were complete, sterile enclosures and one was a downward laminar flow theater without curtains. Conventional theatres were not used.

The body-exhaust system was strictly used for joint replacement—hip, knee, shoulder—but usually not for all other orthopedic surgery.

Out of the 5,600 operations, the following infections occurred:

Shoulder	4	
Arthroscopy knee	4	
Knee ligament	3	
Spine	2	In vertical flow with conventional gowning, cap, and mask 5,227 operations 23 infections = 0.44%
Toe	3	
Hand	1	
Plastic	1	
Fracture fixation	1	
Achilles	1	
Ankle fusion	1	
Peridural catheter	2	
THR, TKR, TSR	2	
Total	25	Infections = 0.44%

Almost all patients had prophylactic antibiotics, either as single shot or for 1–3 days (Cephalosporine 2nd generation, 3×2 g/day). The indication was fear of local infection or a urinary catheter or peridural pain control or a combination thereof.

The senior surgeon (the author) is the only one who refused to administer antibiotic treatment in the absence of a non-orthopedic indication.

One may argue that 0.5% infections is a low infection rate so why change anything?

My personal arguments include:

- Most of our infections could probably have been avoided if all patients had been operated on by the surgical team with a body-exhaust system.
- The infection rate would have been higher if our patients had not had laminar flow facilities.
- Contrary to common sense, the complete Charnley-practice is not used regularly for all types of orthopedic surgery by our group of surgeons. Our behavior is irrational: Personal preference, ie, the non-acceptance of the entire enclosure 'ritual', except for total joint replacement, is a fact.
- When surgeons were patients and as all other informed patients when asked if they wish to be operated on under sterile enclosure or conventional theater conditions, always decided on the safer option. They requested for themselves the highest security against infection—not only the best surgeon!
- When comparing the infection rates in 1999 and 2000, of 0.44% without and 0.536% with the body-exhaust system, the question of whether Charnley's concept is justified surfaces again. The answer is that the types of operation are different: Joint replacement surgery and its infection consequences are more serious, causing more risk than most other orthopedic procedures.

As reported earlier, almost all infections of THR occurred after secondary THR. In primary THR, infection is almost totally prevented by the Charnley clean-air practice—even without antibiotic prophylaxis.

Hematogenetic disseminated infection was in my experience proven only twice (gall bladder, maxillary-dental infection) **[56]**:

1. Late infection of a THR 5 years after surgery immediately following an acute infection of the gall bladder with Coli and Enterococcus.

2. After a THR-revision, immediate infection with Staphylococcus aureus caprae. Hematogenous dissemination from a chronic tooth granuloma with the same germ. The patient is a veterinarian working in South Africa breeding antelopes for consumption.

8 30 years of surgical clean-air conduct

8.1 General

Clean-air surgery depends on the following requirements:

- Effectiveness, ie, prevention of wound airborne contamination.
- Renunciation or at the least reduction of antibiotic consumption down to single-shot administration for medico-legal reasons only.
- Low investment and running costs no higher than for conventional air conditioning.
- Regular testing of the enclosure filters [57] and of all technical equipment.
- A 'ritual' for the surgical team that does not interfere with the well-being of the personnel. The clean-air 'outfit' must be easy to use and should improve and enrich the physical comfort of the users, not the opposite.

8.2 The enclosure and the separating-wall system

Both, the enclosure and the separating-wall systems [29, 30, 58] can be built primarily in a new building or set-up in an existing operating theater.

The clean-air supply for both patterns is focused on the site of surgery. The surroundings take advantage of the overflow of clean air since that air is sterile, filtered rough, then fine, then with high efficient particle absorption HEPA and conditioned (temperature, moistening) [59] (Fig. 1-14).

Depending on the size of the whole operating theater suite, additional conditioned air may be necessary. My partner since 1970, Robert Meierhans [30, 58], who is an engineer, has given copious advice on how to organize these matters. The challenge is to optimize the air conditioning in the whole surgical suite, with priority of the surgeons' working environment.

New in such an operating theater is the implication of more 'ritual' and more discipline. Integral asepsis cannot be bought with equipment. Ultraclean-air operating rooms require corresponding behavior from those who are working in them.

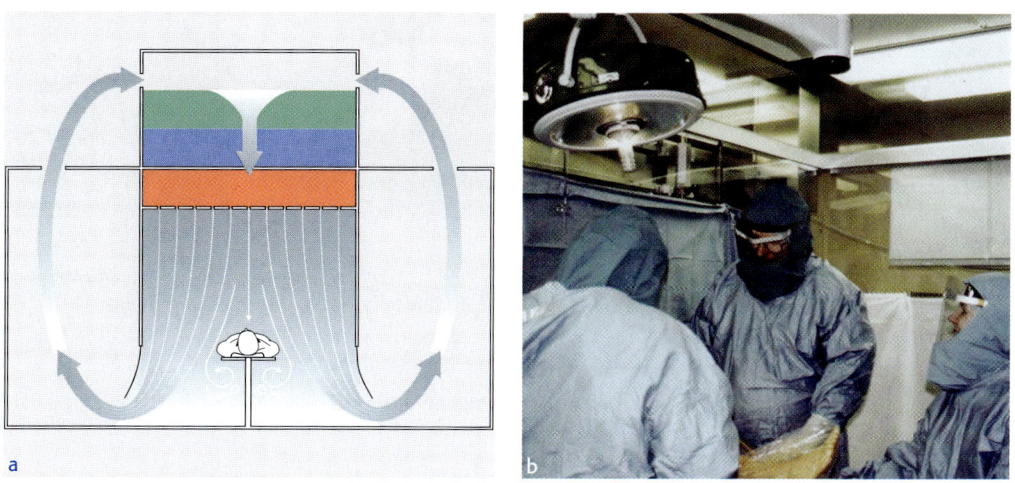

Fig. 1-14a–b Ultraclean-air operating rooms.
a The principal technology: The air circuit is conditioned and then pressurized through rough (green), fine (blue), and HEPA (red) filters. The vertical flow with 0.5 m/sec is conducted by modular curtains to provide an optimal wash-out of potential pollution. The overflow is used for the surrounding and for recycled circuit. Curtains (or stable panels) are mandatory for optimal efficiency.
b The real situation: The team is as small as possible, the enclosure with sterile inner draping, the x-ray view box outside the mobile perspex glass wall.

8.3 The ritual for ultraclean-air surgery

An orthopedic or trauma patient to be operated on in a conventional theater generally undergoes preparation (anesthesia, disinfection of the operation field, draping) in the theater and in absence of the surgeon. The surgeon arrives in the theater only when the operation is ready to begin. The preparation process of surgery under ultraclean air conditions is different. The surgeon has to be in the theater before the patient and must participate in the patient's preparation according to the following protocol [43]:

1. Anesthesia, a first skin disinfection, and provisional draping are performed outside of the enclosure (Fig. 1-15). Simultaneously, the scrub nurse attends to their clothing, unpacking, and arranging the provided instruments and materials inside the sterile enclosure (Fig. 1-16).

2. Meanwhile, the surgeons, as the scrub nurse did before, prepare themselves: In the hand scrub area, they fit the exhaust hose around their necks, disinfect their individual shield with alcohol 96%, put it on and clean and disinfect their hands (Fig. 1-17).

3. The scrub nurse drapes up the inner walls of the enclosure with sterile sheets and is now ready for the surgeons' gowning. They enter one after the other through the side door. The scrub nurse assistant connects the exhaust-hose and helps with the gowning (Fig. 1-18).

4. At this stage, the surgical team puts on a second pair of gloves, the surgeon wears a pair of alcohol-soaked sterile cotton gloves in between the two rubber gloves. The anchorage of the sleeves of the gown according (Fig. 1-16) prevents back-slip and loss of permanent fitting (Fig. 1-19).

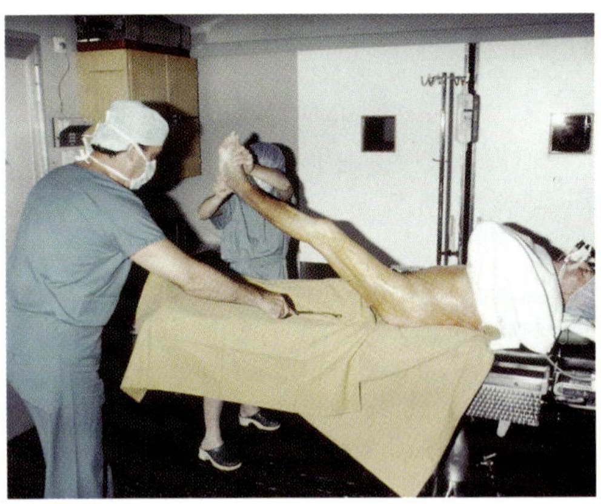

Fig. 1-15 'Outside' preparation of the patient. Positioning, anesthesia, and primary disinfection are performed outside of the clean-air zone.

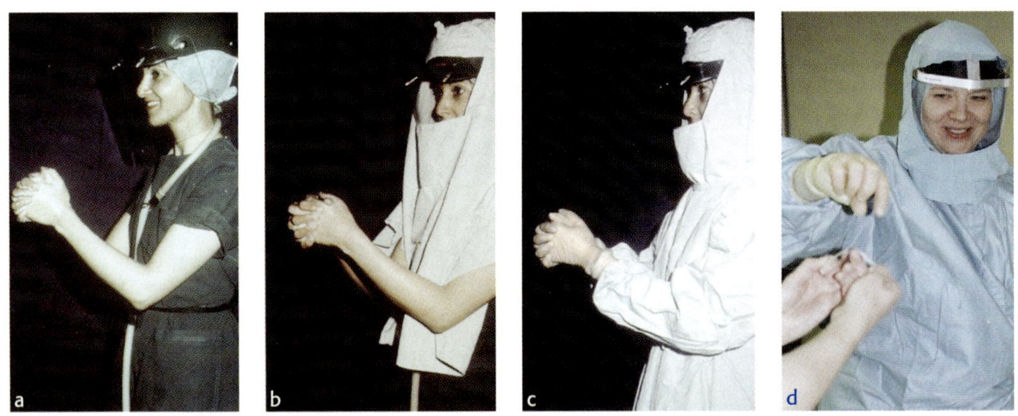

Fig. 1-16a–d The gowning 'ritual'.

a A scrub nurse steps through the inlet of the enclosure with head protection, the shield infection, the exhaust hose around her neck, and her hands washed. The hose is then connected to the pump.

b The sterile hood is 'swung' on to the head by the nurse herself.

c The gown is put on with the help of an assistant nurse.

d A scrub nurse with modern oneway gown preparing the operation material, ie, opening the instrument trays, etc.

5. Only when the whole surgical team is ready is the patient is moved through the inlet of the enclosure. As a team, they perform a second disinfection and draping process with disposable sheets and adhesive plastic iodine draping [53] (Fig. 1-20).

6. The skin incision is instantly disinfected with iodine (Betadine) (Fig. 1-21) to inactivate local staphylococcus albus released from hair bulbs, sebaceous glands, and sweat glands.

7. In operations lasting longer than 1 hour (eg, THR), cotton towels are sutured into the incision and soaked with undiluted Betadine (Fig. 1-22).

With a fresh scalpel surgery then begins.

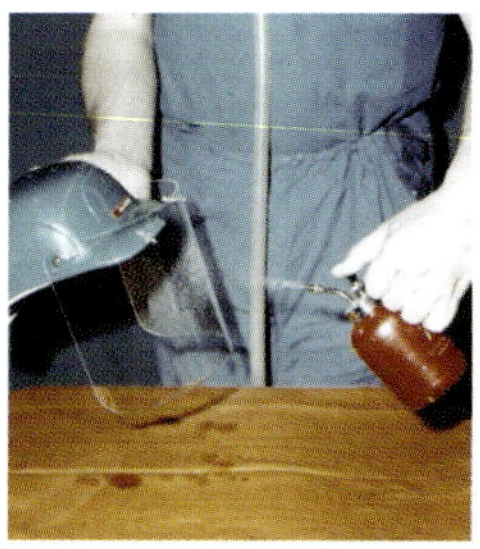

Fig. 1-17 Disinfection of scaphander. The polyacetal shield is sprayed with 96% alcohol.

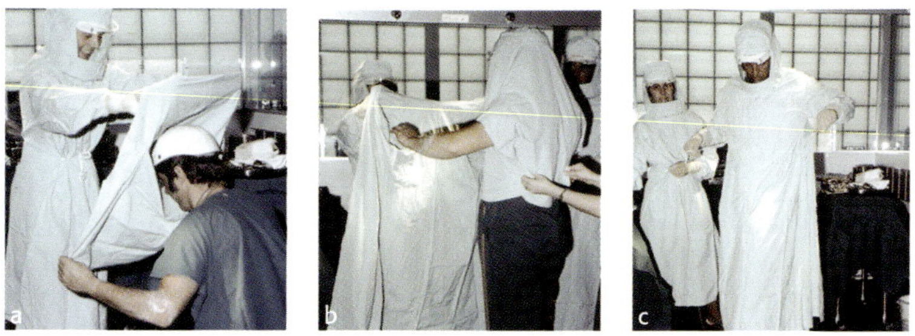

Fig. 1-18a–c The gowning of the surgeons.
a The hood application.
b Gowning with the help of a scrub nurse and an assisting nurse.
c Closure of the wrapped gown.

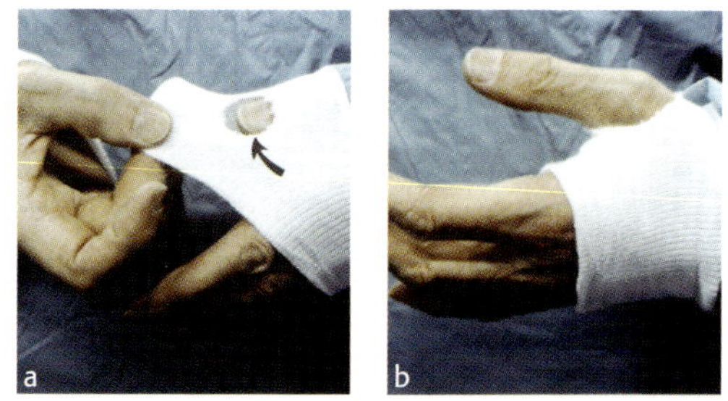

Fig. 1-19a–b Prevention of sleeve slippage.
a The gown sleeve is perforated with a scissors.
b The surgeon's thumb sticks through the sleeve hole. Only then are the hands gloved.

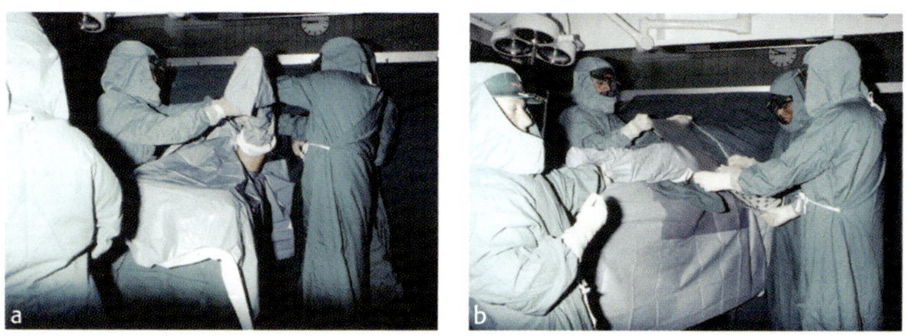

Fig. 1-20a–b The final disinfection after gowning of the operating team.
a The patient enters through the inlet and disinfection is repeated a second time. Draping with disposable material.
b Betadine-impregnated plastic sheets are applied.

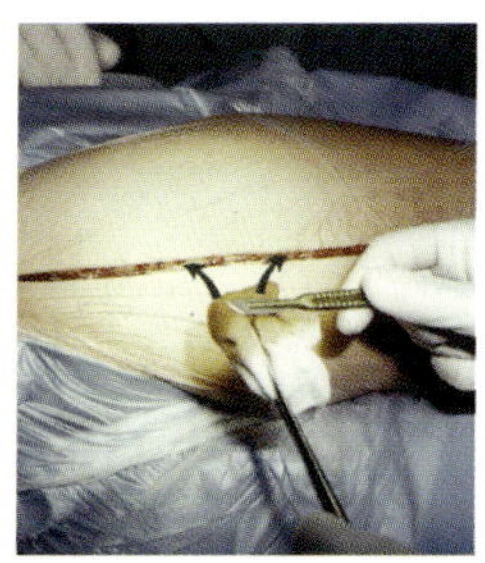

Fig. 1-21 Disinfection of the skin incision. Bacteria released from skin incision and their intracutaneous sites are Betadine-disinfected with a swab as is the knife (arrows).

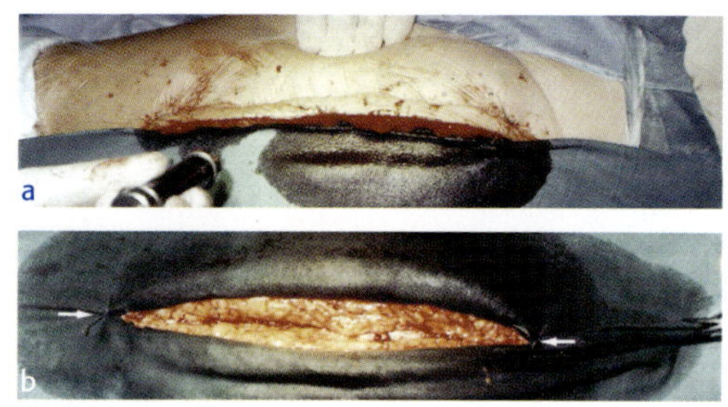

Fig. 1-22a–b Continuous skin incision disinfection.
a One towel is already sutured into the open wound and turned down. Betadine is applied.
b The second towel is sutured onto the ventral incision lip and turned upwards. Stabilizing stitches through the towels and skin keep the coverage stable (arrows).

9 Our body-exhaust equipment

The body-exhaust system needs simplicity to find personal acceptance. It must also be light, and must not disturb the user during surgery. Last but not least, the system must be functionally safe and should not cost more than conventional material [43].

Personal experience with market recommended scaphandering has been disappointing. Functional failures during surgery and discomfort made me opt for Charnley's slightly modified and self-made pattern: It works, it is accepted, and the costs are low (Fig. 1-23).

At the end of surgery, when the patient's wound has been dressed and they have been withdrawn through the enclosure inlet, the surgeons also leave the enclosure, after which they ungown and disconnect the exhaust hoses. The scrub nurse clears away their material, performs a disinfective wash-up of the floor with their assistant and removes the protective sheets along the inner wall of the enclosure. They then leave the enclosure by the side door. The enclosure is then ready for the next surgical procedure.

The exhaust hoses are collected for sterilization, the shields for disinfective cleaning and for storage for subsequent operations.

The textile hoods, which are not disposable, go back to the laundry department, where they are packed and autoclaved for their next use.

The described conduct does not differ much from conventional surgical practice. However, it does require a coordinated performance from the whole team under the goal of integrated aseptic surgery.

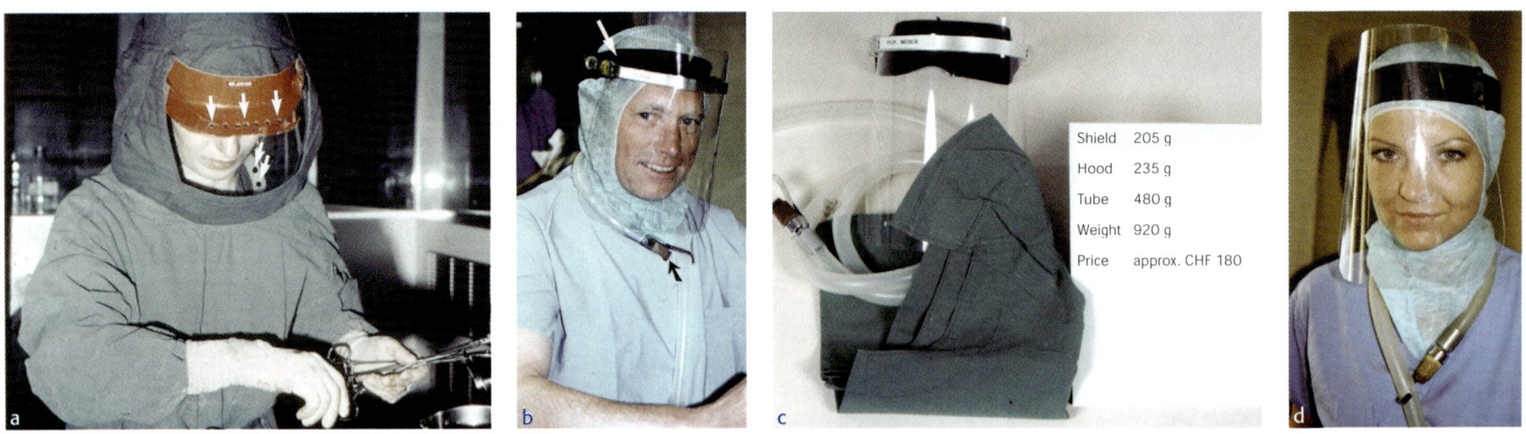

Fig. 1-23a–d The exhaust gear 1970 and 1988.

a The 1970 model: builders' helmet fitted with polyacetal window. Air-inlet in the helmets shield (arrows). Perforated exhaust hose around the neck (arrows).

b The 1988 and current model: helmet is replaced by a lighter neoprene band around the head (arrow). The hose with sound absorption device (arrow).

c The weight and costs of our head gear: gear is much lighter than other systems, 920 g. The real costs are also lower—the green clothhood is the most expensive part. Total costs are USD 100 or CHF 180 approximately.

d The currently last used model true to the maxim: "Reduce to the Maximum".

10 "Nothing learned and everything forgotten" (Wichmann 1992)

Classical asepsis and antibiotic prophylaxis dissimulate the presence of airborne contamination. Increasing antimicrobial resistance will sooner or later impose more attention on airborne infections.

Wichmann was a pessimist regarding our ability to learn from history. Charnley was for us the teacher from whom we have learned in addition to our own experience (Fig. 1-24).

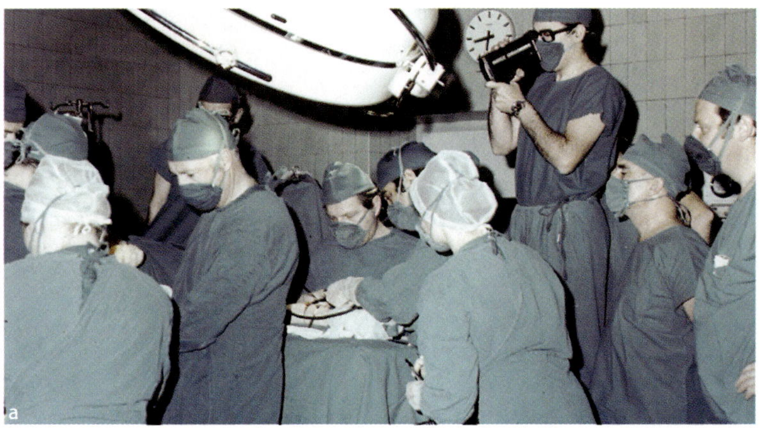

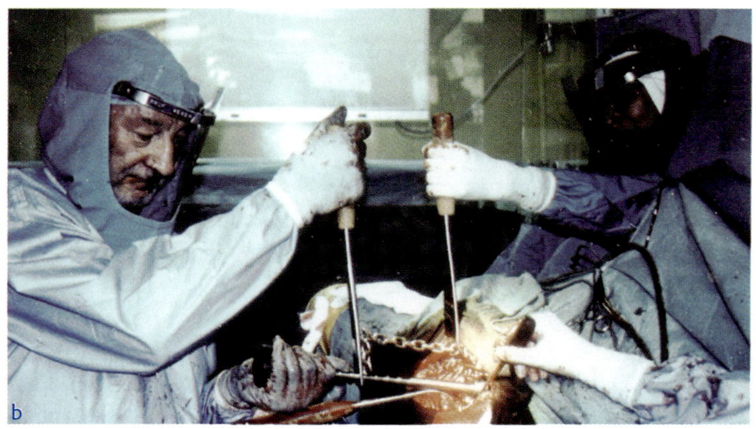

Fig. 1-24a–b "Nothing learned and everything forgotten?"

a At our hospital 1960–1970 asepsis was critical. Such asepsis is still tolerated worldwide due to liberal antibiotic prophylaxis.

b At the Kantonsspital St. Gallen 1970–1993 and the Klinik am Rosenberg, Heiden, 1984 until today, and most orthopedic surgery is performed under ultraclean room conditions, all major surgery with body-exhaust equipment.

11 Conclusions and Summary

For many surgical specialities, conventional asepsis seems to be sufficient. The natural defense of vascularized tissues and prophylactic antibiotics compensate for and resist the inevitable wound contamination during surgery.

Orthopedic and trauma surgery, in contrast, has more work to do with fewer self-defending tissues, bone, ligaments, cartilage, tendons, and with implants. Contamination is not permitted. Integrated asepsis is therefore needed, even mandatory.

Integrated asepsis is the sum of:

1. Conventional asepsis.
2. Ultraclean room conditions.
3. Clean room conduct of the surgical team.

Charnley's concept has encouraged many copies, corresponding investigations and publications. The results agree unanimously that airborne contamination can be avoided with the risk of postoperative infection being lowered.

Without any doubt, ultraclean air operating theaters would not provide the full benefit without all the other improvements in aseptic practice, such as improved clothing, reduced numbers of personnel present in a theater, sealing the patient's skin surface with iodine prepared adhesive plastic sheets, refined surgical techniques and reduced operating time.

One should not forget that under classical asepsis alone, the most important reduction of postoperative infection risk has to be attributed to prophylactic antibiotic administration. A serious question is how long antibiotics will continue to be helpful. The warning from antibiotic resistant bacteria should no longer be ignored.

With the longer operations, the risk of infection increases [60, 61]. This aspect is irrelevant for surgery in the enclosure. There is no hurry to close the surgical approaches. There is no motivation from that aspect for minimal invasive techniques in orthopedic surgery. Open surgery has the benefit of greater technical precision than minimal invasive procedures.

The infection risk, compared with the sterile enclosure, has in our experience since 1970 been:

- 2.5 times higher in a theater with a separation wall and body-exhaust system.
- 6.5 and 7 times higher in conventional theaters when using conventional gowning and masks.

The argument of high costs of clean-air operating rooms is not valid. Surgery in modern hospitals is similar using air conditioning. Conventional air conditioning can easily be converted either into a separating wall suite or into a sterile enclosure with a body-exhaust system. The running costs are the same.

Prophylactic antibiotics are not indicated routinely under integrated asepsis. Aseptic surgery without antibiotics is not only a serious demand, but is also possible.

For everybody working in ultraclean air operating rooms, it is most satisfactory to know they have done the best possible to prevent wound contamination and wound infection—best possible service to the patient.

12 Bibliography

Blue references indicate links to abstracts of articles online available through Medline (www.nlm.nih.gov).

1. **Lister J** (1912) *Joseph Lister's Erste Veröffentlichung über antiseptische Wundbehandlung (1967–1969)*. Leipzig: Johann Ambrosius Barth.
2. **Weber BG** (1969) Die Risiken in der Orthopädie. *Schweiz. Mediz. Wschr.; 99* (1):1–7.
3. **Brown AR, Taylor GJ, Gregg PJ** (1996) Air contamination during skin preparation and draping in joint replacement surgery. *J Bone Joint Surg [Br]; 78* (1):92–4.
4. **Charnley JA** (1964) A sterile air operating theater enclosure. *Brit J Surg;* 51:195–202.
5. **Charnley JA** (1969) La "serre" de Wrightington. *Rev Chir Orthop;* 55:231.
6. **Charnley JA** (1972) Postoperative infection after total hip replacement with special reference to air contamination in the operating room. *Clin Orthop;* 87:167–87.
7. **Charnley JA** (1979) *Low friction arthroplasty of the hip.* Theory and Practice. Berlin: Springer.
8. **Aebi B, Gerber C, Ganz R** (1989) [Prevention of infection in elective orthopedic interventions with special reference to alloplastic joint replacement]. *Helv Chir Acta;* 56 (3):387–97.
9. **Vasey H** (1972) L'infection postopératoire en orthopédie. *Med Hyg;* 30:949.
10. **Whyte W, Lidwell OM, Lowbury EJ, et al.** (1983) Suggested bacteriological standards for air in ultraclean operating rooms. *J Hosp Infect;* 4 (2):133–139.
11. **Gierhake FW** (1975) Antibiotica und ihre Indikationen in der Chirurgie. *Chirurg;* 46 (1):10–15.
12. **Graber P, Zimmerli W** (1999) Antibiotikaprophylaxe in der Chirurgie. *Schweiz. Aerztezeitung;* 80 (50):2921–2926.
13. **Mirimanoff RO** (1979) Utilisation inappropriée des antibiotiques. *Schweiz. Aerztezeitung;* 60 (42): 2089–2092.
14. **Opravil M** (1999) Was ist die Evidenz für den kausalen Zusammenhang zwischen Antibiotika-Gebrauch und dem Auftreten von Resistenzen? (Teil 7). *Schweiz. Aerztezeitung;* 80 (7):409–411.
15. **Pittet D, Sax H** (2000) Alaarm Stufe Eins: Staphylococcus aureus mit verminderter Sensibilität gegenüber Vancomycin! *Swiss-NOSO;* 7 (2):12–16.
16. **Schaffner A** (1999) Antibiotikaresistenz—Mikroben: Sind wir einen Schritt zu spät? *Schweiz. Aerztezeitung;* 80 (50):2899.
17. **Ruef C** (2000) Neue Empfehlungenzur Lüftungstechnik im Spital. Hospitalis; 10:419.
18. **Weber BG** (2000) *Orthopädie an der Schwelle.* Bern, Göttingen, Toronto, Seattle: Hans Huber.
19. **Geiser M** (2000) Die Asepsis nicht vergessen! *Schweiz. Aerztezeitung;* 81 (11).
20. **Geiser M** (2000) Gedanken zur orthopädischen Chirurgie in der zweiten Hälfte des 20. Jahrhunderts. *Schweiz. Aerztezeitung;* 81 (39): 2233–2238.
21. **Zimmerli W, Waldvogel FA, Vaudaux P, et al.** (1982) Pathogenesis of foreign body infection: description and characteristics of an animal model. *J Infect Dis;* 146 (4):487–97.
22. **Müller ME, Allgöwer M, Schneider R, et al.** (1991) *Manual of Internal Fixation.* Berlin Heidelberg New York: Springer-Verlag.
23. **Whitcomb JG** (1969) *Laminar flow devices in critical hospital areas. Technical lecture series on industry and microbial contamination control.* Stanford University, Palo Alto.
24. **Ribbans WJ** (1996) *"Double Jeopardy"? Hepatitis and HIV.* An Orthopaedic Viewpoint Orthopaedic Product News: 30–31.
25. **Moschner C** (1997) Reinraum-Bekleidung Mitte der neunziger Jahre. Schweiz. ges. für Reinraumtechnik, Herbsttagung "Neues in den Reinen Technologien", Basel 1996. *Swiss Med;* 19 (6):11–13.
26. **Merle d'Aubigne R** (1969) L'infection opéeratoire en chirurgie orthopédique. *Rev Chir Orthop;* 55:176.
27. **Hughes SP, Anderson FM** (1999) Infection in the operating room. *J Bone Joint Surg [Br];* 81 (5): 754–755.
28. **Loertscher JJ** (1979) Klinische Infektionsquote bei Hüftgelenkstotalendoprothesen operiert in einer Reinraumoperationskabine. *Med Orthop Techn;* 99:237–239.
29. **Meierhans R** (1975) Raumtrennwand—ein Beitrag zur traditionellen Klimatisierung von Operationsräumen. *Medica;* 3:13–15.
30. **Meierhans R** (1979/1980) Investitions- und Betriebskosten unterschiedlich wirksamer raumlufttechnischer Systeme. *SRRT, Swiss Med;* 33–38.
31. **Stevens DB** (1964) Postoperative orthopedic infections. A Study of etiological mechanisme. *J Bone Joint Surg [Am];* 46:96.
32. **Werner HP** (1984) Forderung und kritische Gewichtung der Hygienemassnahmen durch den Spitalhygieniker. *Swiss Med;* 6 (60).
33. **Williams R, Blowers R, Garrod LP, et al.** (1960) *Hospital infection: causes and prevention.* London, Lloyd-Luke Ltd.
34. **Meierhans R, Weber BG** (1971) Möglichkeiten und Grenzen der Asepsis im Operationssaal. *Medica;* 1 (31).
35. **Wanner HU, Huber G, Meierhans R, et al.** (1980) [Optimum utilization of the ventilation system to reduce airborne bacteria in operating rooms]. *Helv Chir Acta;* 47 (3-4):493–504.
36. **Weber BG** (1979/1980) Der Einfluss der Klimatechnik auf die Chirurgie. *SRRT Swiss Med;* 1 (12).
37. **Weber BG** (1982) Influence of surgical technique and laminar flow on infection rate. Progress in cemented total hip surgery and revision proceeding of a symposium held in Amsterdam. *Excerpta Medica.*
38. **Weber BG** (1982) *Hygieneanforderungen an Operationsabteilungen.* Berlin Heidelberg, Springer-Verlag.
39. **Weber BG, Struehmer G, Meierhans R** (1971) Sterile Operationsboxen. *Z Orthop;* 1009: 803–813.
40. **Weber BG, Blatter R, Stuehmer G, et al.** (1972) Prophylaxe der operativen Infektionen. *Z Unfallmed Berufskrankheiten;* 1:42–46.
41. **Weber BG, Liechti R, Stuehmer G, et al.** (1972) *Periatrite de l'épaule, ostéogenèse et compression, travaux divers.* Bern: Huber.
42. **Weber BG** (1972) *Prophylaxis of infection in orthopedic surgery.* Reprint from Int. Congress Series No. 291. Orthop Surgery and Traumatology, Excerpta Medica, Amsterdam.

43. **Weber BG, Stuehmer G, Meierhans R** (1973) Die Bekleidung des Operationsteams in einer sterilen Operationskabine. *SRRT Reinraumtechnik I;* 132–134.
44. **Weber BG** (1973) *1 1/2 Jahre Erfahrung mit einer Sterilboxe im Operationssaal Ber. über die Unfallmed.* Tagung in Göttingen.
45. **Weber BG** (1973) *Arthroplasty of the hip.* Stuttgart: Thieme.
46. **Bergmann BR, Hobron J, Nachemson A** (1985) Patient draping and staff clothing in the operating theater: A microbiological study. *Scand J Infekt Dis;* 17:421–426.
47. **McLeod GG** (1989) Needlestick injuries at operations for trauma. Are surgical gloves an effective barrier? *J Bone Joint Surg [Br];* 71 (3): 489–91.
48. **Williams TG** (1999) Theater rituals. *Orthopaedics;* 12 (3):49–52.
49. **Stuehmer G, Weber BG, Meierhans R, et al.** (1977) Four and a half years experience with a vertical flow sterile enclosure. *Int Orthop (SICOT);* 1:95–99.
50. **Buerki F, Skripitz W, Van den Wildenberg P** (1985) Die "Kenzone"—das optimierte OP-Konzept. *Hyg And Med;* 10:215–219.
51. **Thomas G** (1979/1980) Luftkeimzahlmessungen als Indikator der Reinheit von Operationseinrichtungen. *SRRT, Swiss Med;* 23.
52. **Thomas G** (1982) *Hygieneanforderungen an Operationsabteilungen.* Berlin Heidelberg: Springer-Verlag.
53. **Le Veen HH, Le Veen RF, et al.** (1993) The Mythology of Povidone-lodine and the Development of self-sterilizing Plastics. *Surgery, Gynecology and Obstetrics;* 176:183–190.
54. **Lidwell OM, Lowbury EJ, Whyte W, et al.** (1982) Effect of ultraclean air in operating rooms on deep sepsis in the joint after total hip or knee replacement: a randomised study. *Br Med J (Clin Res Ed);* 285 (6334):10–4.
55. **Lidwell OM, Elson RA, Lowbury EJ, et al.** (1987) Ultraclean air and antibiotics for prevention of postoperative infection. A multicenter study of 8,052 joint replacement operations. *Acta Orthop Scand;* 58 (1):4–13.
56. **Rees RT** (2000) Infections associated with dental procedures in total hip arthroplasty. *J Bone Joint Surg [Br];* 82 (2):307.
57. **Meierhans R** (1995) Periodic testing of leaks in terminal particulate air filters in the hospital. Hyg Med; 20:140–151.
58. **Meierhans R** (1999) Radical changes in HVAC-planning—also in hospitals. *Hyg Med;* 24 (3):88–97.
59. **Seipp H-M, Schroth A, Besch H** (1998) Operative Reinraumtechnik Teil I: Partikelreduktionsfaktoren zur Bewertung der Schutzfunktion installierter Laminar-Airflow-Zuluftdeckensysteme. *Hyg Med;* 23 (12): 526–540.
60. **Cauchoix J** (1969) [Surgical infection in orthopedic surgery. Technical conditions of the operation]. *Rev Chir Orthop Reparatrice Appar Mot;* 55 (3):205–207.
61. **Decoulx P** (1969) [Surgical infection in orthopedic surgery. Conditions of the operation]. *Rev Chir Orthop Reparatrice Appar Mot;* 55 (3):194–200.

2 The MINIMAX principle for fracture care in adults

1 History, definition, questions

MINIMAX is the trademark of a portable fire extinguisher. MINIMAX means a minimal sized tool with maximal efficiency. Our concept of fracture care in general and of open reduction and internal fixation (ORIF) and the fire extinguisher have similar natures. We therefore adopted the trademark MINIMAX in 1964 for our colloquial clinical usage.

The MINIMAX principle was developed from the original AO (Association for the Study of Internal Fixation) philosophy in the early 1960s [1, 2] by the senior registrars of that time (B.G. Weber, A. Boitzy, Ch.F. Brunner) at the orthopedic department of County Hospital, St. Gallen, Switzerland (Head Prof. M.E. Müller, 1960–1967).

The subsequent department heads (B.G. Weber, 1967–1986, and F. Magerl, 1986–1994) continued to follow the principle in St. Gallen. It was also transferred to the University of Bern by A. Boitzy, who became an ordinary professor there, after following M.E. Müller. Our ideas have been published several times [3–9] and are still practiced now.

The introduction to our book "Special Techniques in Internal Fixation" [3], encapsulates our ideas as: "Every internal fixation should achieve maximum effect with a minimum of material and effort. In all the techniques described the basic biomechanical principles remain the same. The reader may be surprised to learn that almost all the implants used have been derived from the standard instrumentarium. It is unnecessary to manufacture a special plate for every conceivable fracture situation; the AO principles, the basic implants and the corresponding operative skills are sufficient for almost any situation that may arise." By the phrase "With a minimum of material and effort", we meant a well-judged expenditure of metal and limited surgical invasion to avoid additional vascular insult to fragments.

The "Special Techniques" and other publications from St. Gallen [6, 9–11] received little attention. Only with time was the message spread across Europe and the world by the St. Gallen and Berne trainees. It has received remarkable attention in the last few years, although it has also been interpreted differently than we intended. For instance, our 'biological fixation' is different from what is currently promoted under the same key word.

An impressive development from the MINIMAX principle is the book "Planning and Reduction Technique in Fracture Surgery" by Jeff Mast et al [12]. While Mast was on an AO fellowship in St. Gallen and Berne in 1979, he became 'infected' by the MINIMAX virus. He is currently the promoter of an AO group in the USA developing fracture care based on ideas close to our old MINIMAX principle.

What is the difference between the AO and the MINIMAX principles

- Anatomical open reduction (OR).
  Modification: anatomical open or closed reduction.
- Rigid internal fixation (IF).
  Modification: rigid or elastic internal or external fixation.
- Care for blood supply of the fragments.
  Modification: first priority.
- Functional after treatment.
  Modification: continuous active function (CAF).

The AO principles [1, 2] remain unchanged; they are, at most, slightly modified by MINIMAX:

Within the AO principles, open reduction with internal fixation is the most attractive feature for surgeons gaining familiarity with surgical fracture treatment. Open reduction and internal fixation are active, "fixation is fun", as Graham Apley [13] used to say when warning them to resist unqualified fracture surgery. The fixation technique, the 'doing', stood at the centre of the early AO movement and teaching. Care for blood supply was always cited, but enjoyed less attention than the handicraft, although the 1963 AO handbook [1] page 19 (translated) states: "Stable fixation asks not only mechanical skill, but also biological understanding. It is essential that the surgeon is alert to the blood perfusion during the whole procedure."

In 1983, R. Orozco [14] stated in his book "Fracturas diafisarias" (monografias de la Fundaciòn Maurice E. Müller—Espana): "La Révision de nuestros casos nos ha decidido a dar prioridad al componente mécanico sobre el vascular." Translated: "The follow-up of our cases has urged us to prioritize the mechanical component over the vascular component."

Peri- and endostial callus following open reduction with internal fixation was considered a disturbance of primary union and an index of failed rigid fixation. Only in 1991 did the term 'biological fixation' appear in the AO Manual of Internal Fixation (page 108), although 'biological fixations' had been presented from St. Gallen since the mid-sixties. The term 'biological fixation' and its definition was published in 1981 [3].

The discussion on priorities, either rigid fixation or blood supply, is different today. Over the last 20 years, the pendulum of opinion has gradually swung from rigid fixation in the direction of blood supply. Terms like 'biological fixation', 'minimal invasive technique', 'electronic navigation', and 'robotic' for the placement of nails, screws, and subcutaneous bridging plates are the predominant subjects in the current academic trauma scene. There are fewer and fewer meeting programs dealing with anatomical reduction and stable fixation. Today, 'modern' fracture care is scared of open reduction and internal fixation; minimal invasive procedures are advocated and promoted. We suspect that failures with open reduction with internal fixation, infections and their consequences have caused this change of opinion and such defensive surgery.

The origin of the MINIMAX principle in the 1960s was based on our own clinical observations. Enforced anatomical reduction of simple and complex fractures, following periosteal stripping and heavy rigid fixation were sometimes harmful and became a deplorable lesson for us senior registrars at that time in St. Gallen (Fig. 2-1a–b; 2-2a–d): Devitalized fragments did not unite. The surgery-related loss of blood perfusion of fragments was underrated. The periosteum elevator stripper was, for us, an instrument that created more harm than benefit and its 'peeling' use was abandoned forthwith. In retrospect, the 'maximal invasive' fracture fixation of the early AO deserved criticism.

The consequence of such failures was the challenge to minimize surgical vascular insult without giving up our strive for a maximal result according to the original AO objective, ie, full anatomical and functional restoration.

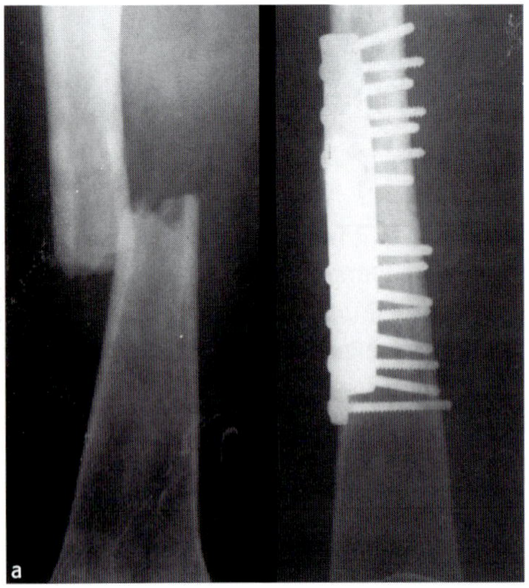

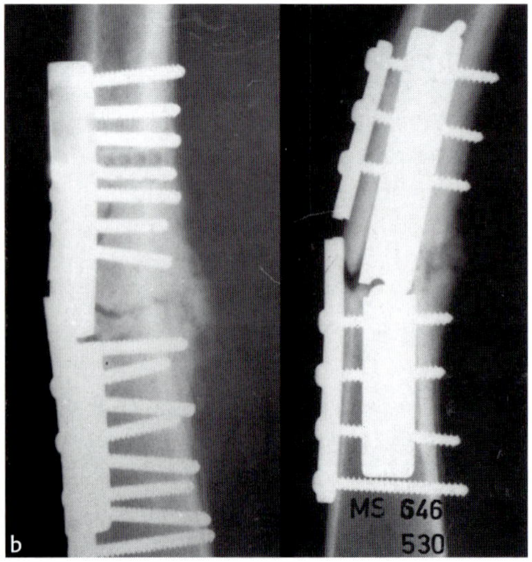

Fig. 2-1a–b Damage to blood supply by periosteal stripping and by double plating.

a The denuded bone is splinted with two heavy plates, fixed with 15 screws. Periosteal and endosteal blood supply are hampered.

b Fatigue fracture 17 weeks later, necrotic bone under the plates, only small amount of callus opposite the necrotic cortex.

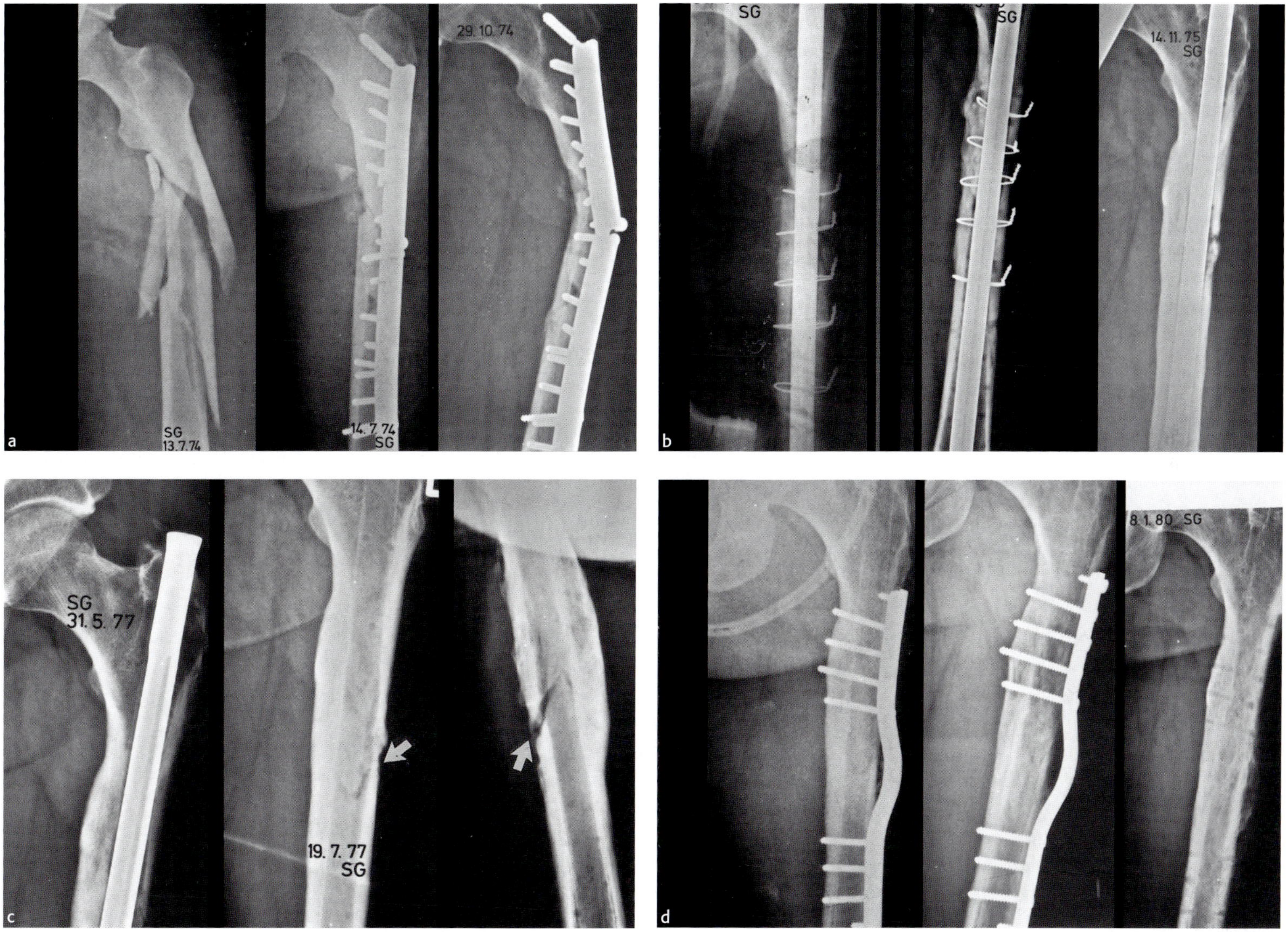

Fig. 2-2a–d Bone necrosis following periosteal stripping and plating.

a Preprogrammed course of events with fatigue fracture of the plate after 16 weeks, after failure of fracture healing process.

b Next step of damage to the blood supply: Replacement of the broken plate by intramedullary nail and wire cerclages. Some revascularization, but persistent necrosis of the lateral cortex 1 year later.

c 3 years after the fracture, the nail is removed. Fatigue fracture 7 weeks later arising from the necrotic lateral cortex (arrows).

d Salvage procedure for bone necrosis: waveplate plus corticocancellous pelvic graft. Removal of the plate 2 1/2 years later.

MINIMAX—What to do and what not to do

- Anatomical reduction of all fragments is not enforced at the price of damage to the blood supply of fragments. Normal length, axis, torsion after shaft fractures must be restored nevertheless. 'Waterproof' reduction, however, is mandatory in joint fractures.
- Plates are applied upon and no longer under the periosteum. Stripping of the periosteum is reduced to the absolute minimum along the fracture gaps for accurate reduction. Peeling of bone like a banana is strictly prohibited.
- Screws in plates and lag screws are inserted only in necessary numbers and where it makes sense mechanically. The AO rule: one screw for every screw hole in a plate, as a minimum number, has been abandoned.
- Double plating of tibia and femur fractures is considered a most serious surgical mistake.
- Cerclage of denuded bone is also banned.
- Medullary reaming for nailing is reduced to the minimum.
- Metal is used as much as necessary and as little as possible: Reduce to the maximum.
- Fracture care for youngsters and children was also included. Closed and open fracture treatment are described elsewhere [11].

With the refinement of the original AO fixation techniques, some points of fracture care gained new impulses and further development:

- The external fixator [8] is finding more and more application. No longer is it a preliminary first step fixation, but it is a new first and single fixation for the whole fracture healing period. For that challenge and for infected nonunions [6, 8] further refinement of the threaded-rod fixator system was necessary.
- In complex fractures, minimal local fixations (screw, antigliding plate) must be reinforced with an unilateral fixator.
- To stabilize comminuted shaft fractures, bridging plates or the external fixator were applied, leaving the zone of fragment comminution all by itself [3, 8].
- In case of missing blood supply or loss of fragments, the primary or early-secondary autogenous cancellus bone transplant became standard.
- Last but not least Sarmiento's functional bracing [15] and traditional closed fracture treatment were practiced, when preferable.

Since the 1980s, 'minimal invasive' fracture treatment has been in use at numerous AO centers and biomechanical institutions, and all sorts of new implants have been designed: dynamic hip screw (DHS), dynamic condylar screw (DCS), proximal femural nail (PFN), unreamed tibial nail (UTN), cannulated tibial nail (CTN), unreamed humeral nail (UHN), gamma nail, less invasive stabilization system (LISS), limited contact dynamic compression plate (LC-DCP), point contact fixator (PC-Fix), specific devices for many bone areas, for the left and the right side, cannulated or not cannulated, in steel or titanium. The following questions need answers to explain this change from open reduction with internal fixation to minimal invasive fixations. There is no doubt, however, that most of the new implants are also suitable for classical open reduction with internal fixation and are used in that way by surgeons that use theater facilities that allow open surgery. Implants in steel, however, have stood the test of time. The 'modern' implants are more expensive and 'fashionable'. Most of them are unnecessary in the hands of a skilled surgeon who is familiar with open reduction and internal fixation.

Questions

1. Why 'minimal invasive'? Is it fear of infection or/and of failure of open reduction and internal fixation?
2. Are the classical open reduction with internal fixation and MINIMAX procedures too difficult to perform?
3. Are the 'biological' and 'minimal invasive' fixations easier and quicker? This is persistently promoted by the implant makers and by surgeons as a specific progress and advantage of so-called modern fracture care.
4. What role do the implant makers play? Who finally creates the new fracture treatment fashion, the surgeons, the biomechanics, the engineers, or the businessmen? What is the motive for all the hectic activity, for the innovation fever? Is market expansion part of so-called progress of surgery?
5. Has fracture treatment lost the challenge of 'back to normal' in our changing society with its gradually shorter training of orthopedic and trauma surgeons? Is the market asking for fast surgery like the saturated society for fast food?

2 Ideas behind the MINIMAX principle

The MINIMAX principle has several roots:

- The MINIMAX principle is widespread in engineering, ie: "The great art in construction technology consists in the omission of parts" (Brown Ch Sr., 1827–1905) [16].
- Even more impressive is the MINIMAX principle in living nature. Bone is saving material to the maximum (Roux W, 1881) [17].
- Bone preserves, adjusts, and transforms its inner and outer shape according changing strains and load (Wolff J, 1892) [18].
- Fracture healing occurs along two patterns:
  - indirectly by means of callus formation (Pauwels, F., 1940) [19],
  - directly by angiogenetic osteonformation, which bridges and bolts the fracture gap (Krompecher 1937 [20], Danis 1932, 1949, Perren 1972, 1979 [21, 22], Perren and Boitzy 1978 [23]).
- "Bone tissue is made of two components of material, with different properties to resist deformation: The tensile resistant collagen fibres and the pressure resistant anorganic calcium apatit. Both components are interlocked according to a compound structure. The rules of the prestrained compound technology (ferro-concrete) may not be easily transferred on bone" [24]. Knese's conclusions are at least a suitable concept for ostheosynthesis [5, 6, 25].

3 The AO principles and the MINIMAX principle

The classical AO and MINIMAX principles have the same goal, full recovery after a fracture. Every compromise of success is considered a failure—or at least as a successful failure when circumstances were against a full recovery back to normal.

The principles of the AO standard bearers have remained unchanged since 1958 (foundation of the AO) [1, 2]: Open anatomical reduction, rigid stable fixation, care for the blood supply, and function after treatment.
For many more or less simple fractures, these four principles are of ideal utility. With rigid fixation, the bone has instantly regained its capacity as a load carrier, the fracture is virtually healed and painfree a long time before direct angiogenic ossification has occurred. Restitutio ad integrum, ie, full recovery occurs within 3–4 months and the fixation material may be removed one year after the injury without leaving any negative repercussions.

In complex fractures, in presence of significant soft-tissue damage, in polytrauma, when multiple fractures are present, or when the treatment has not started early within the first 6–8 hours, the same treatment, suitable for simple fractures, is critical. The complexity of each individual case needs customized decision making.

General considerations in fracture care: ask questions first, operate later. The following questions must be asked prior to treatment:

1. Is it best for the patient to operate on their fracture?
2. Does the patient's general health permit surgery on the fracture?
3. Are the necessary surgical requirements present to operate: asepsis, instruments, anesthesia, staff, aftercare, etc?
4. Am I, as a surgeon, competent to do such surgery?
5. Can the fracture be treated with minimal risk along the original AO rules or along the MINIMAX principle or is closed treatment the safer alternative?
6. If I myself, as a surgeon, were the patient: What treatment would be the right one for me and, therefore, also for the patient?

The MINIMAX principle is fracture care between maximal and minimal invasive surgery—change of priorities

First priority: blood supply

Of utmost interest is the blood supply of fragments and of soft tissues. A trauma-generated vascular insult must not be increased by surgery.

Second priority: reduction and stability

For simple shaft fractures and joint fractures, anatomical reduction and rigid fixation is preferred. In complex shaft fractures, open reduction is not enforced. Anatomical axial-torsional alignment and length are restored and maintained with 'biological, elastic, bridging' plating, nailing, or an external fixator to allow at least restricted function after treatment. Articular fractures are, as far as is possible, reconstructed anatomically with open reduction and internal fixation.

Third priority: regain of function

Whatever site, type of fracture and treatment, the greatest amount of early function favors the healing process. This rule stands for surgical fixation as well as for functional bracing.

The stability of fracture fixation results in case-dependent full or restricted load transmission, ie, a reamed nailed transverse femur midshaft allows full weightbearing and a bridging plated compound femur fracture only restricted. Operated on fractures of the upper limb must permit performance of manual practice.

The better the repair of bone and soft tissues, the sooner spontaneous permanent pain subsides and the sooner the patient will fearlessly use the injured limb. Function-linked pain will also soon vanish with resorption of swelling and fracture disease, ie, posttraumatic Sudeck-dystrophy will not develop. In bone lesions combined with injured ligaments (knee, ankle), temporary cast-splinting will not impair the healing result at all as long as progressive loading of the leg is performed. Weightbearing—restricted, progressive to full—is essential for successful fracture healing, the treatment being by bracing alone or by surgical fixation. The worst scenario would be: Unstable fracture fixation, additional cast-splinting and prohibition of loading and joint and muscle function—'fracture disease' would be programmed.

Cartilage benefits from continuous passive motion (CPM) and from continuous active motion (CAM). Bone healing is activated by continuous active function (CAF).

The MINIMAX principle—the role of metal

For the healing process of a fracture, it is irrelevant if the standard AO implants are made of stainless steel or titanium. Essential is that the surgical fracture fixation respects the blood supply of the fragments and soft tissues.

- When the blood supply is normal or hardly disturbed: The metal must leave the blood supply undisturbed. No surgical vascular insult can be permitted!

- When the blood supply is impaired, but still present: The metal cannot be allowed to impair the blood supply further.

- When the blood supply is absent: The metal, ie, its arrangement, must favor the restoration of the blood supply. When shaft fragments are deprived of periosteal blood flow, the intramedullary blood supply should not be destroyed with a nail. The medullary flow route is kept open by using a bridging plate or an external fixator.

Tricks and hints

1. Less is sometimes more. Take advantage of intrinsic stability of openly reduced fragments.
2. Keep fixation simple, but not too simple. Fixation should be 'economic'.
3. Surgery is not better than closed treatment per se.
4. Use the fragments as building material in simple fractures or leave them by themselves in complex, comminuted fractures with impaired blood perfusion.
5. The medullary cavity as a blood supply route to the fracture area. Use medullary nails only when periosteal perfusion is undisturbed.

The MINIMAX principle—the role of quality of asepsis

- Fracture treatment according to the AO and MINIMAX rules is open redution and internal fixation: it depends on real asepsis—if not, wound contamination and infection would be regular. Open reduction and internal fixation allows debridement of damaged tissues, decompression of compartments, it facilitates reduction and fixation by visual navigation and manipulation, reduces x-ray exposure, shortens the time of surgery and lowers the risk of wound infection due to closure of 'dead space'. Under 'normal' operating room conditions without real asepsis, all open wounds become contaminated.

- Under conventional theater conditions, with bacteria count levels of more than $100/m^3$ air, systemic antibiotic prophylaxis is mandatory, because all wounds are contaminated through the air [8, 26]. Such generally accepted practice is of high economic interest for the antibiotics chemical industry. However, the increasing resistance of bacteria [26] is the major problem of surgery in the near future.

- Since 1970, all our fracture and selective orthopedic surgery has been performed under clean-air conditions. Charnley's [28], our own [8, 26] and Lidwell's [29] experience in total hip and knee prosthesis surgery, applies identically to trauma and to fracture surgery: Infection has become almost nonexistent. From that viewpoint, there is no demand for so-called minimal invasive surgery. Single shot prophylactic antibiotics may be given for medico-legal reasons only. Prolonged antibiotic prophylactic protection, however, is obsolete and unnecessary.

- Why is Charnley's clean-air concept of asepsis [28] a wallflower in contrast to all sorts of spectacular contemporary achievements in surgery? Apparently, antibiotic medication is better accepted by surgeons than clean-room behavior. Awareness of the problem is mostly ignored except by orthopedic surgeons who were trained in it.

4 Cases—examples of MINIMAX fixations

The examples on the following pages (Fig. 2.3–2.14) illustrate these facts:

- The MINIMAX principle dates back to the 1960s. Most examples have been selected from the first two decades (note the dates). The same principle has stood the test of time till now and is routine for all those who were trained in it (see the last two examples).

- Only standard implants were used. Up to now there has not been any need for canulated screws, dynamic hip screws, dynamic codylar plates, low contact plates, interlocking nails, etc.

- Intraarticular and simple shaft fractures were reconstructed anatomically and rigidly fixed according to original AO rules (lag screws, compression plates, reamed nails).

- Complex comminuted shaft fractures were treated with biological, elastic, bridging fixations (plate, external fixator).

- X-ray control and navigation during surgery are not required—open reduction with internal fixation allows direct visual control (with rare exceptions).

- The examples have been selected from endless possible variations. However, they all fulfill the MINIMAX principle.

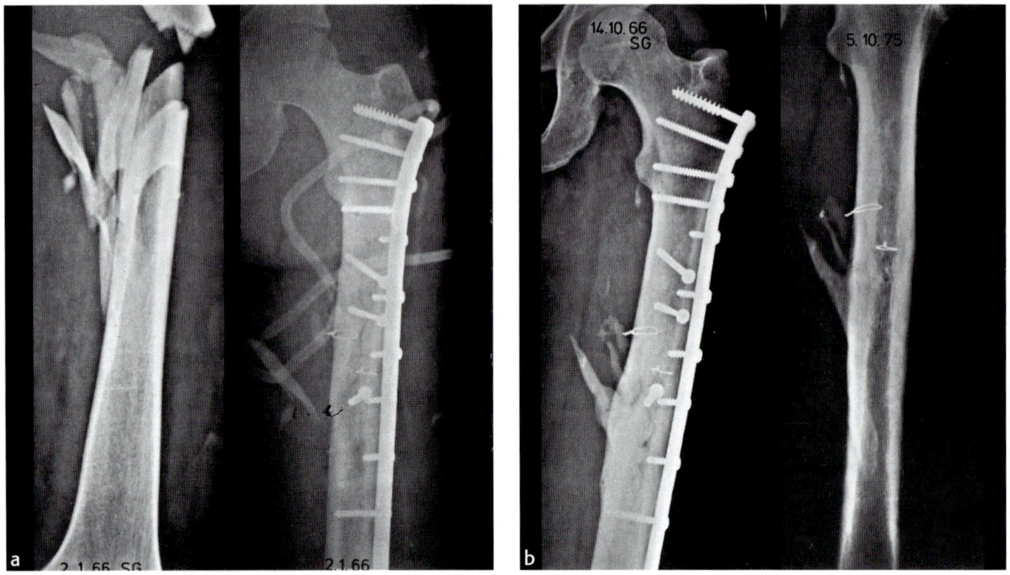

Fig. 2-3a–b Complex fracture. Bridging plate.

a Gentle open reduction and internal fixation, minimal periosteal stripping.

b Undisturbed periosteal and mainly endosteal bony union.

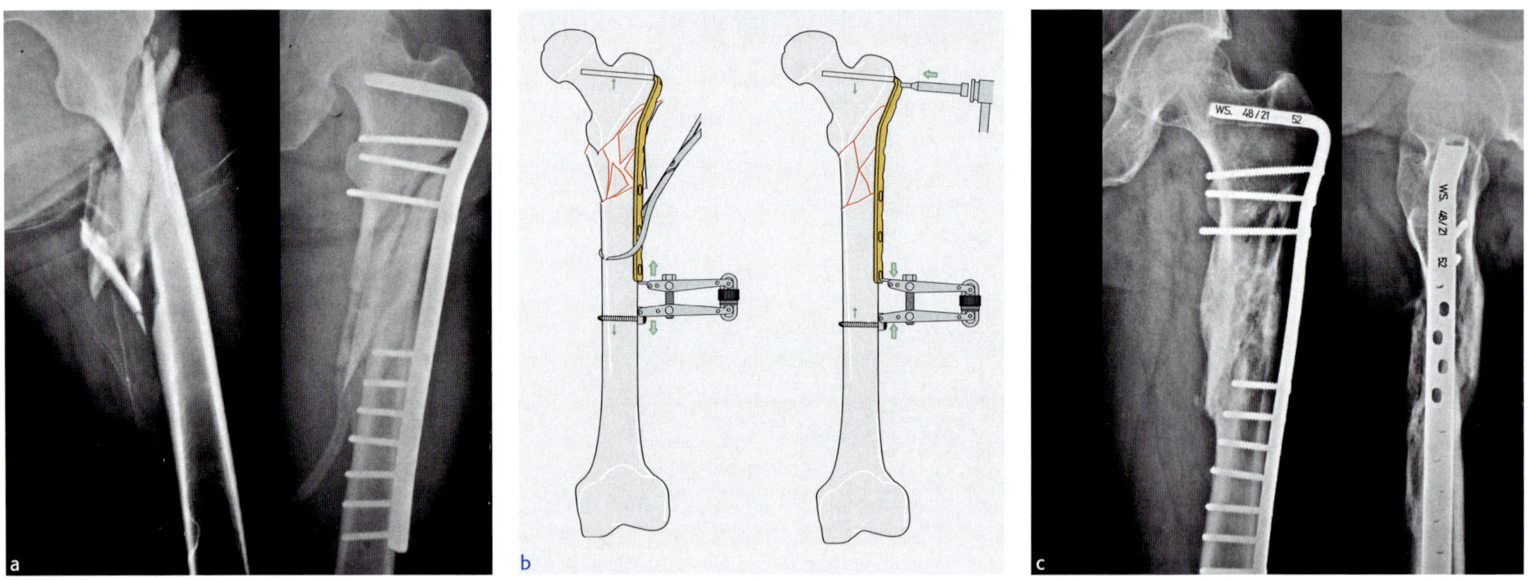

Fig. 2-4a–c Complex fracture. Indirect alignment. Bridging plate.

a Fracture bridged with plate (1967).

b Alignment with indirect distraction, with the plate-tensioning device.

c 'Biological' fracture healing after 52 weeks.

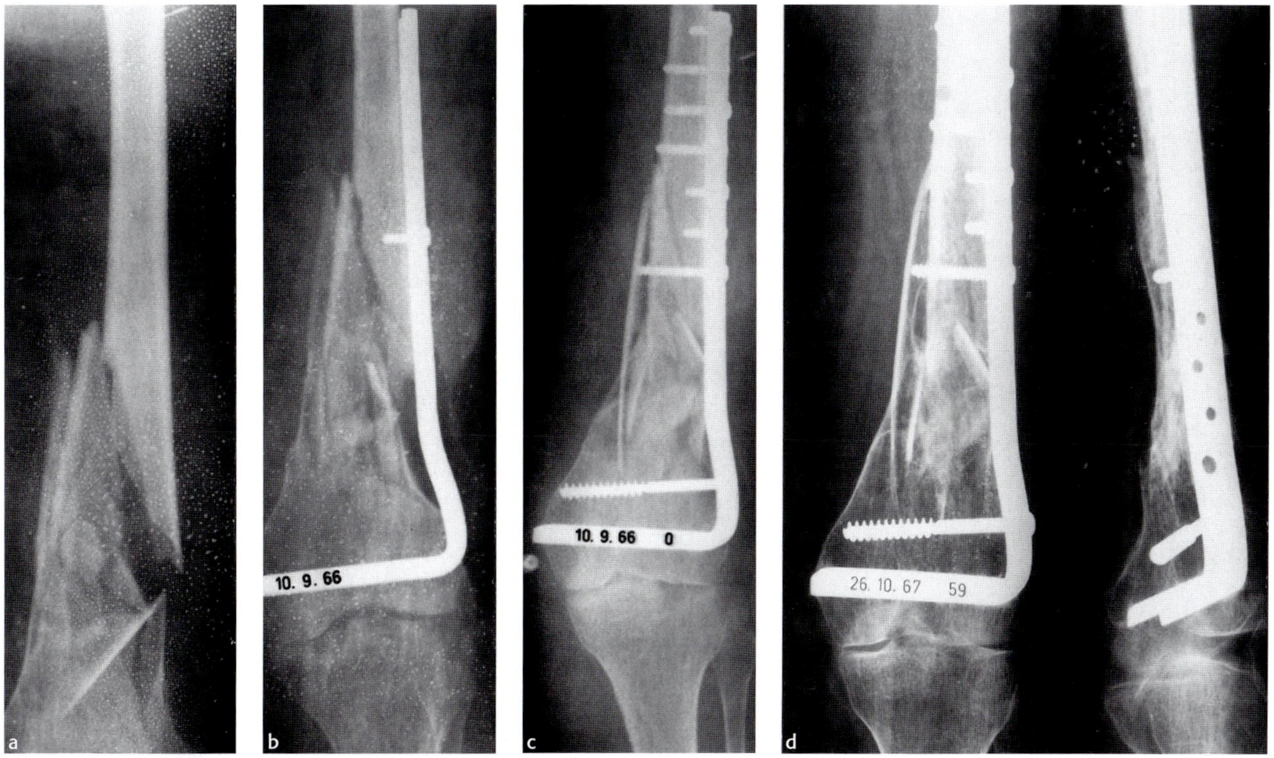

Fig. 2-5a–d Bridge plating without anatomical reduction, using opposite fragments as medial buttress.

a Multifractured osteoporotic bone.

b Bridging plate.

c One long opposite fragment is drawn near with a lag screw to work as medial buttress.

d 59 weeks since injury: uneventful 'biological' fracture healing.

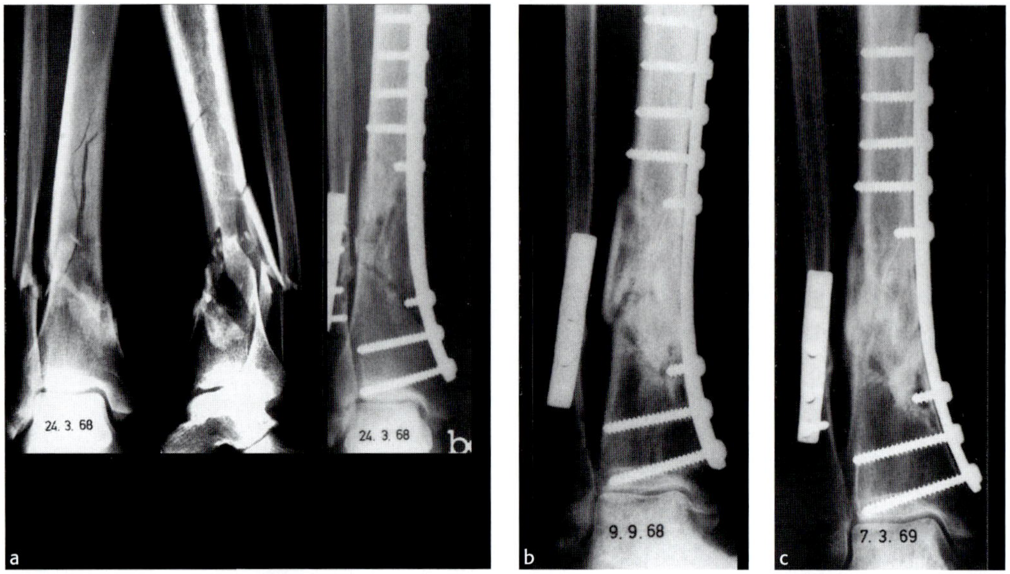

Fig. 2-6a–c Bridge plating without anatomical reduction. Auxiliary plating of the fibula.

a The fracture and the primary reduction fixation: First plating of fibula, second epiperiosteal reduction fixation of medial tibial cortex with a contoured bridging plate.

b 6 weeks later: small fragments behave like pedicled bone grafts.

c 12 months since injury: 'biological' and anatomical fracture healing.

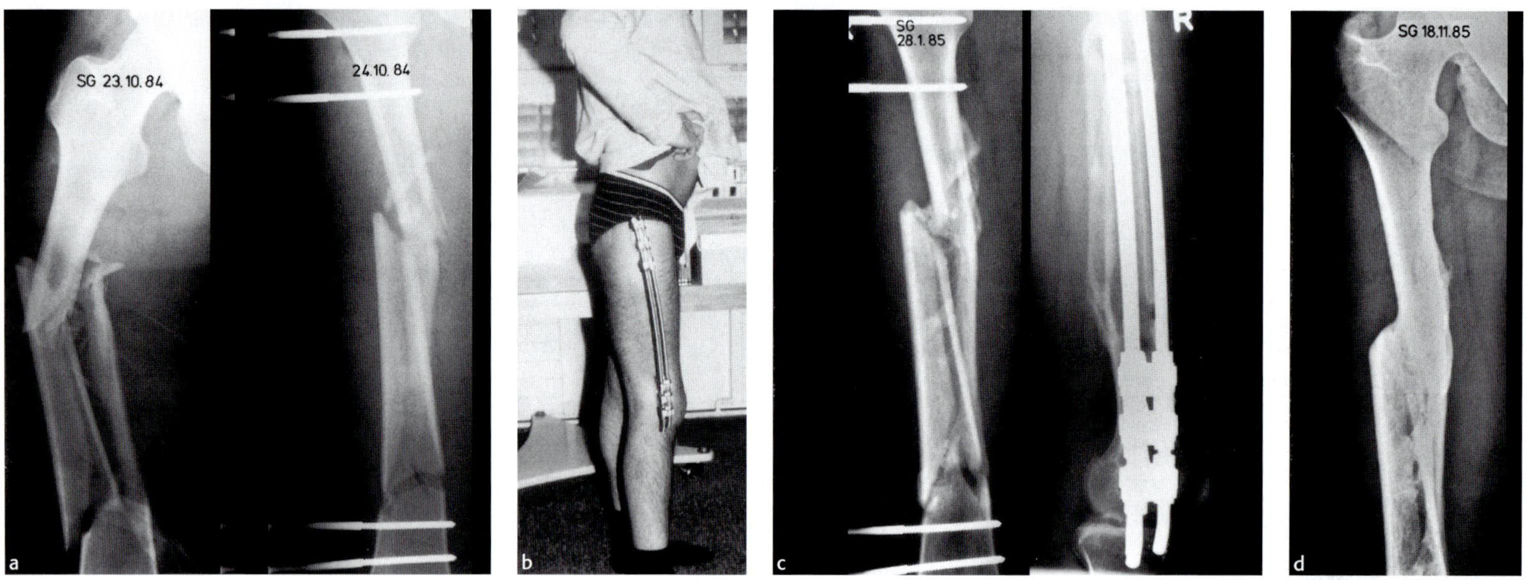

Fig. 2-7a–d Unilateral bridging external fixator, closed application.

a The fixator restores the malposition and the shortening by distraction.

b 8 weeks later: unsupported weightbearing.

c At 3 months: the fixator is removed.

d 13 months after the fracture: full restoration after 'biological' healing.

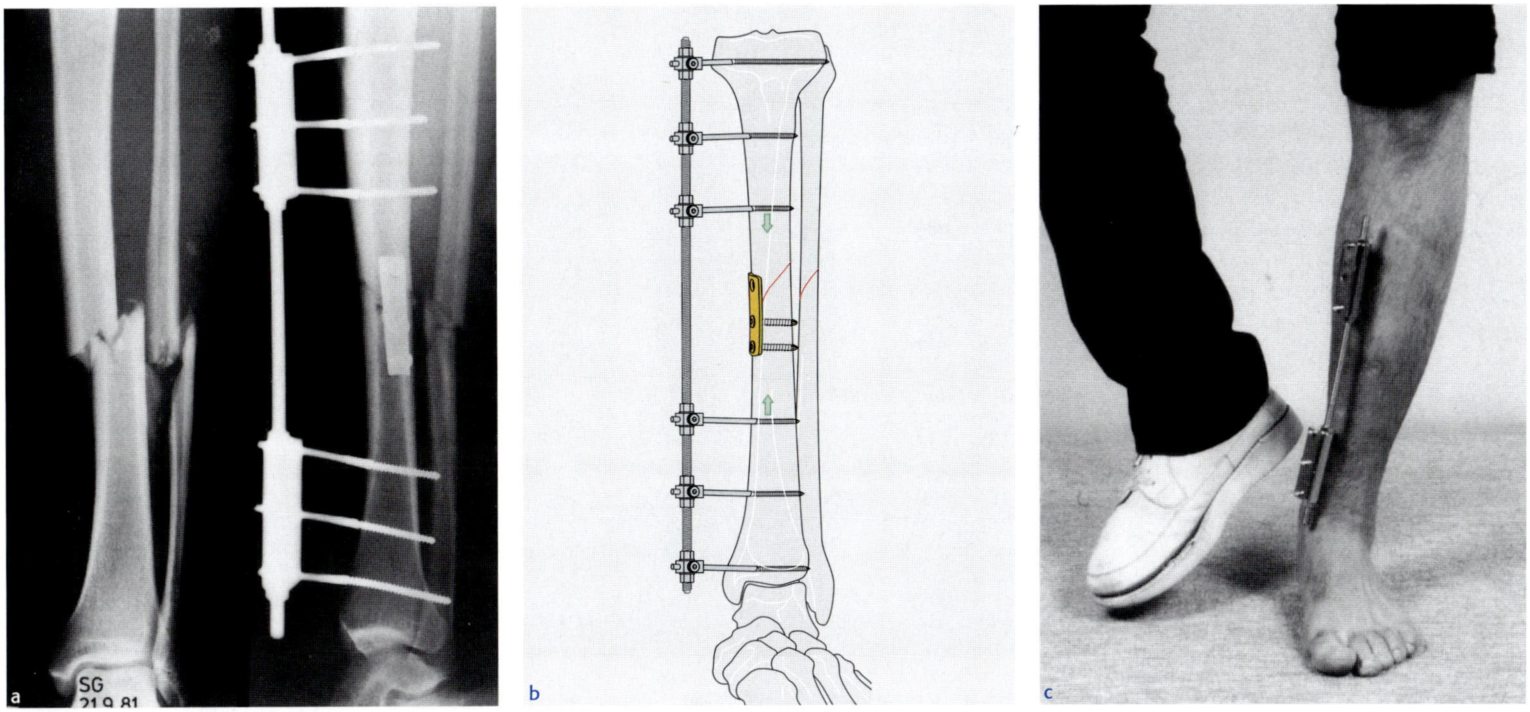

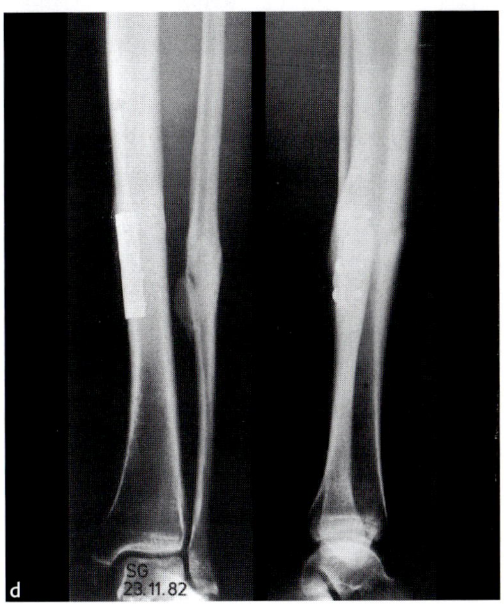

Fig. 2-8a–d Antigliding plate plus unilateral external fixator.

a The fracture is protected from displacement by a small antigliding plate. The tibia is protected from angulation by the prestrained-prestressed unilateral 90° fixed angle fixator.

b Antigliding plate and external fixator.

c The compound fragment-fixation system allows full weightbearing. 7 weeks later, removal of the fixator 8 weeks after injury.

d 14 months after surgery: full recovery.

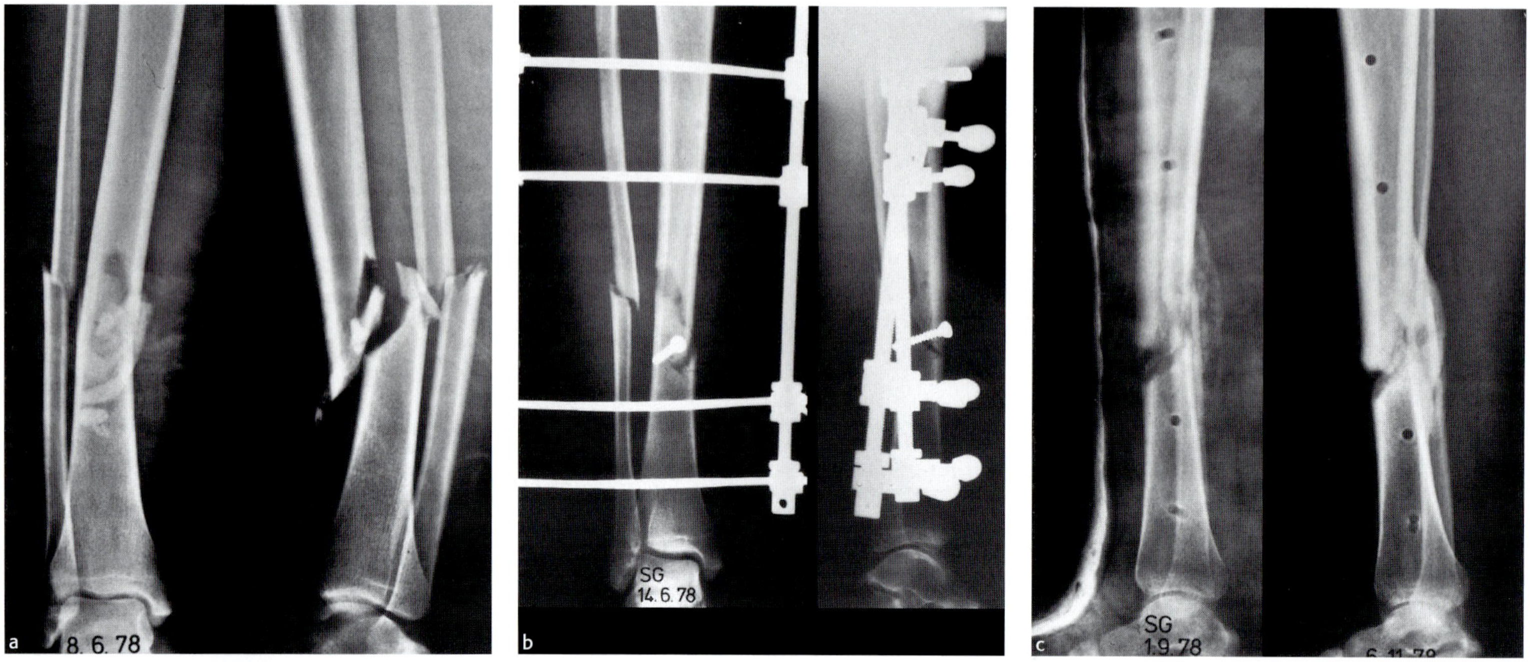

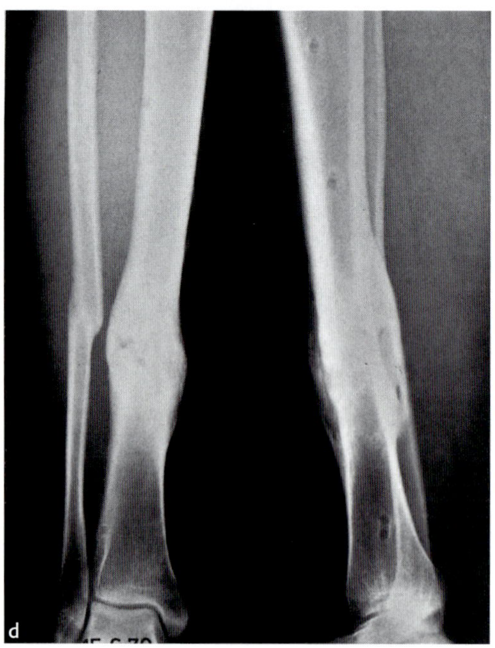

Fig. 2-9a–d Minimal direct fixation and frame external fixator. Staged secondary autogenous bone grafts.

a The unstable open fracture.

b The denuded, devitalized small cortical fragments are removed. One screw fixation. In view of such limited stability, application of a full frame fixator for 3 months.

c 6 weeks after injury autogenous bone grafting on the posterior plane of the tibia, at 3 months second grafting on the front and removal of the external fixator followed by a functional brace for another 3 months.

d 1 year after the injury: full recovery.

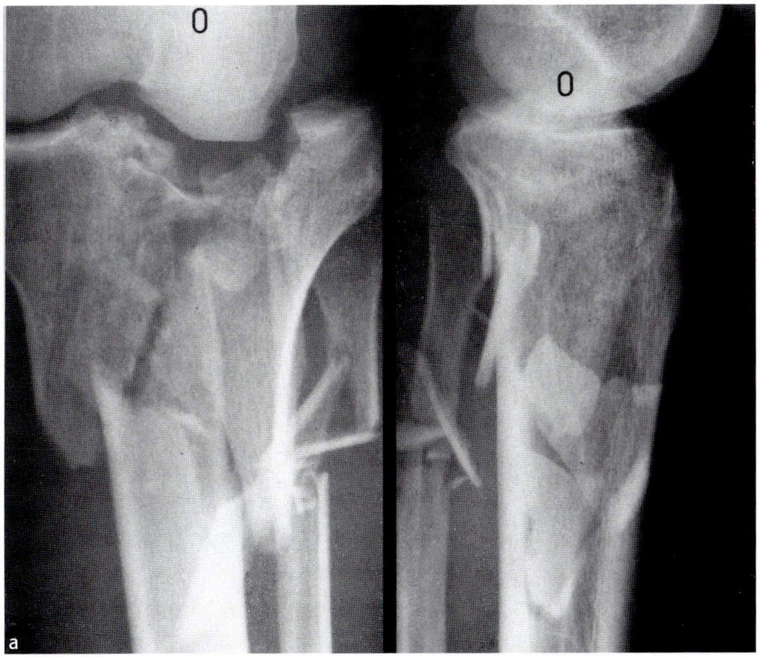

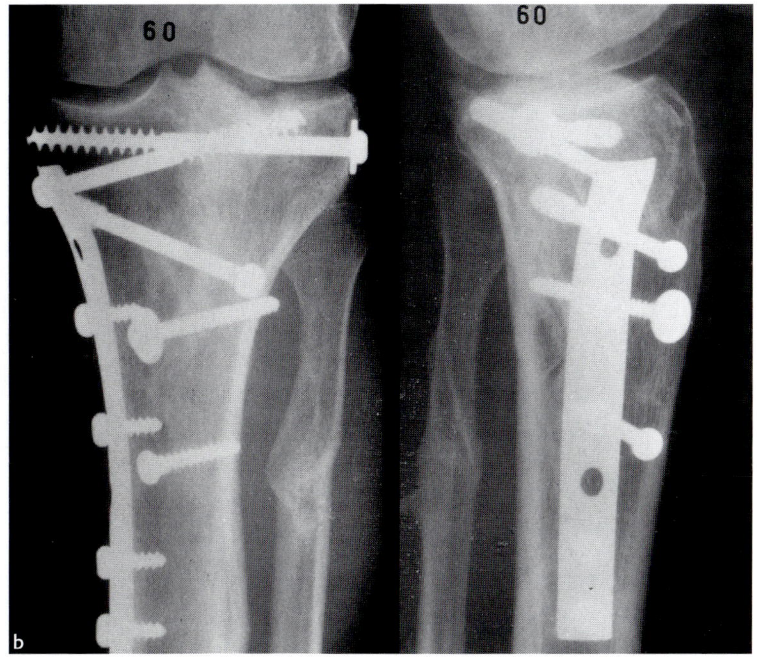

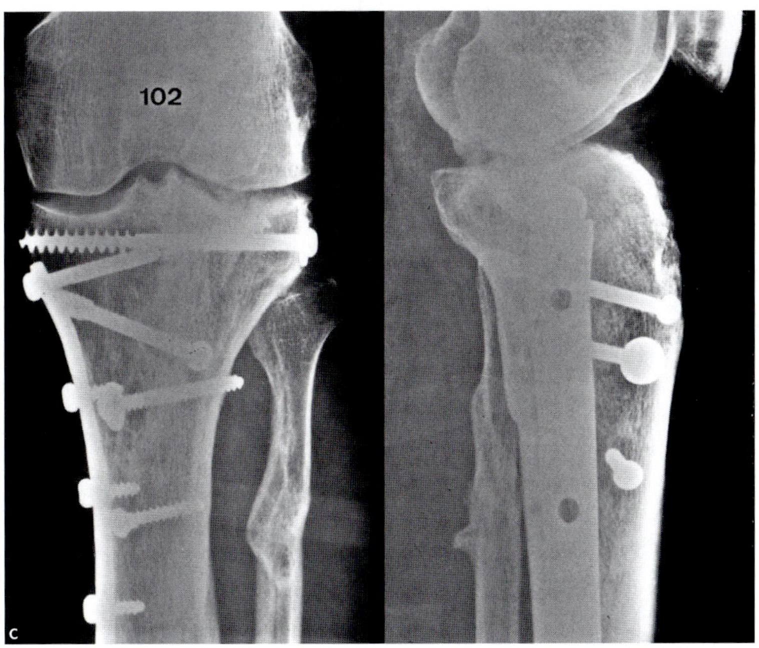

Fig. 2-10a–c Anatomical reduction and stable fixation with small amount of metal. Corticocancellous pelvic bone graft to compensate bone crush adjacent to the joint surface.

a The complex fracture with crush in the epiphysis (1965).

b 60 weeks later: fracture gaps are healed with bone density in the area of grafting.

c At 102 weeks: full recovery at that time.

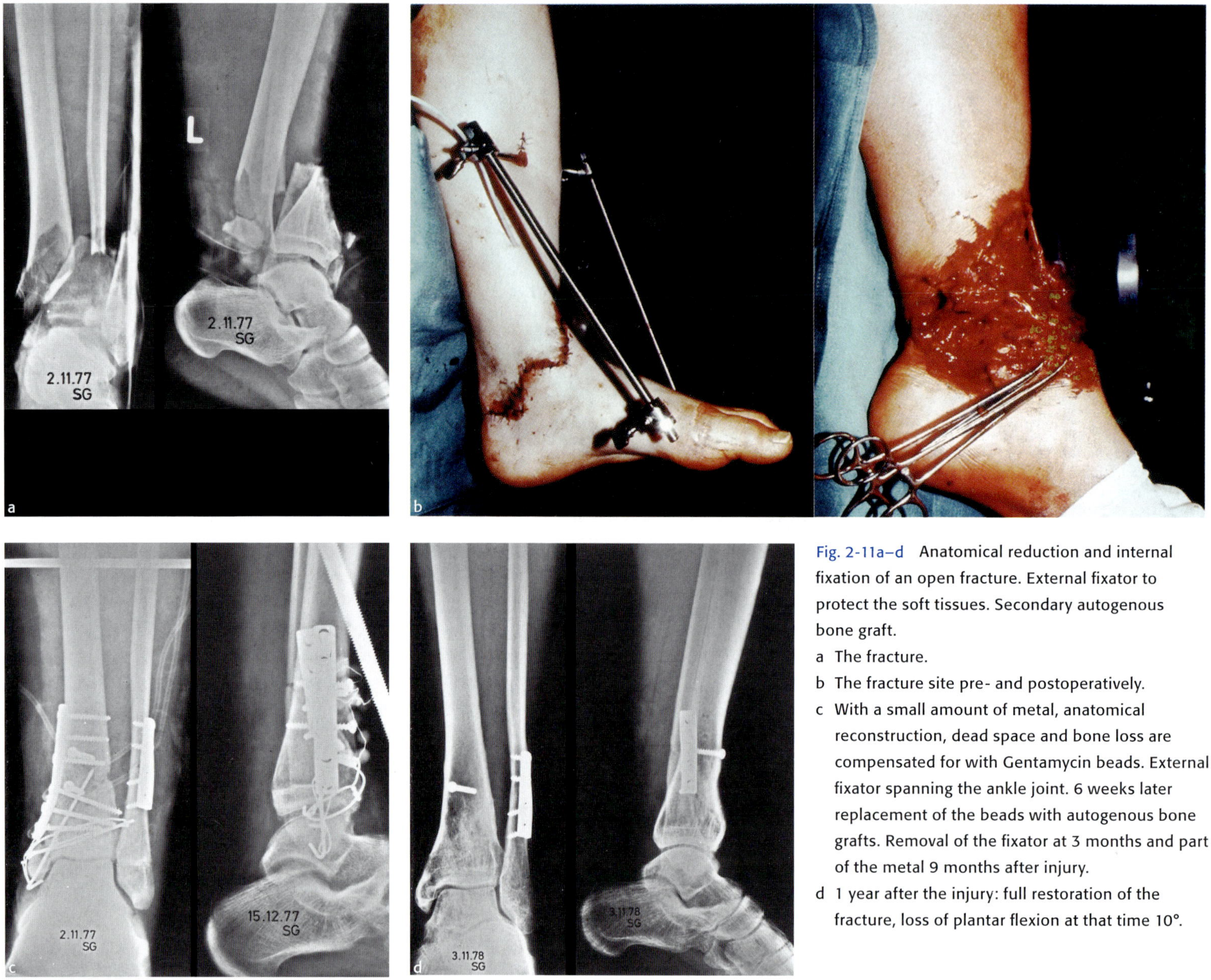

Fig. 2-11a–d Anatomical reduction and internal fixation of an open fracture. External fixator to protect the soft tissues. Secondary autogenous bone graft.

a The fracture.

b The fracture site pre- and postoperatively.

c With a small amount of metal, anatomical reconstruction, dead space and bone loss are compensated for with Gentamycin beads. External fixator spanning the ankle joint. 6 weeks later replacement of the beads with autogenous bone grafts. Removal of the fixator at 3 months and part of the metal 9 months after injury.

d 1 year after the injury: full restoration of the fracture, loss of plantar flexion at that time 10°.

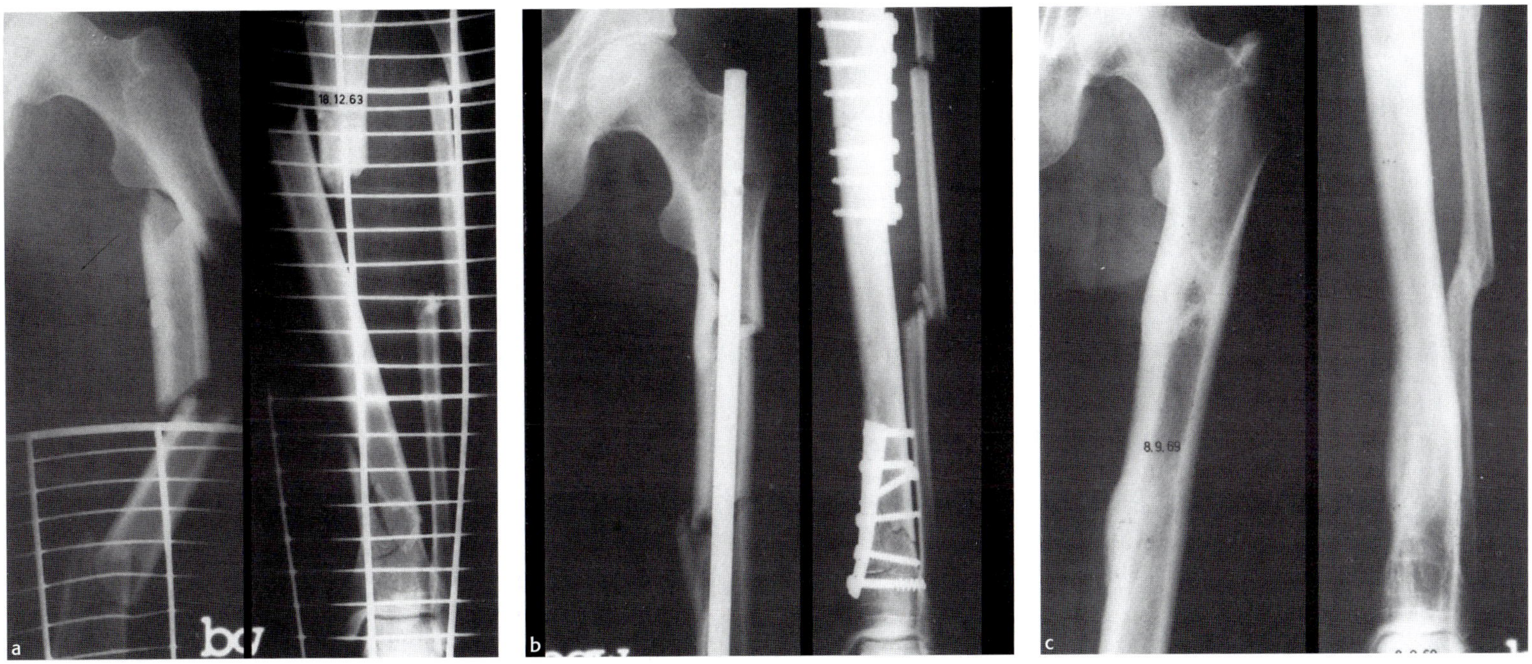

Fig. 2-12a–c Gently reamed medullary nailing and situation-adapted plating.

a Ipsilateral fractures of femur and lower leg.

b The three femur fractures are exposed and reduced through skin and fascia without additional periosteal elevation. Reaming of the proximal and adjacent fragment to 9 mm and nailing. Nailing of the next two fragments without reaming. Tibia: proximal plate is 'sheltered' by muscles, distal fracture is stabilized with a contoured semitubular plate applied atop the periosteum.

c Metal was removed one year after injury. The late result at 6 years: full recovery.

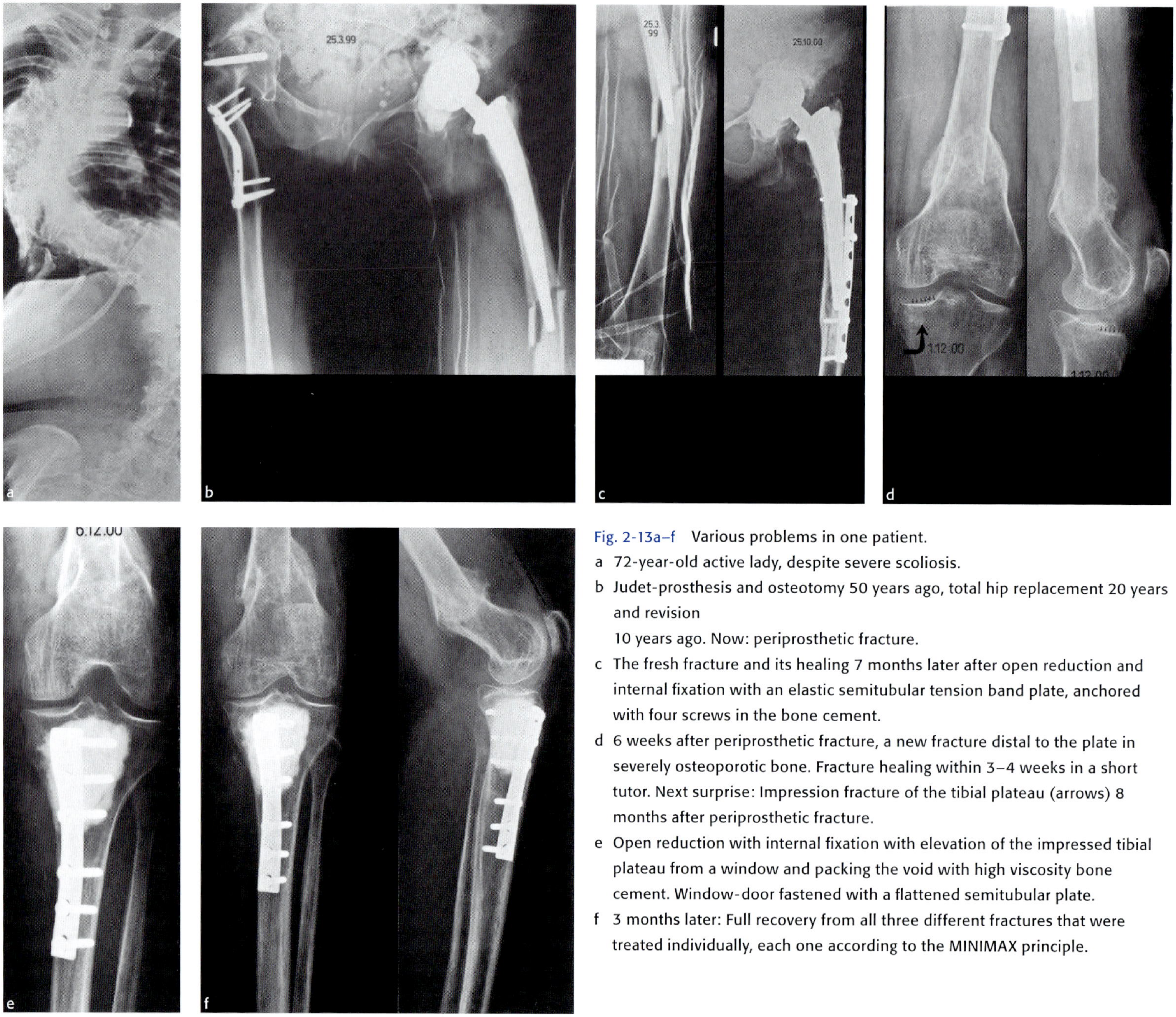

Fig. 2-13a–f Various problems in one patient.

a 72-year-old active lady, despite severe scoliosis.

b Judet-prosthesis and osteotomy 50 years ago, total hip replacement 20 years and revision 10 years ago. Now: periprosthetic fracture.

c The fresh fracture and its healing 7 months later after open reduction and internal fixation with an elastic semitubular tension band plate, anchored with four screws in the bone cement.

d 6 weeks after periprosthetic fracture, a new fracture distal to the plate in severely osteoporotic bone. Fracture healing within 3–4 weeks in a short tutor. Next surprise: Impression fracture of the tibial plateau (arrows) 8 months after periprosthetic fracture.

e Open reduction with internal fixation with elevation of the impressed tibial plateau from a window and packing the void with high viscosity bone cement. Window-door fastened with a flattened semitubular plate.

f 3 months later: Full recovery from all three different fractures that were treated individually, each one according to the MINIMAX principle.

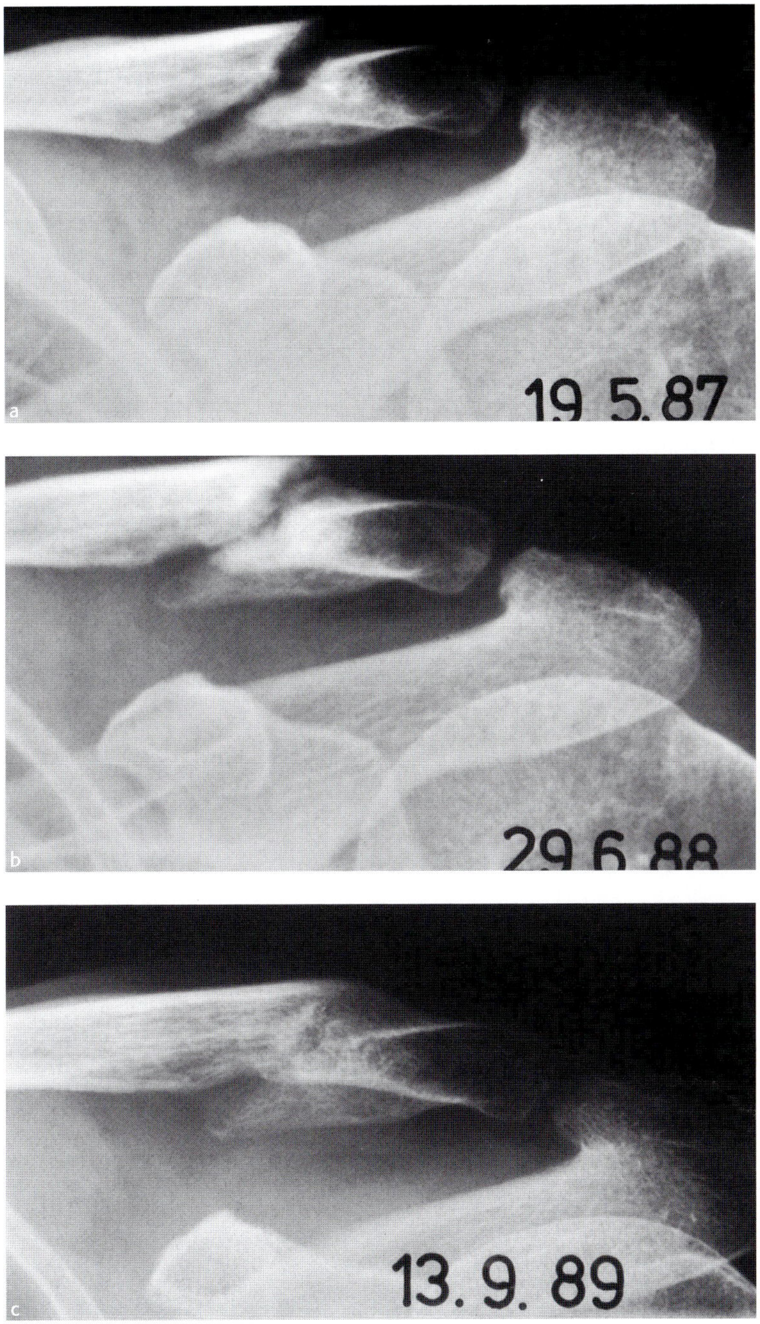

Fig. 2-14a–c MINIMAX treatment of a nonunion of the clavicula.

This final example documents how important blood perfusion of fragments and protection of a fracture or nonunion from mechanical strains are for the healing process.

a 60-year-old lady suffers from a painful nonunion that is 2 years old.

b At admission: Hypertrophic painful pseudoarthrosis with false mobility, but with a secondary frozen shoulder joint.

c 15 months after admission and treatment: the pseudarthrosis is healed without any local intervention. No drugs, no osteogenetic-bioactive medicaments, no electric or magnetic stimulation were administred. What was done: Eliminiation of mechanical strains to the nonunion from the stiff shoulder joint to the pseudarthrosis. Under general anesthesia, the stiff shoulder was mobilized by manipulation in 5–10 sec. Thereafter the nonunion healed spontaneously within 3 months.

5 Summary

Confrontation of different fixation concepts:

- Maximal invasive
  Tendency towards too much metal. Open reduction after periostial stripping.
  Risk: fragment necrosis, avital nonunion.

- MINIMAX principle
  Economic, but enough metal. Biological fixations with care for blood perfusion of fragments.
  Risk: vital nonunion.

- Minimal invasive
  Not enough metal stability for true functional aftercare.
  Risk: deformity, incongruency, dystrophy, vital nonunion.

MINIMAX fixations take pronounced care of the blood supply of bone and soft tissues. This care modifies the pattern of the original AO fixation techniques. Bone necrosis after MAXIMAL invasive fixations is difficult to treat. Should MINIMAX surgery fail, the fragments are perfused. Such nonunions are a much smaller problem and even easier to cure than fresh fractures.

For simple shaft and articular fractures, the classical AO principles have never lost any restriction. In complex problem fractures, however, a more differentiated approach for fixation is adequate. The MINIMAX principle is between rigid maximal fixation by all means and minimal invasive procedures.

When today's fashion for 'biological' and 'minimal invasive' procedures with an expanding arsenal of implants, the question remains: Is that better for the patient or better for the doctor or best for the implant industry?

The pendulum has swung too far away from the rules of open reduction and good fixation. It seems that the new products themselves are the core problem of fracture care and the procedure itself enjoys more attention than the patient's injury.

MINIMAX fixations are all 'biological'

Biological fracture fixations—Vascularity of bone and soft tissues		
Normal	>	Preserve
Impaired	>	Take care
Absent	>	Restore

Fracture fixations must be customized

Metal devices
1. Amount
2. Application
3. When not?

Internal fracture fixations may be good or bad

Internal fixation with metal devices		
Minimal	>	Insufficient
Adequate	>	Beneficial
Excessive	>	Destructive

"...überhaupt hat der Fortschritt das an sich, dass er viel grösser ausschaut, als er ist".

"...in general progress has something about it that it looks much bigger than it really is."

Johann Nepomuk Nestroy, 1801–1862 [30].

6 Bibliography

Blue references indicate links to abstracts of articles online available through Medline (www.nlm.nih.gov).

1. **Müller ME, Allgöwer M, Willenegger H** (1963) *Technik der operativen Frakturenbehandlung.* Berlin Göttingen Heidelberg: Springer-Verlag.
2. **Müller ME, Allgöwer M, Schneider R, et al.** (1991) *Manual of Internal Fixation.* Berlin Heidelberg New York: Springer-Verlag.
3. **Brunner Ch F, Weber BG** (1981/1982) *Besondere Osteosynthesetechniken, Special Techniques in Internal Fixation.* Berlin Heidelberg New York: Springer-Verlag.
4. **Weber BG** (1972) *Die Verletzungen des oberen Sprunggelenkes.* Bern Stuttgart Wien: Huber.
5. **Weber BG** (1972) L'ostéosynthèse à compression au niveau des diaphyses. In: Boitzy A, editor. *Périarthrite de l'épaule. Ostéogénèse et compression.* Berne Stuttgart Vienne: Huber: 192–193.
6. **Weber BG** (1976) *Pseudarthrosis.* Bern Stuttgart Wien: Huber.
7. **Weber BG** (1979) *Die Verletzungen des proximalen Femurendes.* Chirurg. Operationslehre Breitner IV/2. Ergänzung 33: 22–56. München Wien Baltimore: Urban und Schwarzenberg.
8. **Weber BG** (1984) Reinraumtechnik in der orthopädischen Chirurgie. In: Draenert K, Rütt A, editors. *Erfahrungen mit dem operativen Gelenkersatz.* München: Art and Science: 117–123.
9. **Weber BG, Magerl F** (1985) *The external fixator.* Berlin Heidelberg New York Tokyo: Springer.
10. **Boitzy A** (1971) *La fracture du col du fémur chez l'enfant et l'adolescent.* Paris: Masson.
11. **Weber BG, Brunner Ch, Freuler F** (1980) *Treatment of Fractures in Children and Adolescents.* Berlin Heidelberg New York: Springer-Verlag.
12. **Mast J, Jakob R, Ganz R** (1989) *Planning and Reduction Technique in Fracture Surgery.* Berlin Heidelberg New York London Paris Tokyo: Springer-Verlag.
13. **Apley AG** (1997) cited from Murphy L. Movement is life. *AO Dialogue;* 10 /(4-5).
14. **Orozco Delclos RuL** (1983) *Fracturas diafisarias Objetivos de la técnica AO. Criterios quirurgicos. Fundamentos clinicos e Histologicos.* Monografias de la Fundacion Maurice E. Müller—Espana.
15. **Sarmiento A, Latta LL** (1981) *Closed functional treatment of fractures.* Berlin Heidelberg New York: Springer.
16. **Brown Ch Sen.** (1992) cited from Lang N. *Schweizer Pioniere der Wirtschaft und Technik.* Gründer eines Weltunternehmens Charles EL Brown Walter Boveri Verein für wirtschaftliche Studien, CH-8706 Meilen, 1992.
17. **Roux W** (1881/1965) cited from Pauwels F. *Gesammelte Abhandlungen zur funktionellen Anatomie des Bewegungsapparates.* Berlin Heidelberg New York:Springer.
18. **Wolff D** (1892) *Das Gesetz der Transfermation der Knochen.* Berlin: A. Hirschwald.
19. **Pauwels F** (1965) Grundriss der Biomechanik der Frakturheilung In: Pauwels F, editor. *Gesammelte Abhandlungen zur funktionellen Anatomie des Bewegungsapparates.* Berlin Heidelberg New York: Springer: 139–182.
20. **Krompecher S** (1937) *Die Knochenbildung.* Jena: Gustav Fischer.
21. **Perren SM** (1972) Biomécanique de la compression interfragmentaire. In: Boitzy A, editor. *Périarthrite de l'éaule. Ostéosynthèse et compression.* Berne Stuttgart Vienne: Huber: 136–145.
22. **Perren SM** (1979) Physical and biological aspects of fracture healing with special reference to internal fixation. *Clin Orthop;* (138):75–196.
23. **Perren SM, Boitzy A** (1978) Cellular Differentiation and Bone Biomechanics During the Consolidation of a Fracture. *Anatomia Clinica;* 1:13–28.
24. **Knese K-H** (1958) *Knochenstruktur als Verbundbau.* Stuttgart: Thieme.
25. **Weber BG** (2000) MINIMAX-Prinzip für Osteosynthesen beim Erwachsenen. In: Dubs L, editor. *Orthopädie an der Schwelle.* Bern Göttingen Toronto Seattle: Huber: 19–133.
26. **Weber BG** (1982) *Influence of surgical technique and laminar flow on infection rate Proceedings Symposium.* Geneva Hongkong Princeton Tokyo: Excerpta Medica Amsterdam: 43–46.
27. **Bernasconi E, Francioli P** (2000) Empfehlungen zur perioperativen Antibioticaprophylaxe. *Swiss-NOSO;* 7 (9).
28. **Charnley J** (1979) *Low friction arthroplasty of the hip.* Berlin Heidelberg New York: Springer-Verlag.
29. **Lidwell OM, Lowbury EJL, Whyte W, et al.** (1982) Effect of ultraclean air in operating rooms on deep sepsis in the joint after total hip or knee replacement: A randomised study. *Br Med J (Clin Res Ed);* 285 (6334):10–14.
30. **Nestroy JN** (1997) In: Bankl H, editor. *Der Pathologe weiss alles... aber zu spät.* Wien: Verlag K & S; 88.

3 Lower leg fractures with and without involvement of the ankle joint

1 Introduction

Fracture classifications are helpful in several ways:

1. Anatomical description of all possible and observed fractures, like a stamp collection, striving for completeness, eg, Cooper 1842, Helferich 1903.

2. Identification of fractures of long bones in a comprehensive system that allows dialogue studies on frequency, severity, adequate treatments, and results, eg, Classification AO des fractures (1987) [1] and the AO manuals 1991, 2000 [2, 3].

3. Description of specific joint fractures and their ligament injuries, eg, for the ankle joint, Danis 1949, Weber 1966 [4].

In the following sections, the problem of which patterns of lower leg fractures are more or less likely to be accompanied by additional lesions of the ankle joint and which patterns not, will be discussed. About 800 fractures of the lower leg (shaft and ankle), documented in my slide collection, were analyzed.

In the AO literature, ankle lesions, fractures of the tibial head and of the tibial pilon are classified and discussed separately from lower leg shaft fractures.

The author's ankle and pilon classifications and treatment continue to have validity within the AO. In contrast, shaft fractures are no longer systematically and openly reduced and internally fixed. So-called biological fixations are 'en vogue' (indirect reduction, minimal invasive procedures), which is not, however, without negative and underrated consequences:

With interlocking nailing and subcutaneous bridging plating, precise anatomical reconstruction is impossible. For lower leg fractures, associated with lesions of the ankle joint, precise repair is mandatory. Such fractures are more than just a fractured tibia. The ankle lesion is the lesion with the higher priority and it needs attention for 'waterproof' reduction and rigid fixation, ie, for restoration of normal anatomy.

The original classification of ankle fractures (Fig. 3-1a–c) is the layout of what may be associated with a leg fracture. Flake fractures of the talar dome (Fig. 3-2) and lesions of the tibial pilon fractures (Fig. 3-3) also deserve attention.

In absence of positive x-ray findings at the ankle joint in a lower leg fracture, but in presence of local injury suspicion, precise x-rays will give diagnostic answers (Fig. 3-4a–b, 3-5a–b), mostly without the need for additional imaging (MRI, CT-scan, arthrography).

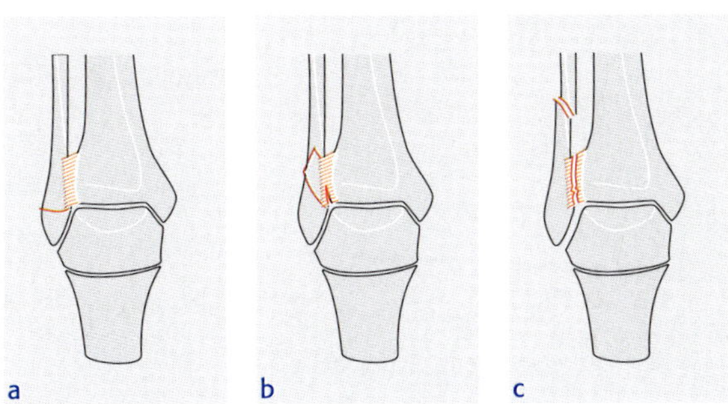

Fig. 3-1a–c Ankle fractures.
a Fibula fractured below the syndesmosis.
b Fibula fractured at the level of the syndesmosis.
c Fibula fractured above the syndesmosis.

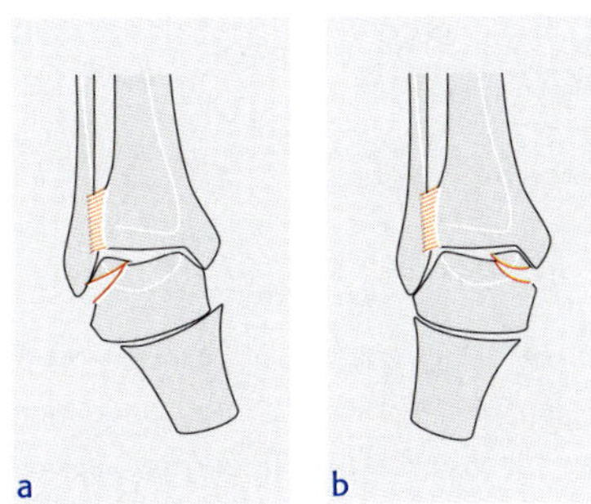

Fig. 3-2a–b Talar dome fractures.
a Lateral flake.
b Medial flake.

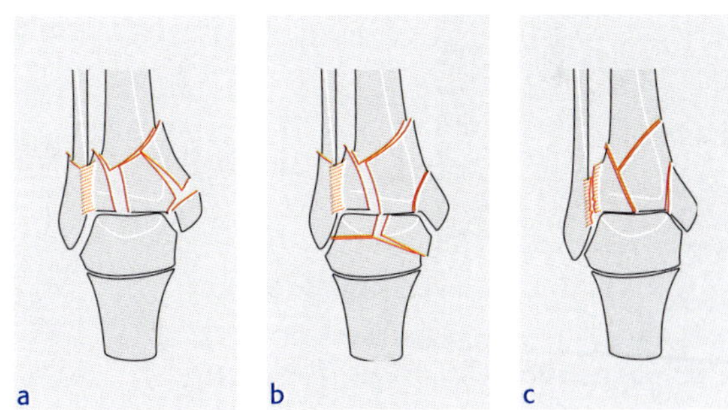

Fig. 3-3a–c Classification of tibial pilon fractures.
a Fibula and pilon fractured.
b Fibula, pilon, and talus fractured.
c Fibula, not pilon fractured.

2 General points on lower leg fractures and associated lesions of the ankle joint

The 'forearm' chapter of the AO Principles of Fracture Management [3] 2000, describes the fractures of both bones, their treatment and stresses the importance of the interosseous membrane.

Not only the forearm, but also the lower leg, the tibia, the fibula, and the interosseous fibrous-ligamentous elements need full recovery to be part of fracture treatment. Though the fibula is much smaller than the tibia, it needs utmost attention in cases of lower leg fractures. The final result may be more controlled by the fibula than the tibia. Pol Le Coeur's statement has lost nothing since 1938 [6]: "Dans les fractures de jambe, seul l'état du péroné permet d'expliquer l'état fonctionnel de la tibio-tarsienne. C'est au péroné que doivent se juger ces fractures. Leur thérapeutique doit éviter les alterérations de la fonction tibio-péronière." Translated: "In leg fractures, only the state of the fibula allows us to judge the state of the ankle joint. Leg fractures must be judged on the fibula. Their treatment must avoid any alteration of the tibio-fibular function."

The purpose of the following section is to establish the severity of different lower leg fractures from that standpoint. In addition, the question should be answered as to fractures should be treated with open reduction and internal fixation and which ones can be treated 'biologically'.

The tibia and fibula are tied together by a complex structure, by the syndesmotic ligaments and by the interosseous membrane (SLIM) (Fig. 3-6a–b).

Whenever SLIM is ruptured downwards into the ankle joint, the ankle fork becomes widened and unstable. The ankle joint then becomes incongruent and undergoes posttraumatic osteoarthritis.

When SLIM is intact, the ankle fork is normal. There may be damage in the ankle joint of a different nature. A broken fibula and downward ruptured SLIM therefore has treatment priority, not only in typical ankle fractures, but also in all lower leg fractures.

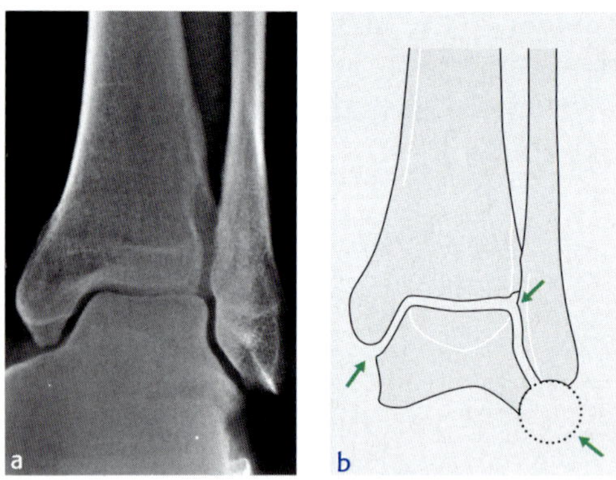

Fig. 3-4a–b X-ray of a normal ankle joint.

a Parallel joint space all the way.

b Normal length of fibula: parallel joint space, unbroken subchondral line from fibula to tibia, virtual ball fitting the distal fibula and the talus (arrows).

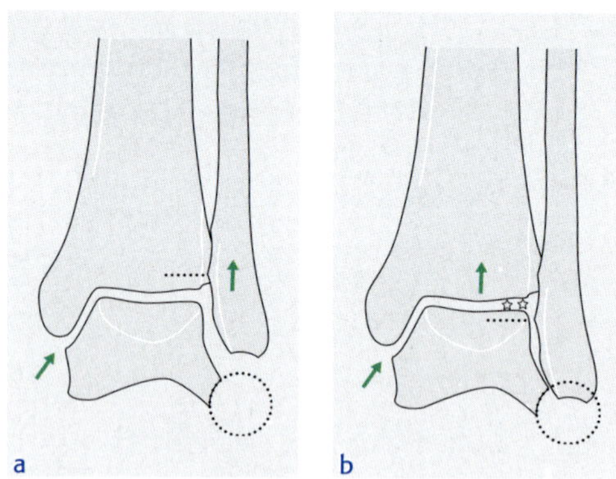

Fig. 3-5a–b Length misfit.

a Shortened fibula: widened joint space medially, broken subchondral line, fibula elevated from the virtual ball.

b Shortened tibia: no widening of joint space medially, but occasionally widening next to the fibula (starlets), broken subchondral line in the other direction, fibula impacted into the virtual ball.

3 Classification of lower leg fractures

The following classification does not compete with the AO classification of long-bone fractures. It is an additional one for the ankle joint that might be included into the injury of the lower leg.

Classification of fractures in the lower leg:

Type F: Fractures of the fibula
Type T: Fractures of the tibia
Type F+T: Fractures of the fibula and the tibia

The diagrams are labeled with literal notation and the SLIM lesions are expressed schematically with a red dot.

The illustrations are briefly annotated regarding the fracture pattern and ankle joint involvement and illustrated stepwise with clinical examples. The x-rays are dated with time of injury, treatment, and follow-up.

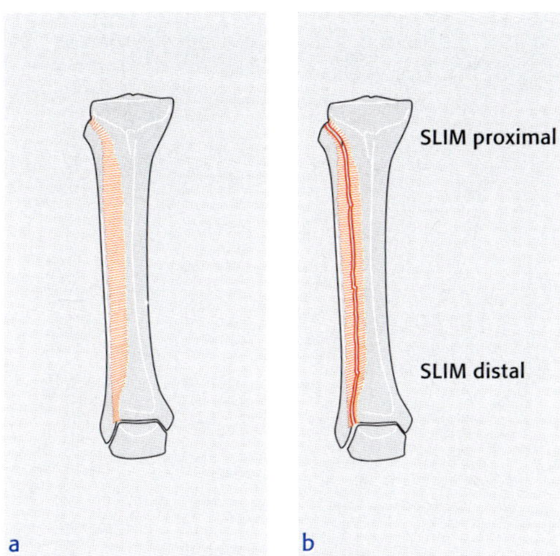

Fig. 3-6a–b The fibulotibial compound structure.
a Fibula and tibia are tied together by the proximal and the distal syndesmotic ligaments and the interosseous membrane, the SLIM.
b All degrees of SLIM rupture are possible, either total or proximal or distal.

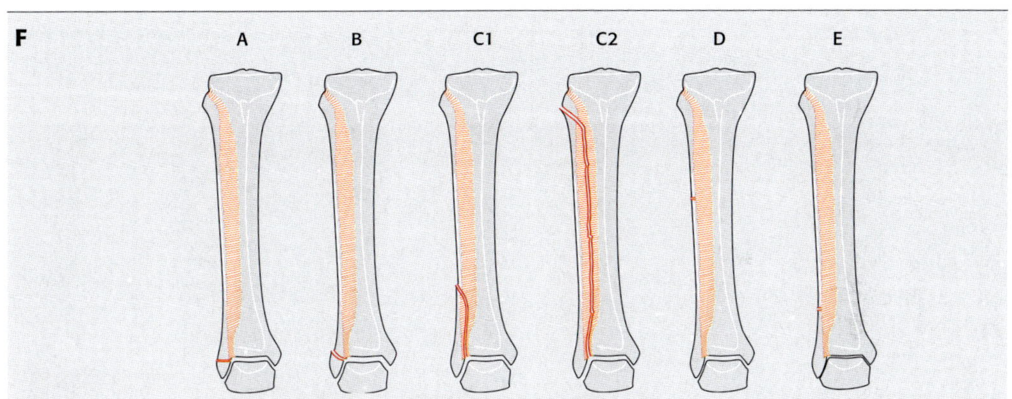

	A	B	C1	C2	D	E
SLIM proximal	○	○	○	●	○	○
SLIM distal	○	◐	●	●	○	○
Ankle joint injury	●	●	●	●	○	○

Fig. 3-7 Type F fractures of the fibula A–E.
A, B, C are the classical ankle fractures according to Danis and Weber . Their variations are seen in Fig. 3-1–3-3.

Clinical examples are described in Fig. 3-8–3-14.

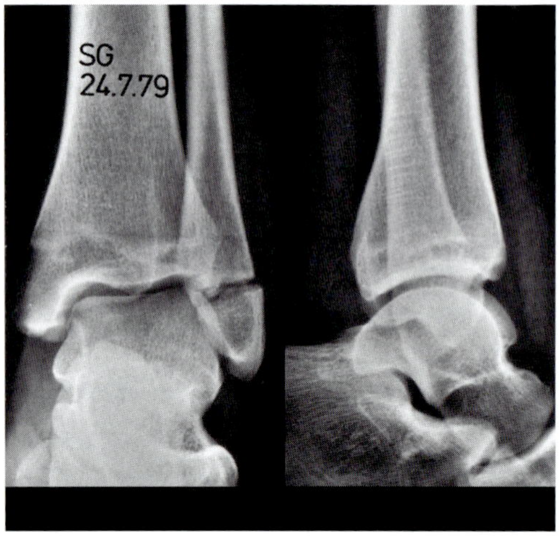

Fig. 3-8 According to Fig. 3-7 A.
Fracture below SLIM.

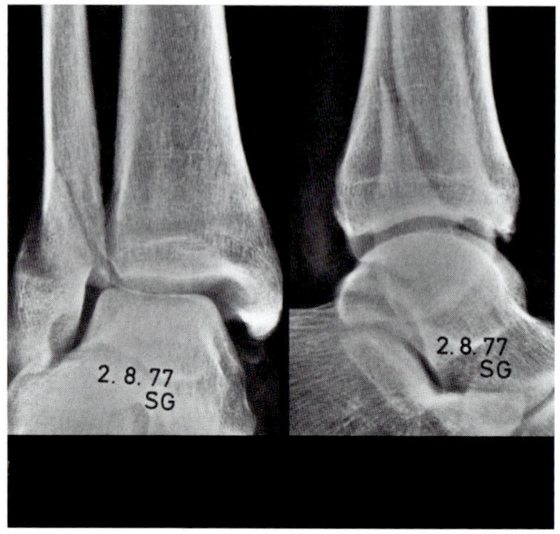

Fig. 3-9 According to Fig. 3-7 B.
Fracture at the level of distal syndesmotic ligaments.

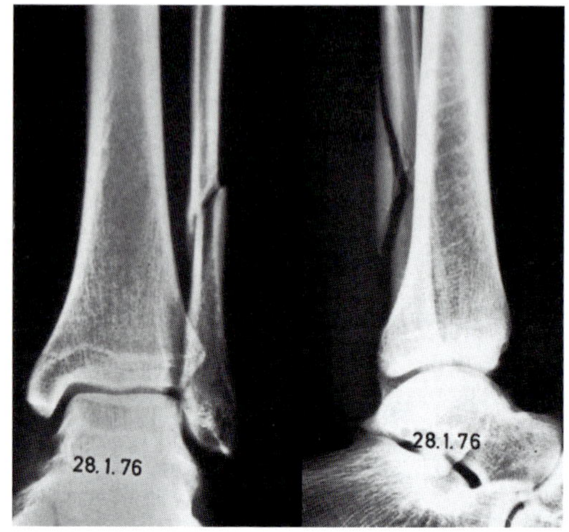

Fig. 3-10 According to Fig. 3-7 C1.
Fracture above of distal syndesmotic ligaments.

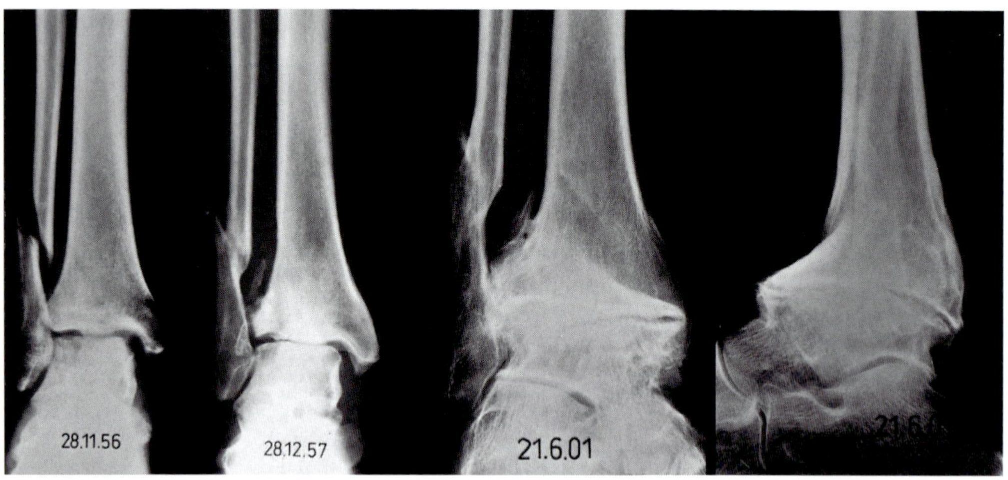

Fig. 3-11 According to Fig. 3-7 C1.
Neglected injury and secondary osteoarthritis.

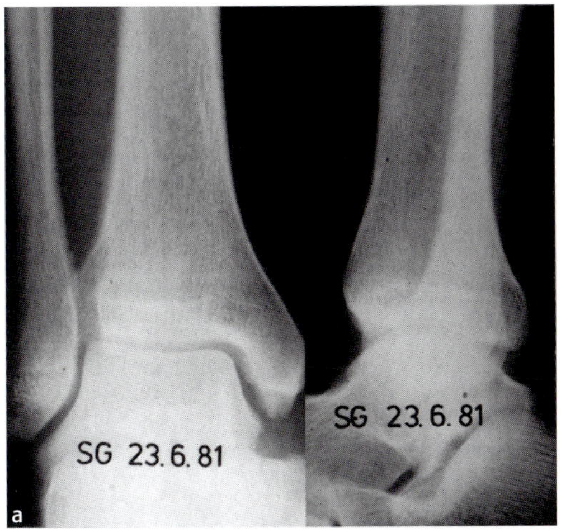

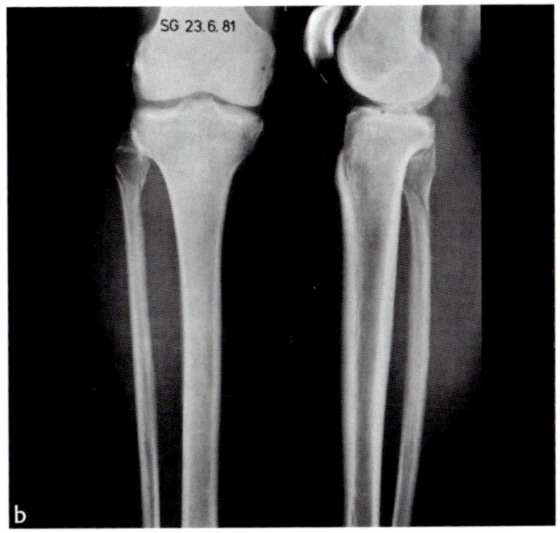

Fig. 3-12a–c According to Fig. 3-7 C2.
a Swollen ankle, x-ray normal.

b Subcapital fracture: Maisonneuve lesion.

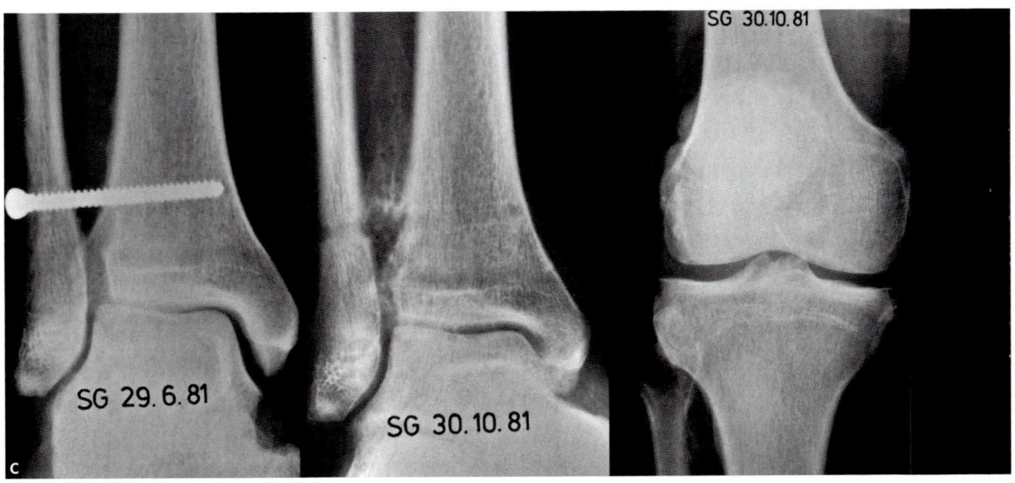

c Positioning screw. Ossification of interosseous membrane. Fracture healed.

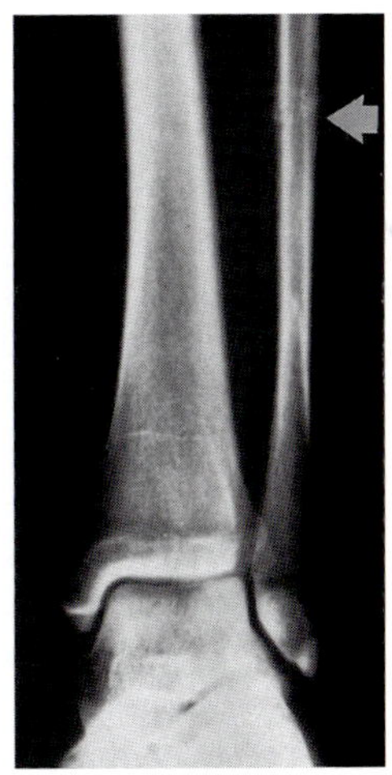

Fig. 3-13 According to Fig. 3-7 D.
Fatigue fracture in a runner (arrow).

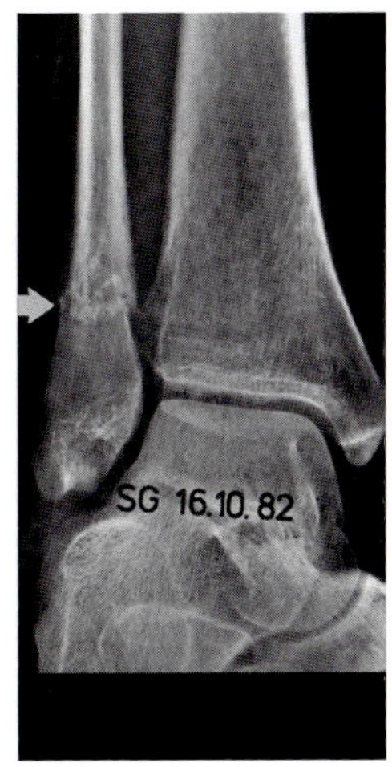

Fig. 3-14 According to Fig. 3-7 E.
Direct blow fracture in a woodchopper (arrow).

Type T fractures A–F with clinical examples (Fig. 3-16–3-30).

The level and the degree of displacement of the fracture determines the severity of injury (Fig. 3-15).

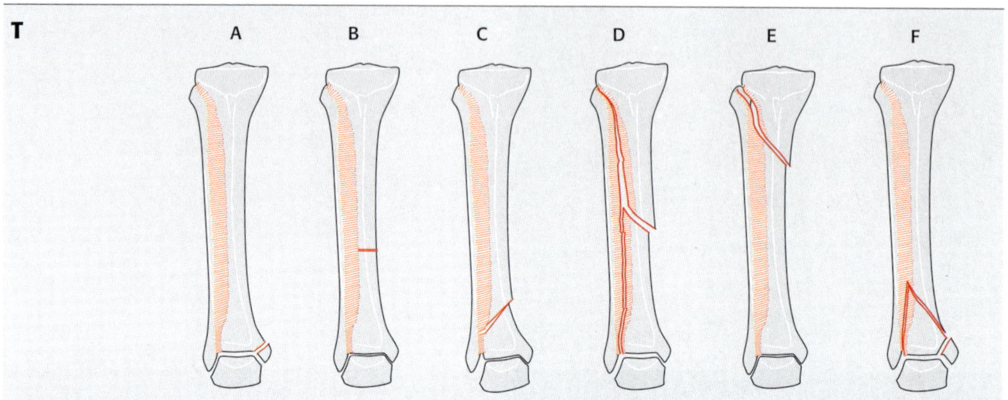

T	A	B	C	D	E	F
SLIM proximal	○	○	○	●	●	○
SLIM distal	○	○	○	●	○	●
Ankle joint injury	●	○	○	●	○	●

Fig. 3-15 Type T fractures A–F.

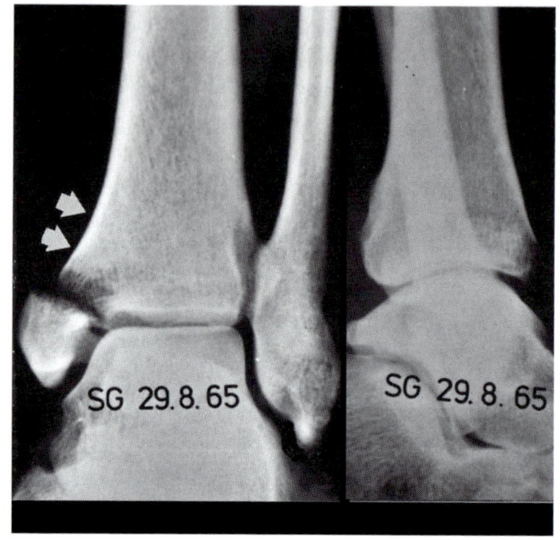

Fig. 3-16 According to Fig. 3-15 A.
Direct blow (arrows) fracture in a soccer player.

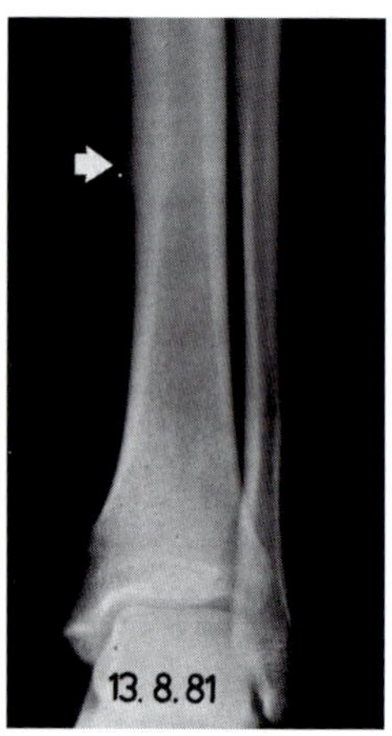

Fig. 3-17 According to Fig. 3-15 B.
Fatigue fracture in a ballet dancer (arrow).

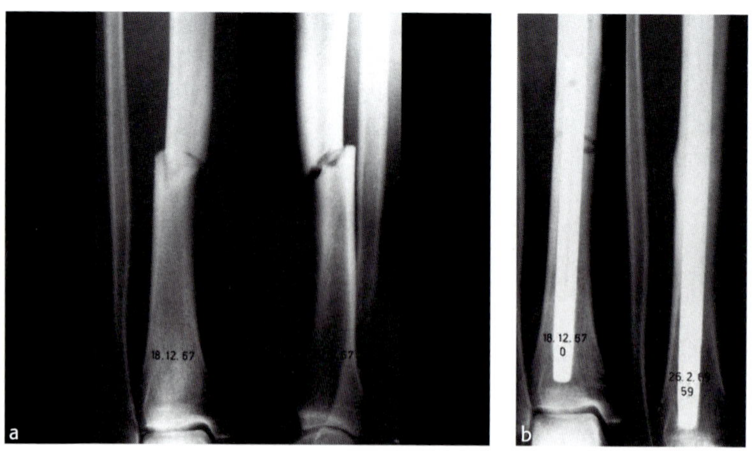

Fig. 3-18a–b According to Fig. 3-15 B.
a Slightly displaced transverse-short oblique fracture.

b Open reduction and internal fixation with nail and healing x-ray 59 weeks later.

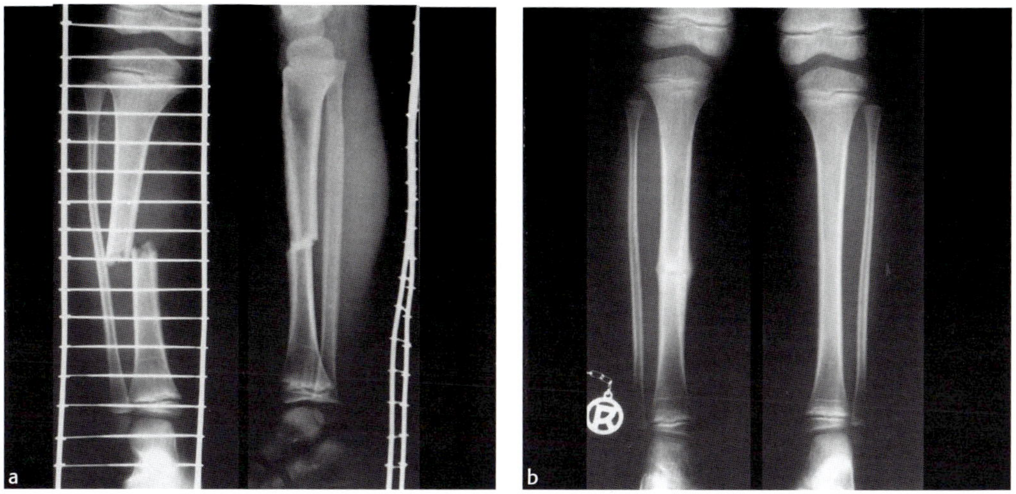

Fig. 3-19a–b According to Fig. 3-15 B.
a Displaced fracture in a child.
b Healing after closed reduction. Slight overgrowth (see Harris lines) at fracture site.

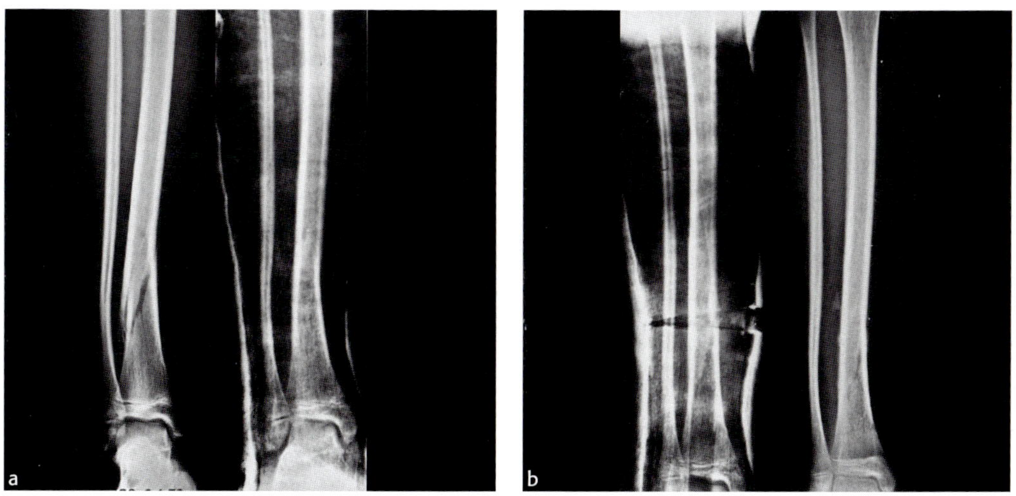

Fig. 3-20a–b According to Fig. 3-15 C.
a Varus bowing in a child's fracture.
b Cast wedging and anatomical healing after 8 weeks.

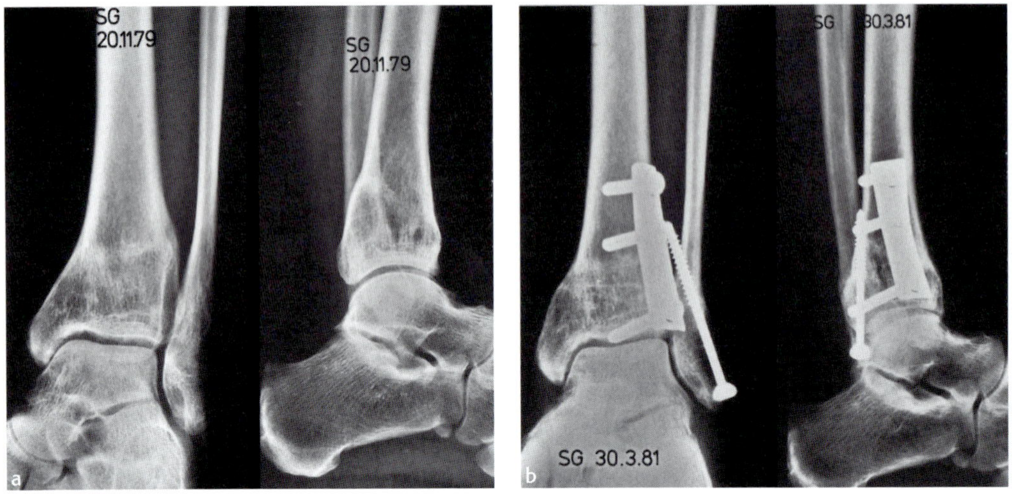

Fig. 3-21a–b According to Fig. 3-15 C.

a Varus and bowing of fibula 4 years after fracture.

b Malalignment corrected with osteotomy.

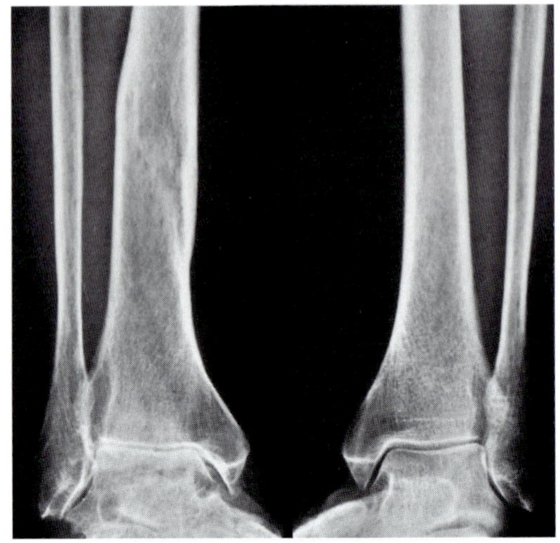

Fig. 3-22 According to Fig. 3-15 D.
Fracture healed with tibia shortening and relative overlength of fibula. Secondary osteoarthritis (compare with left side).

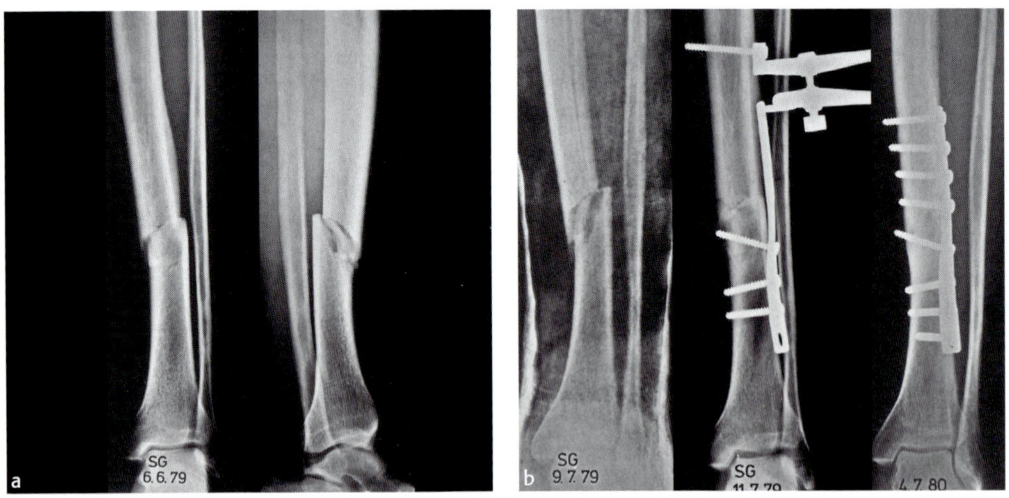

Fig. 3-23a–b According to Fig. 3-15 D.

a Slight varus and shortening of tibia. Fibula not bowed, but straight and too long.

b Correction of deformity in favor of the ankle joint 5 weeks after bracing: lengthening of tibia with open reduction and internal fixation. Result after 1 year: normal ankle joint.

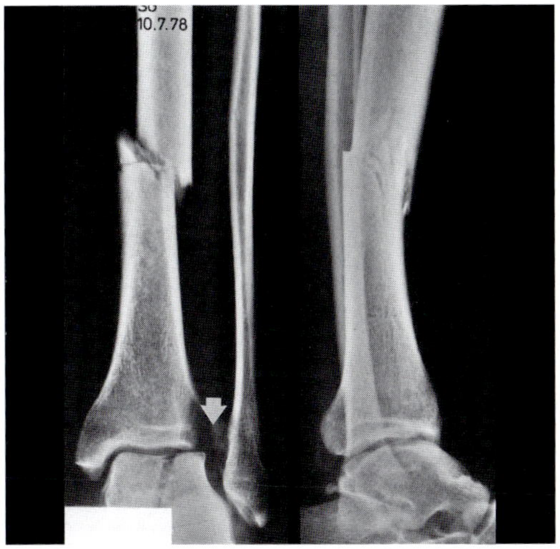

Fig. 3-24 According to Fig. 3-15 D.
Evident tibial shortening, rupture of distal SLIM and fibula overlength (arrow), sagittal talus splitting under the axial impaction trauma.

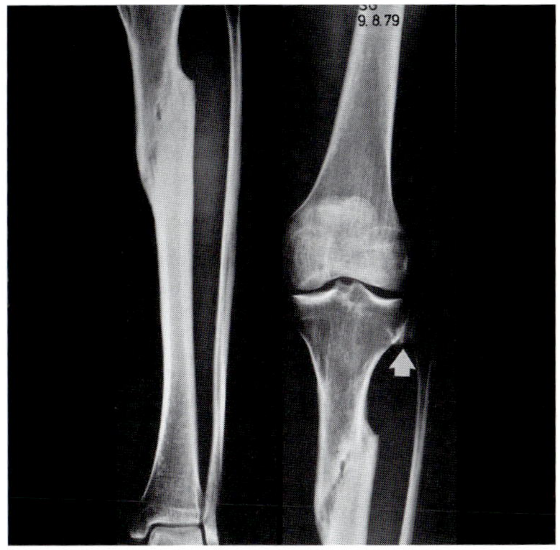

Fig. 3-25 According to Fig. 3-15 E.
Tibial shortening, rupture of proximal SLIM, overlength of fibula and dislocation of fibular head (arrow).

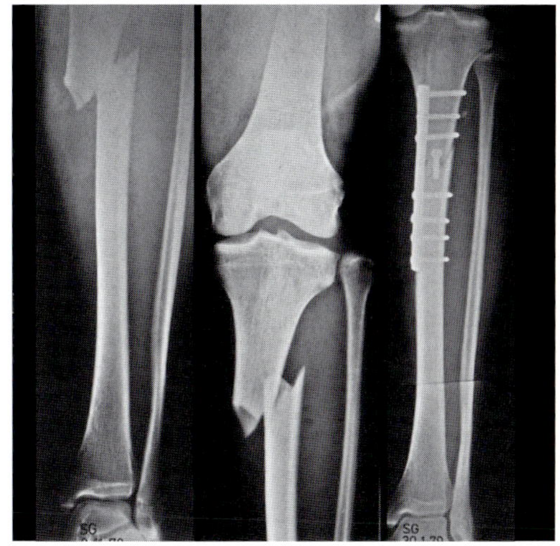

Fig. 3-26 According to Fig. 3-15 E.
Identical lesion to Fig. 3-3–25, but open reduction and internal fixation of the tibial fracture reduces the dislocated fibular head automatically.

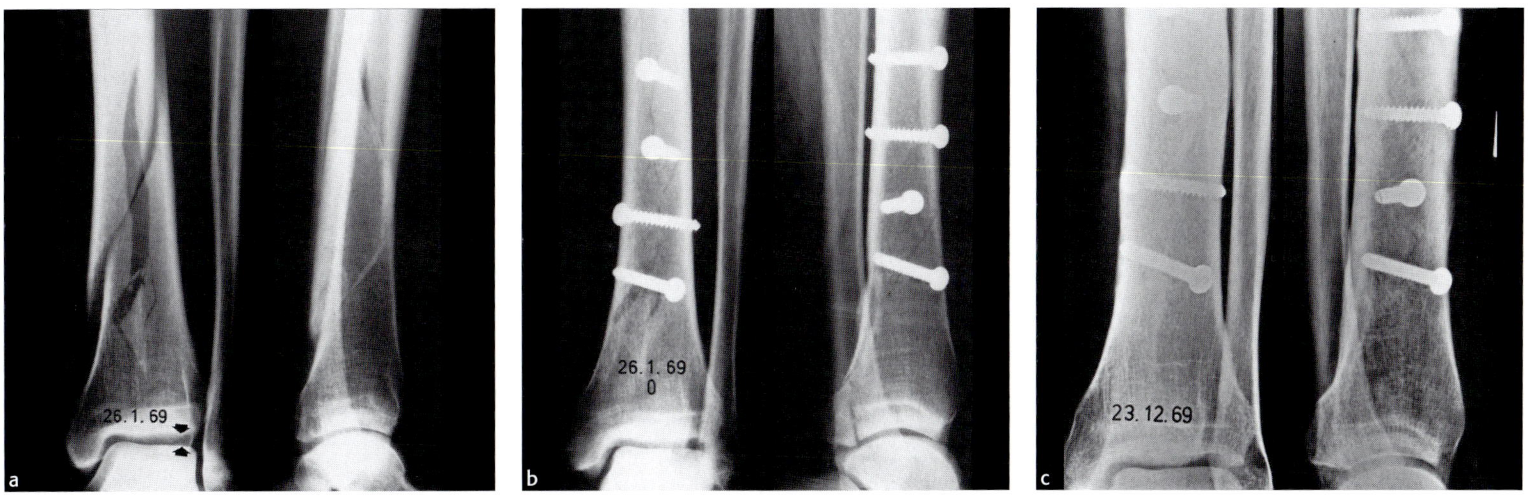

Fig. 3-27a–c According to Fig. 3-15 F.

a Spiral tibial fracture with shortening. Note widened joint space (arrows).

b Only now manifest after open reduction and internal fixation: The posterior lip fragment, linked with the fibula by the posterior syndesmotic ligaments, pushes down the talus since it is not reduced anatomically.

c The lip fragment is correctly healed under functional aftercare and the joint space is normal.

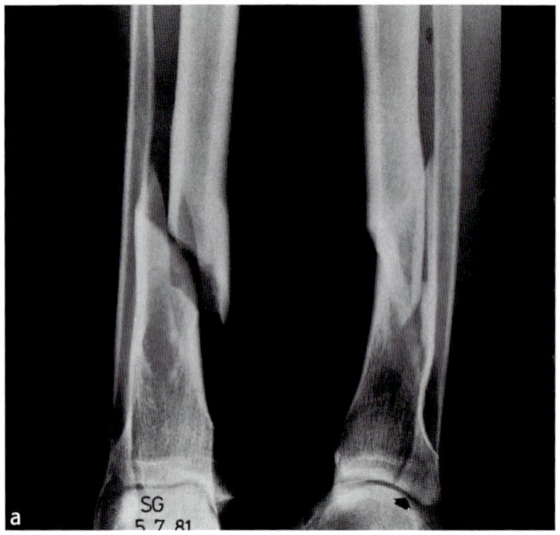

Fig. 3-28a–b According to Fig. 3-15 F.

a A large posterior lip fragment linked with the fibula (arrow). The tibia is shortened by varus.

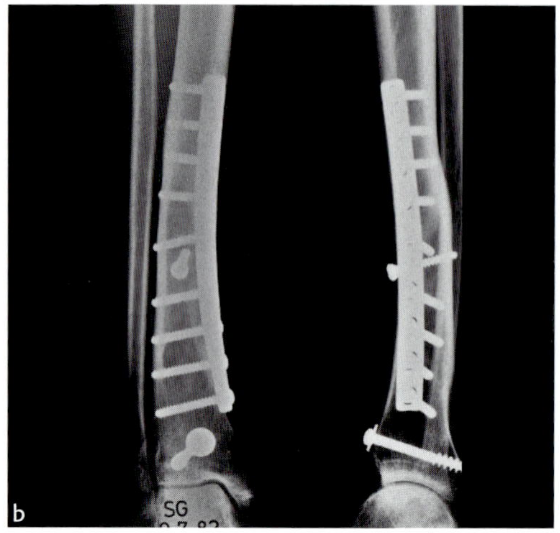

b Anatomical healing 1 year after open reduction and internal fixation.

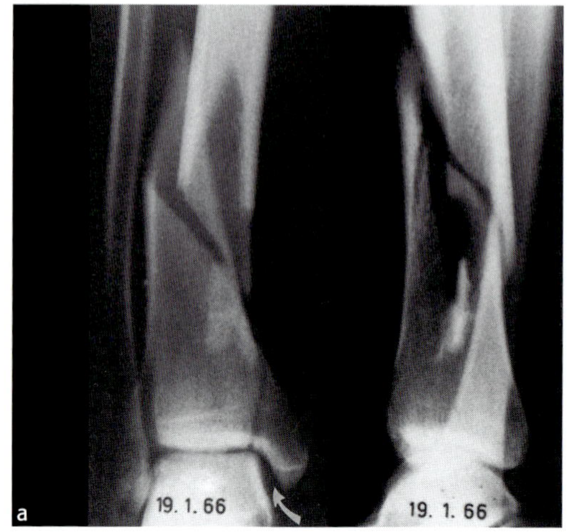

Fig. 3-29a–b According to Fig. 3-15 F.

a Shortened tibia, bowing of fibula, medial malleolus pushed medially, widening of joint space (arrow).

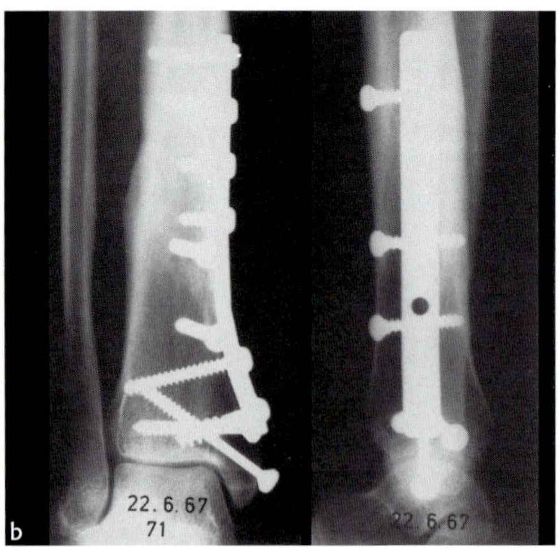

Fig. 3-29a–b

b 71 weeks after injury and osteosynthesis: back to normal, note parallel joint space.

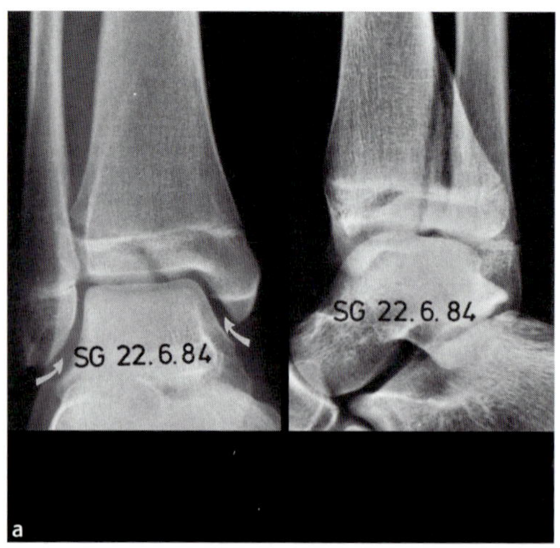

Fig. 3-30a–b According to Fig. 3-15 F.

a Three-plane fracture in a youngster. Widened ankle fork (arrows).

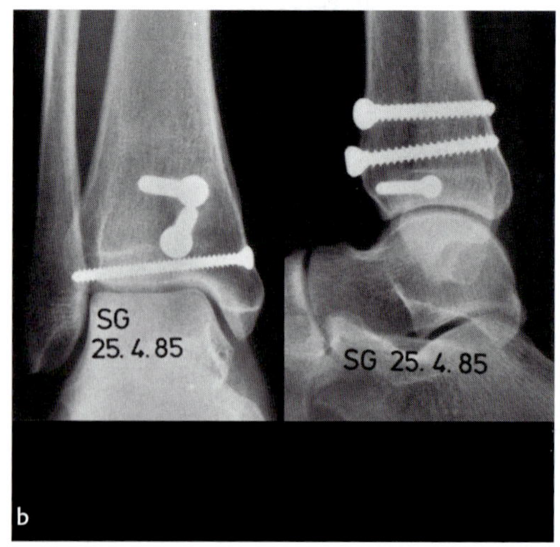

b Joint space parallel-normal 10 months after open reduction and internal fixation.

Type F+T fractures of fibula and tibia with clinical examples described in Fig. 3-32–3-38.

When both lower leg bones are broken, either transverse, spiral, or complex, typical fracture patterns result in relation to the ankle joint and to SLIM.

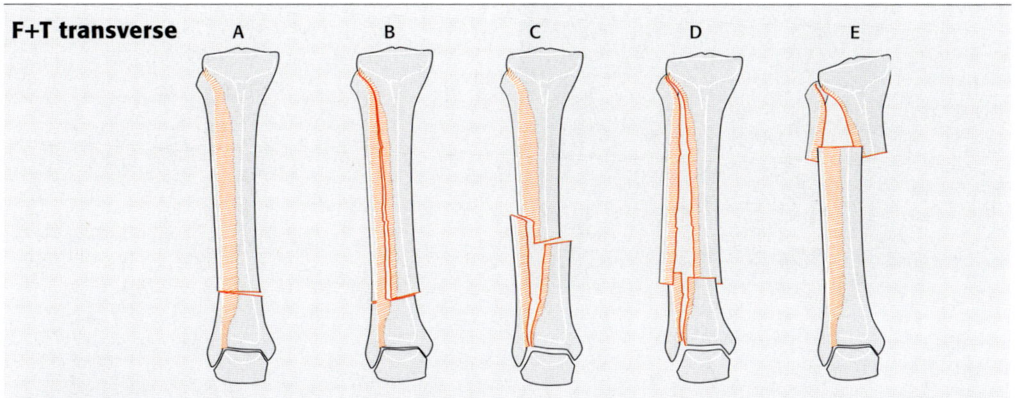

	A	B	C	D	E
SLIM proximal	○	●	○	●	●
SLIM distal	○	○	●	●	○
Ankle joint injury	○	○	●	●	○

Fig. 3-31
Type F+T transverse fractures A–E.

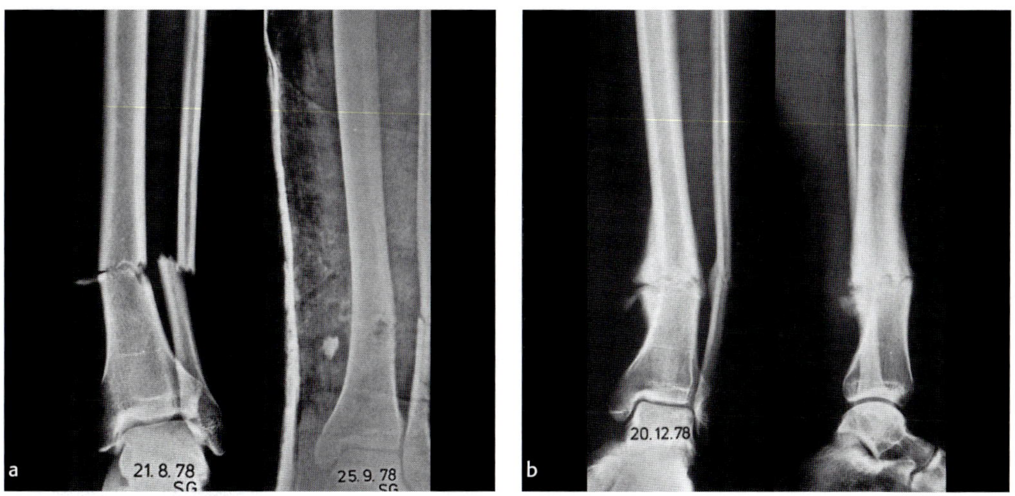

Fig. 3-32a–b According to Fig. 3-31 A.
a Closed reduction and functional bracing.
b After 4 months, slightly delayed healing with varus deformity.

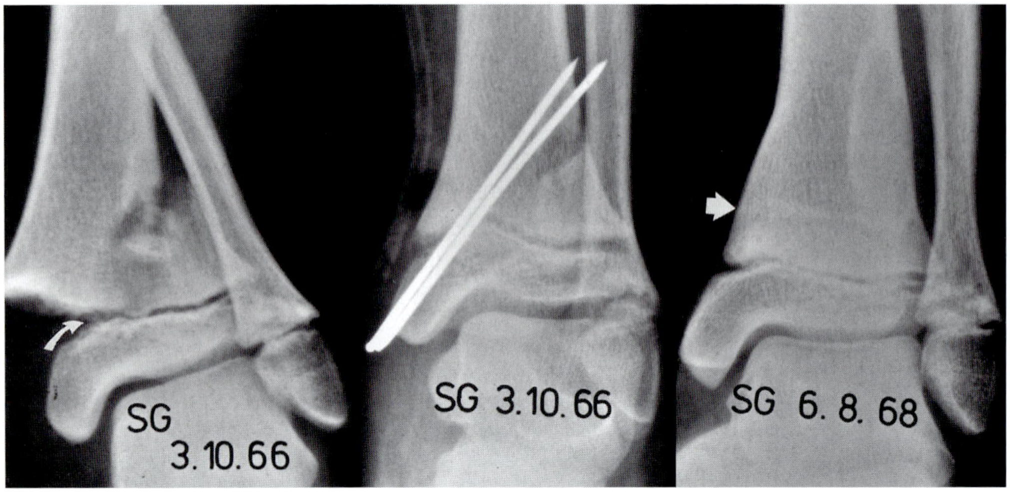

Fig. 3-33 According to Fig. 3-31 A.
Lysis-metaphyseal fracture entrapment of periosteum (arrow). Open reduction and internal fixation and anatomical healing, normal growth, see Harris line (arrow).

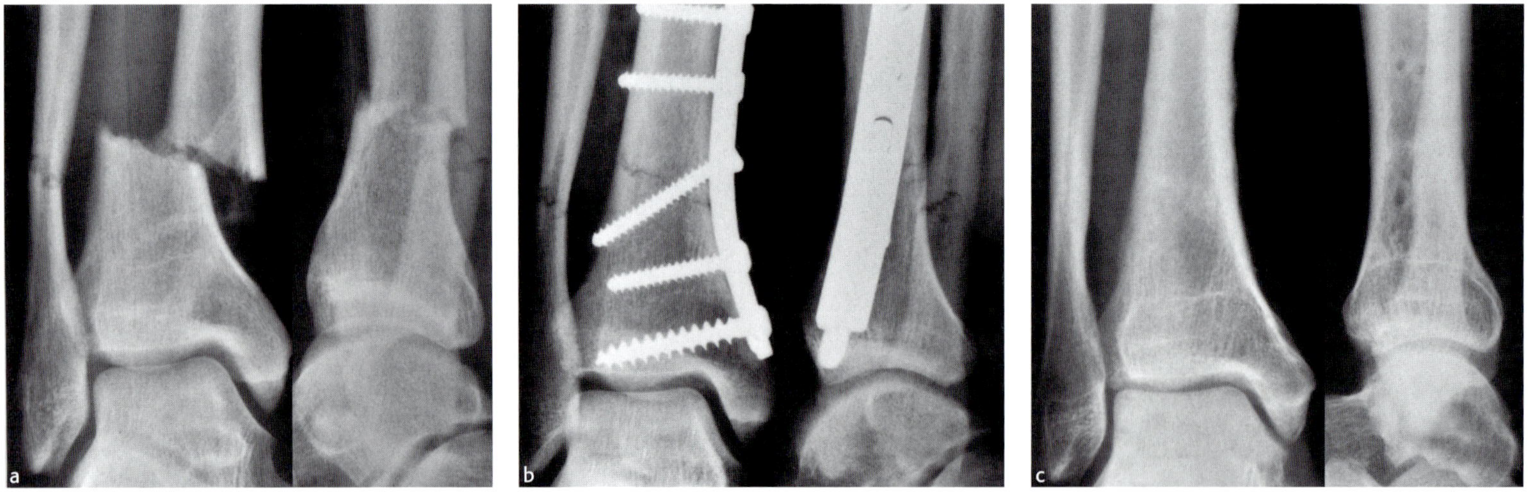

Fig. 3-34a–c According to Fig. 3-31 B.
a Fibula broken, but buttressed varus of tibia. Joint space normal.
b Open reduction and internal fixation.
c Back to normal 52 weeks after injury.

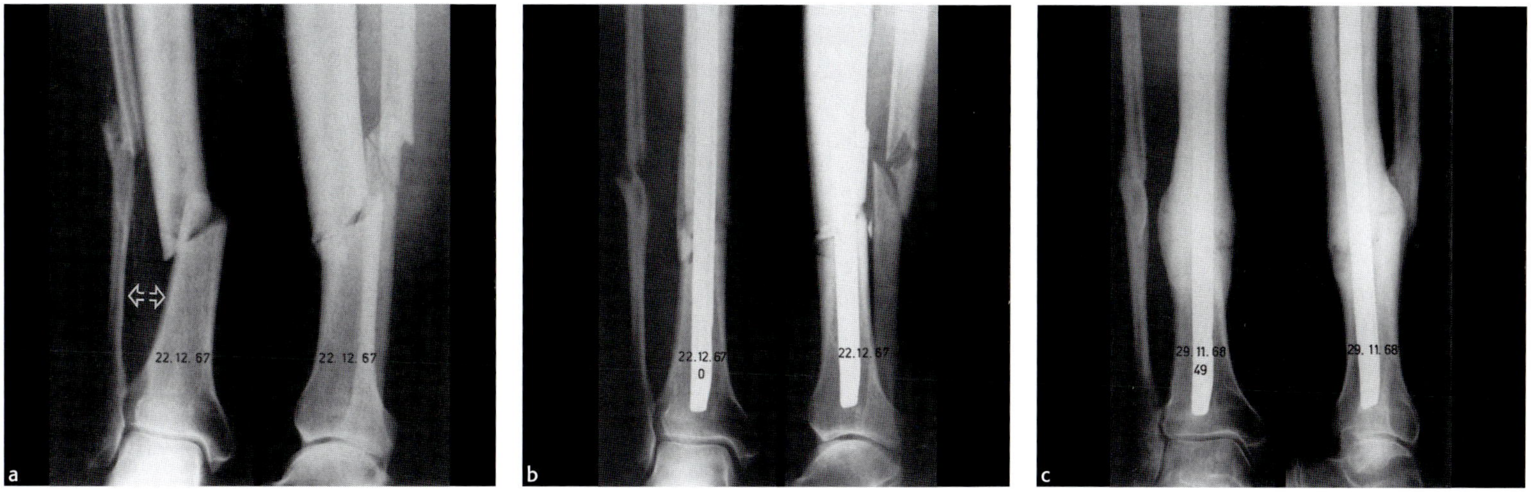

Fig. 3-35a–c According to Fig. 3-31 C.

a Transverse-short oblique tibial fracture. Distal fibula tilted away from the tibia (arrows), distal interosseous membrane ruptured, the distal syndesmotic ligaments intact, acting as a hinge.

b Open reduction and internal fixation, fibula 'hinged' back into place.

c Healed back to normal 49 weeks after fracture. Note: massive callus after disruption of Interosseous membrane.

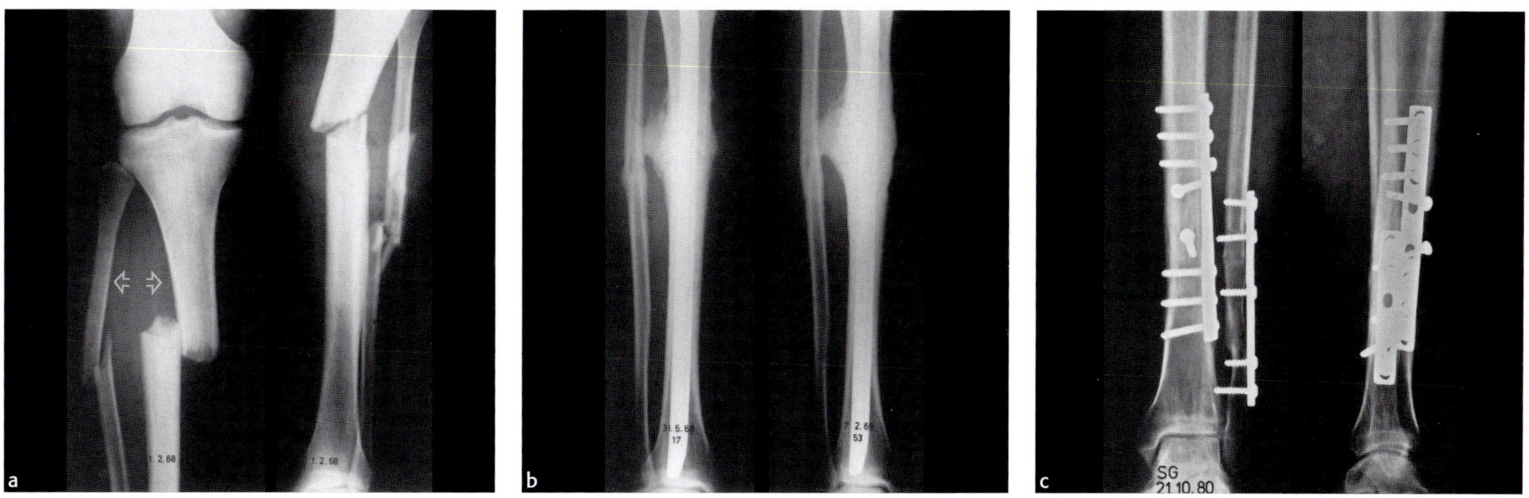

Fig. 3-36a–c According to Fig. 3-31 D.

a Telescoping-shortening, distal fibula displaced more proximally than the tibia.

b After open reduction and internal fixation of tibia: fibula still short (see Fig. 3-4 and 3-5). After secondary open reduction and internal fixation of fibula: ankle joint normal again.

c Final result: back to normal.

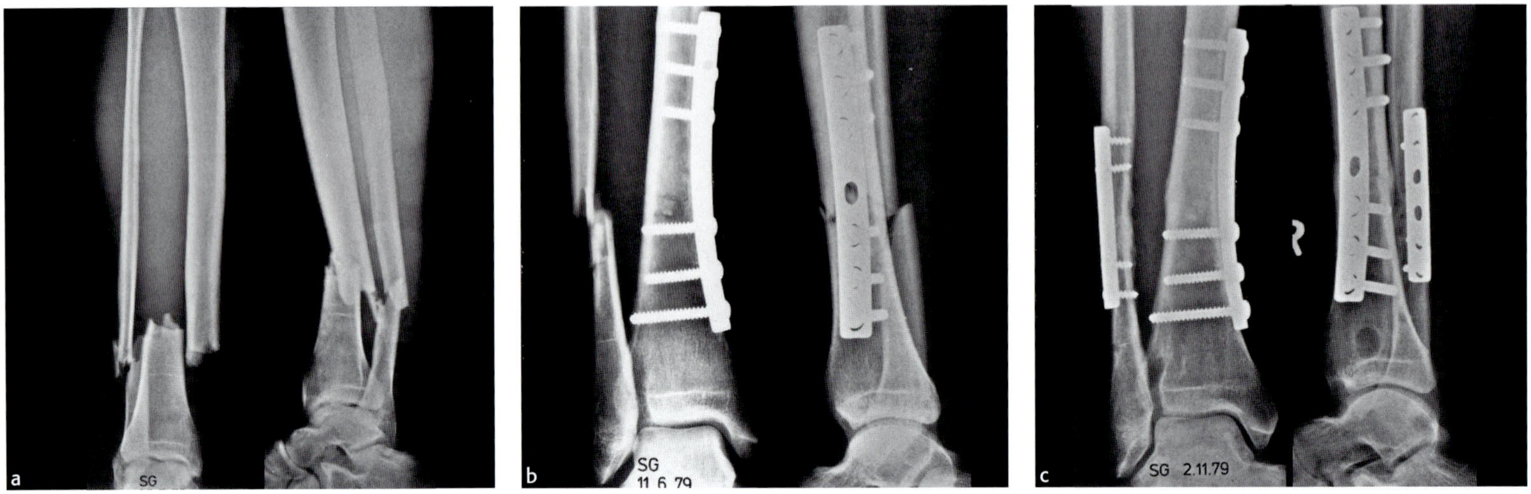

Fig. 3-37a–c According to Fig. 3-31 D.

a Telescoping-shortening.

b After open reduction and internal fixation of tibia: fibula too short (see Fig. 3-4 and 3-5).

c Secondary open reduction and internal fixation of fibula: normalized ankle joint.

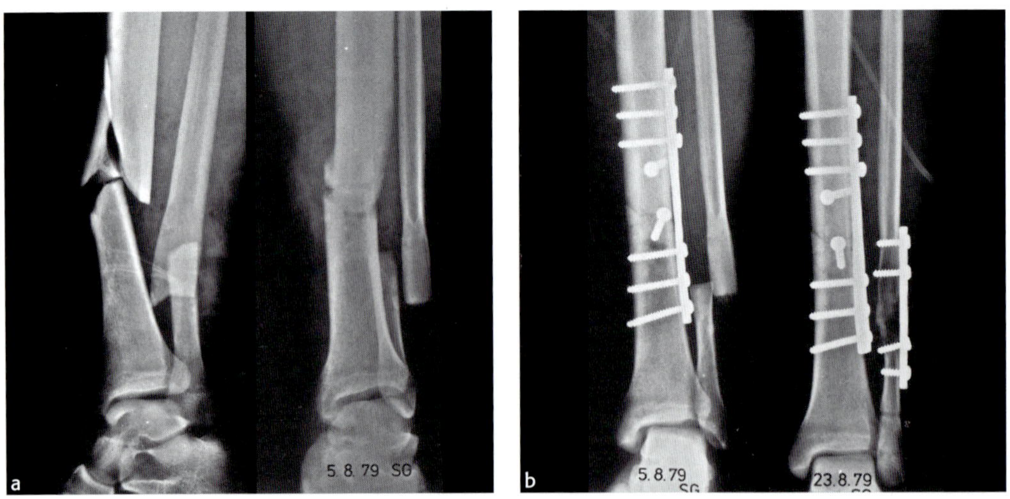

Fig. 3-38a–b According to Fig. 3-31 E.

a Telescoping-shortening. The proximal fibula tilted away from the tibia, with the syndesmotic ligaments as a hinge.

b Open reduction and internal fixation of the tibia fracture has automatically reduced the fibula fracture. Note: interosseous membrane callus after disruption.

Type F+T spiral fractures A–C with clinical examples (Fig. 3-39–3-45).

The fibula is broken proximally, distally, or at the same level as the tibia.

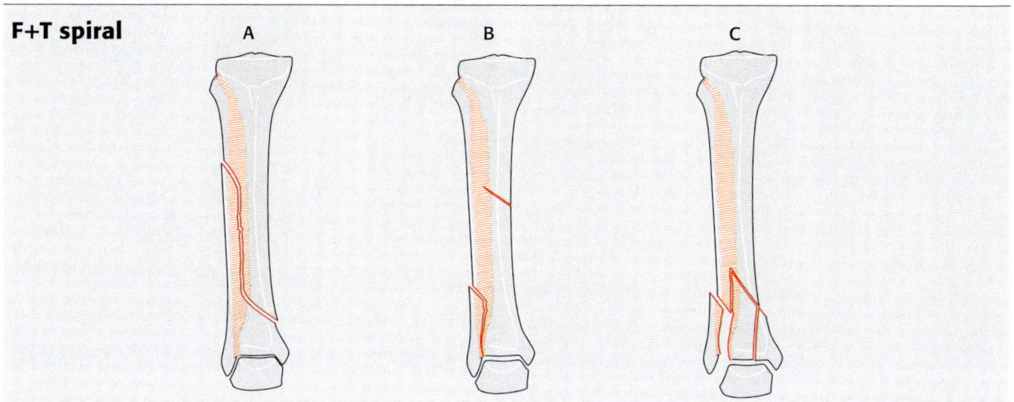

	A	B	C
SLIM proximal	○	○	○
SLIM distal	○	●	●
Ankle joint injury	○	●	●

Fig. 3-39 Type F+T spiral fractures A–C.

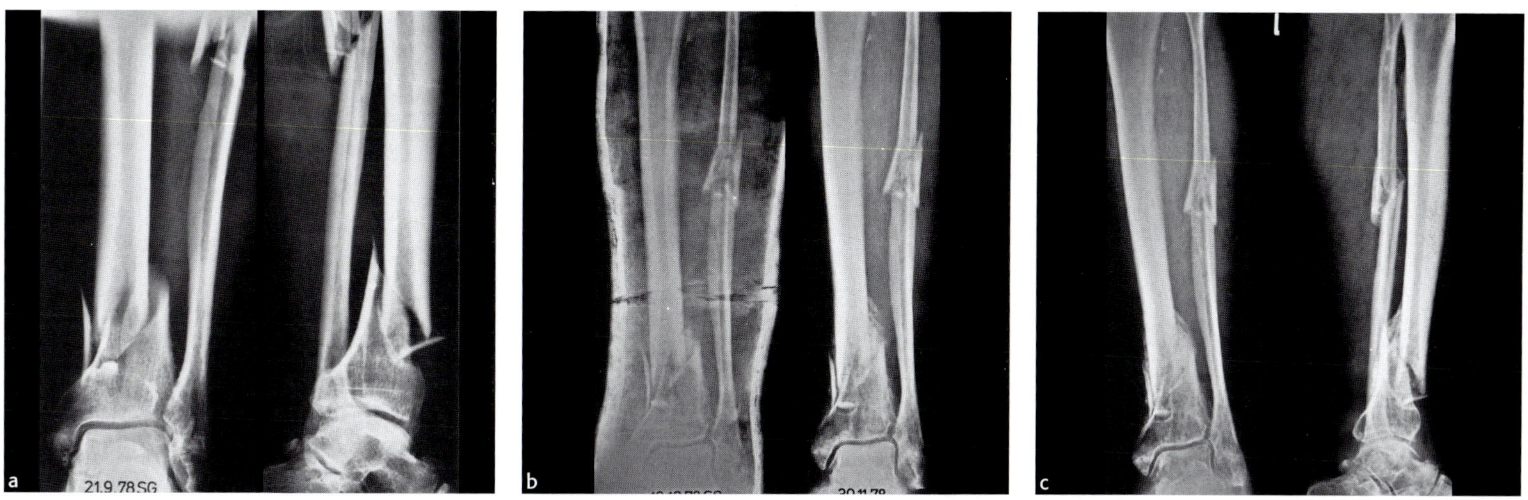

Fig. 3-40a–c According to Fig. 3-39 A.

a Telescoping-shortening. Fibula fracture is proximal to the tibia fracture. Ankle fork is undisturbed.

b Fragments aligned, 8 mm shortening. Wedged functional brace.

c Fracture united with undisturbed ankle joint, with shortening, 4 months after injury.

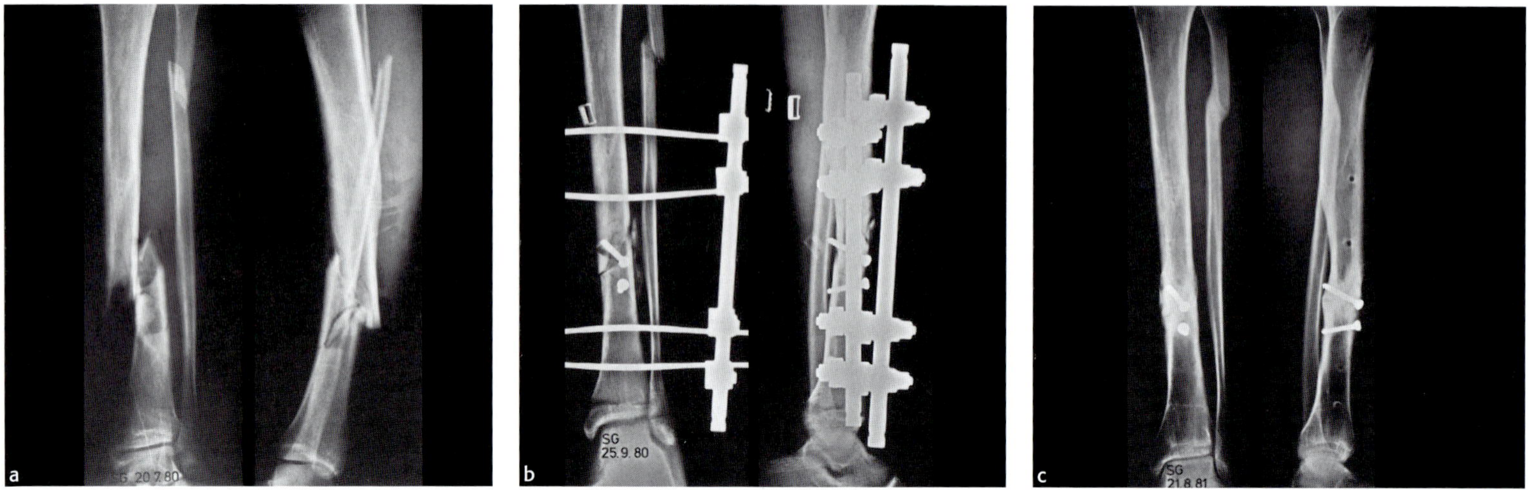

Fig. 3-41a–c According to Fig. 3-39 A.

a Telescoping-shortening. Fibula fracture is proximal to the tibial fracture. Ankle joint spared from injury.

b Minimal internal fixation plus external fixator.

c Anatomical healing, ankle joint normal.

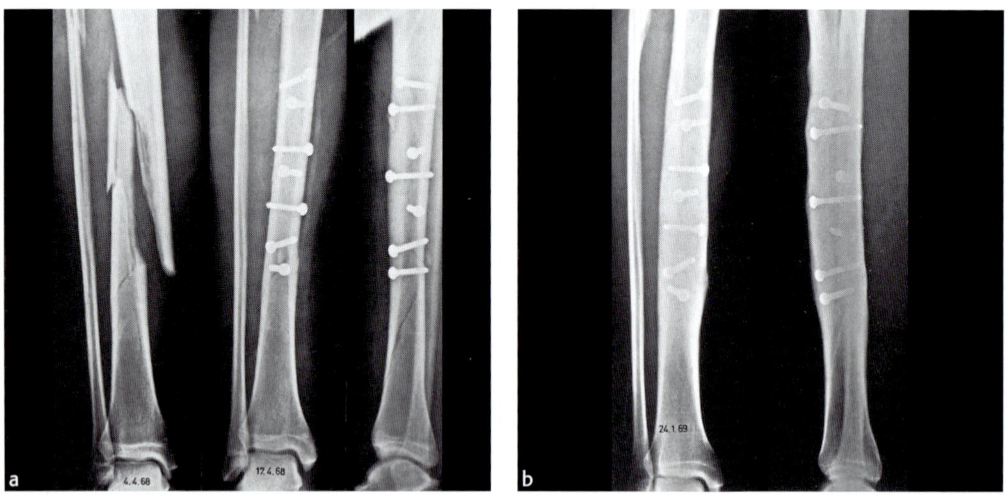

Fig. 3-42a–b According to Fig. 3-39 A.

a Shortening, fibular fracture is proximal to the tibial fracture, distal fibula is not displaced from the tibia. Open reduction and internal fixation.

b Anatomical healing. Ankle joint normal 9 months after injury.

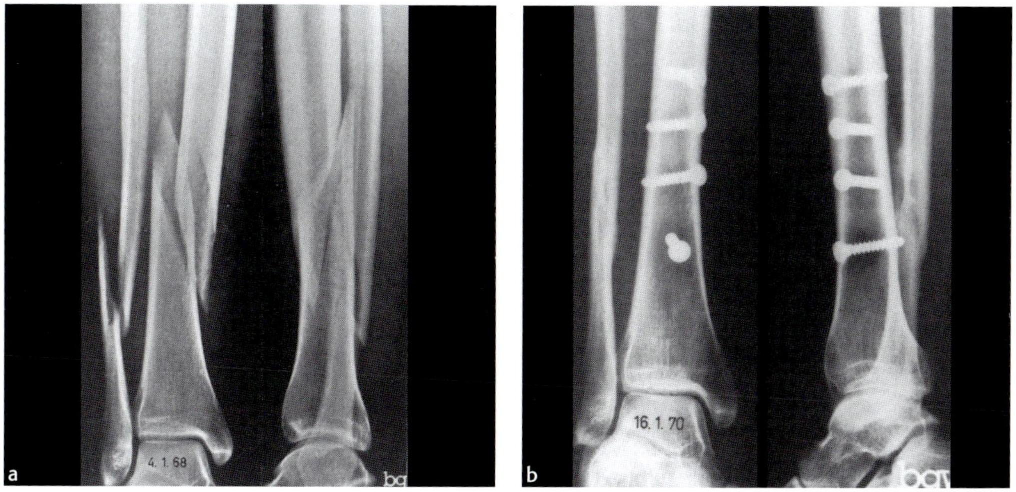

Fig. 3-43a–b According to Fig. 3-39 B.

a Fibular fracture below tibial fracture, distal interosseous membrane is ruptured, but syndesmotic ligaments still present as a hinge.

b Distal fibula was hinged back into place by open reduction and internal fixation of tibia, 2-year result.

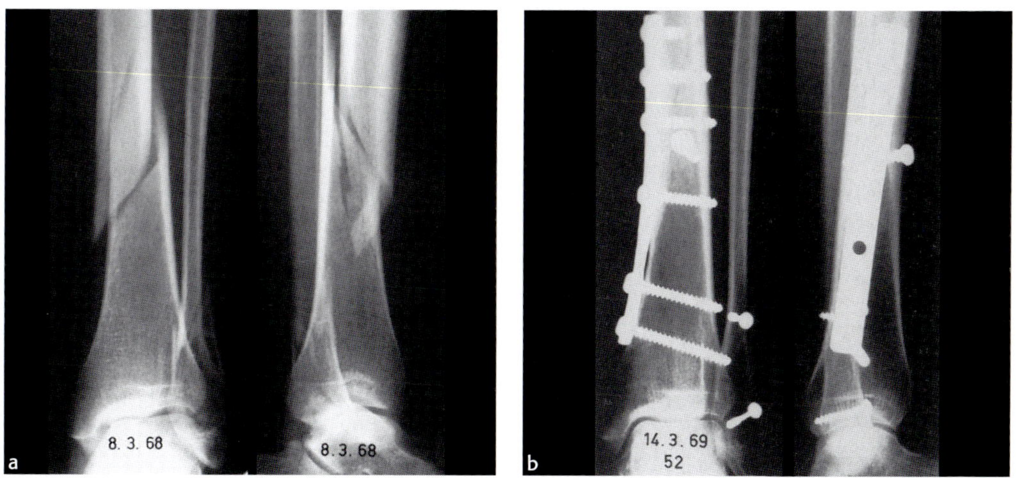

Fig. 3-44a–b According to Fig. 3-39 B.

a Fibular fracture below tibial fracture, syndesmotic ligaments at risk.

b Both fractures and ankle joint are back to normal following osteosynthesis 52 weeks after fracture.

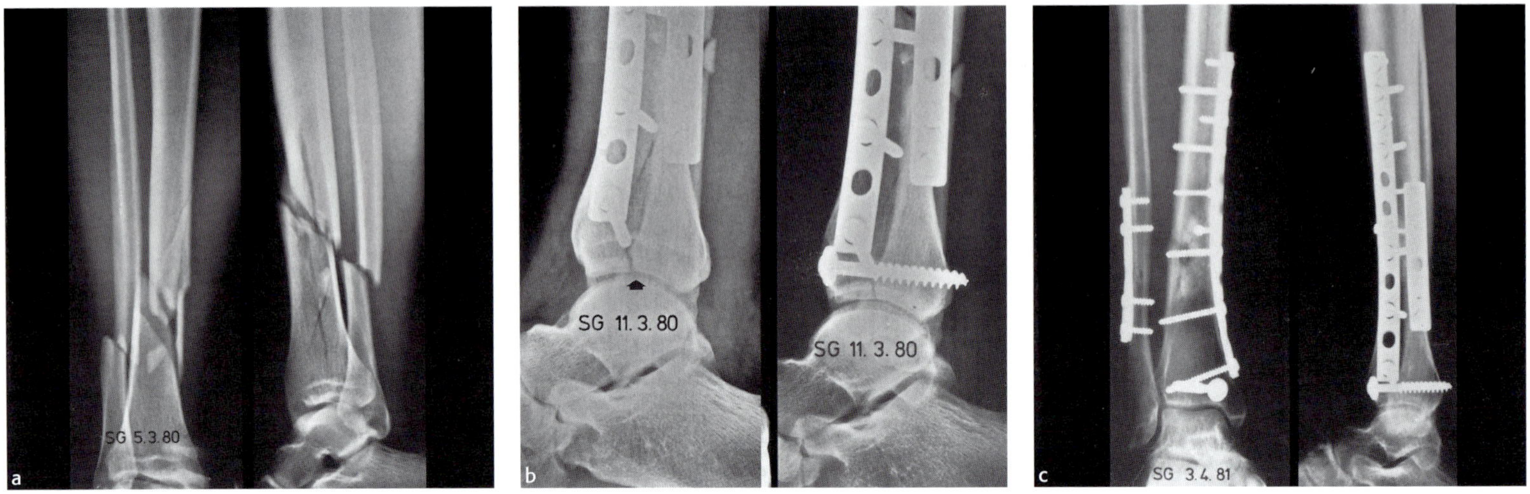

Fig. 3-45a–c According to Fig. 3-39 C.

a Fibular fracture below tibial fracture, syndesmotic ligaments and ankle joint at risk.

b Open reduction and internal fixation has restored the shaft fractures. The long frontal split in the tibia (arrow) was missed. Therefore, instant screw fixation.

c Anatomical healing, back to normal 1 year later.

Type F+T complex fractures A–D with clinical examples shown in Fig. 3-47–3-51.

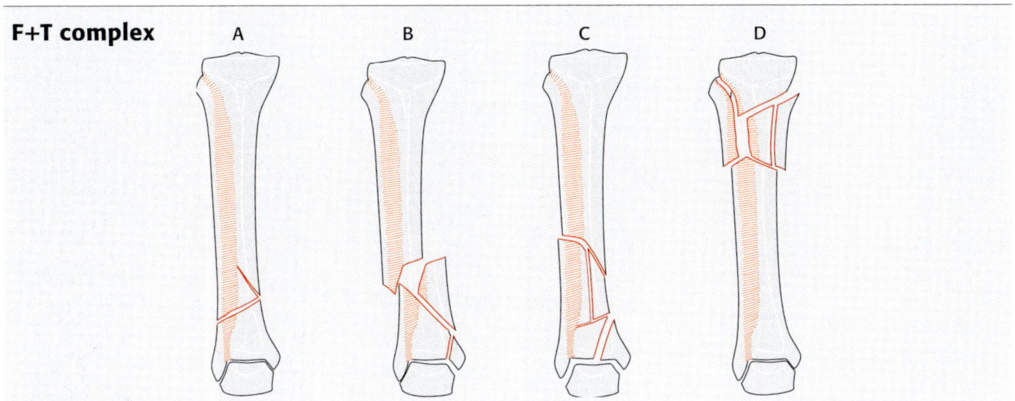

	A	B	C	D
SLIM proximal	○	○	○	●
SLIM distal	○	○	○	○
Ankle joint injury	○	●	●	○

Fig. 3-46 Type F+T complex fractures A–D.

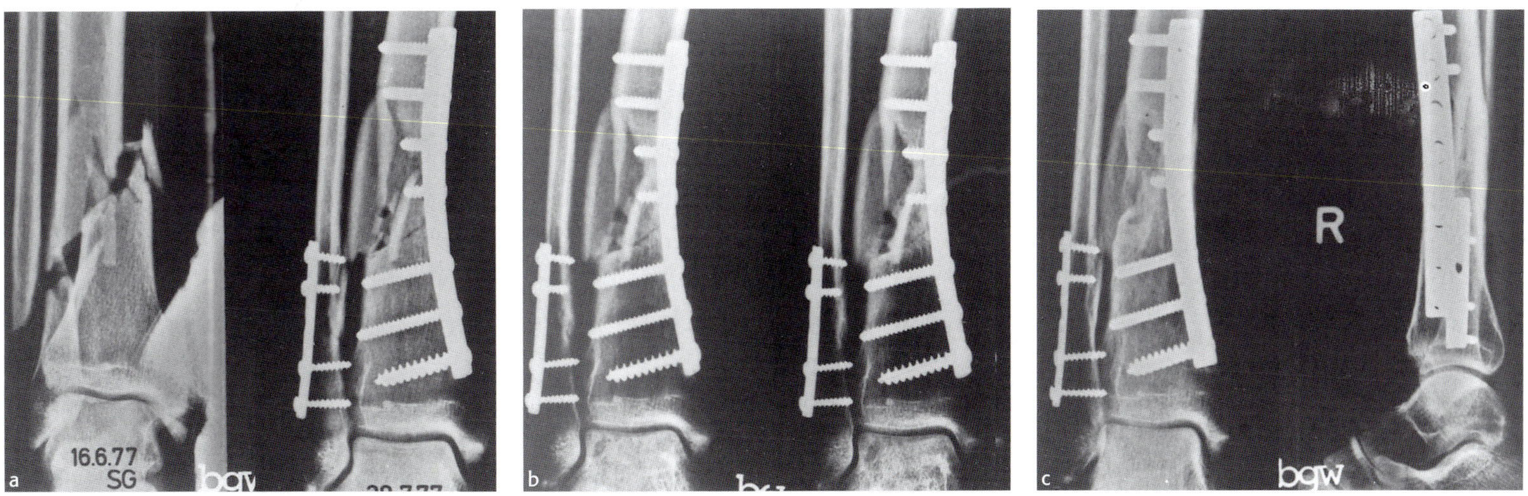

Fig. 3-47a–c According to Fig. 3-46 A

a Short distal fibular fragment, distal SLIM intact. ORIF (bridging plate for the tibia, 'supporter'-plating of fibula).

b 'Biological' healing mode. Ankle joint normal.

c 1-year result with anatomical healing.

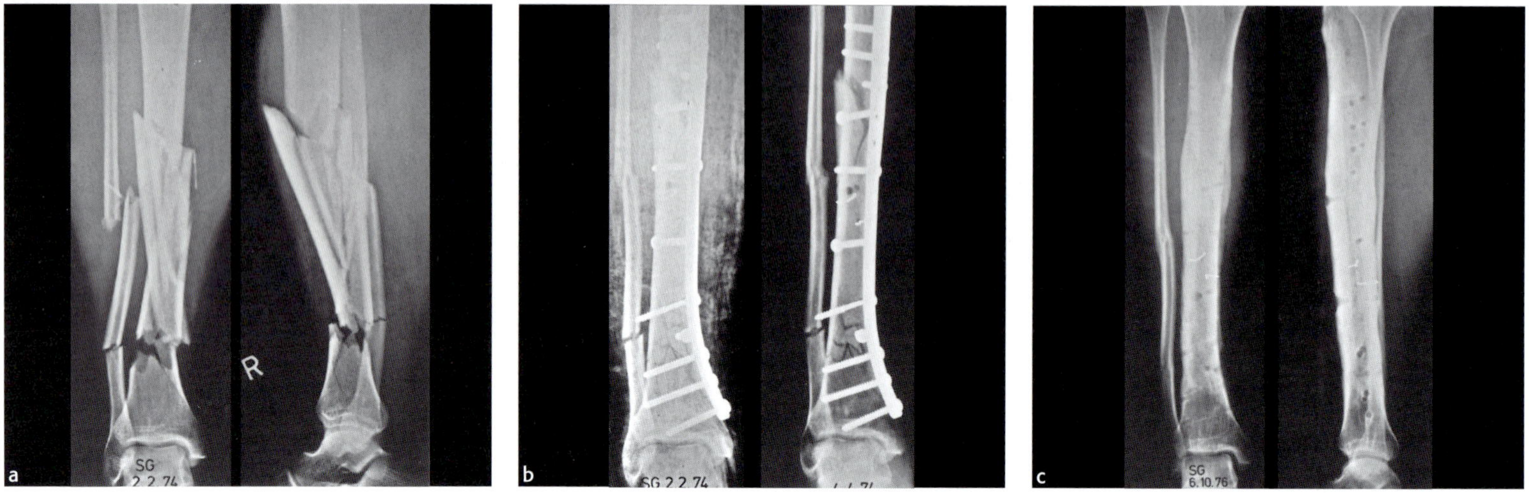

Fig. 3-48a–c According to Fig. 3-46 A.

a Shattered bones, but distal SLIM uninjured.

b Immediately and 2 months after ORIF (bridging plate).

c 2 years and 8 months after injury and after metal removal: normal leg and ankle joint.

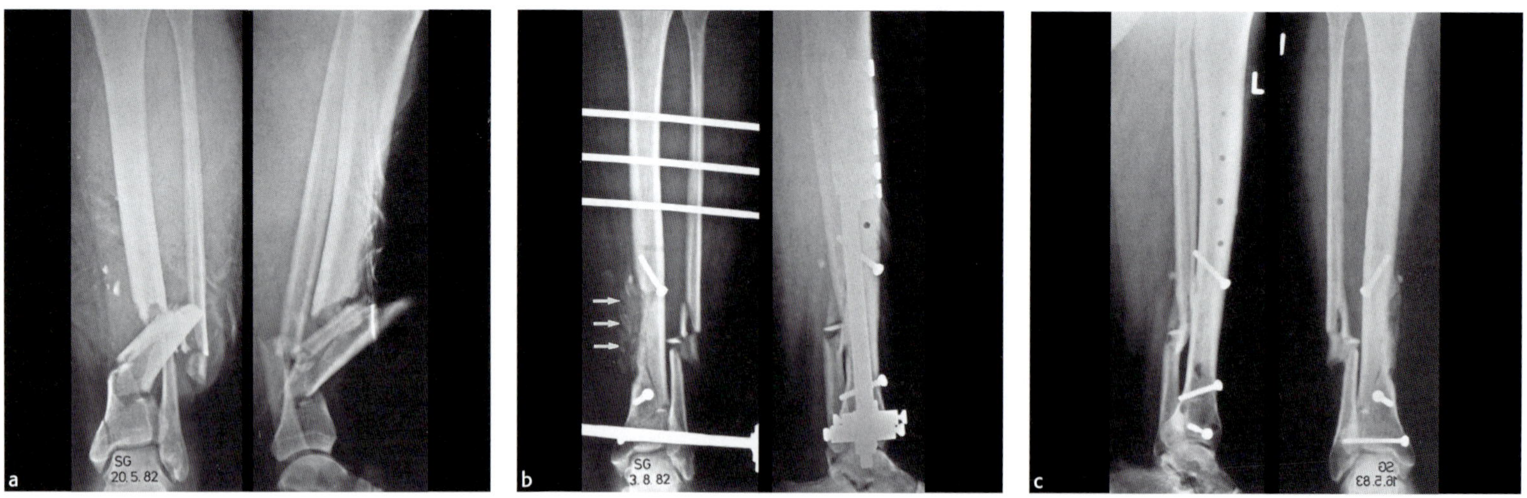

Fig. 3-49a–c According to Fig. 3-46 B.

a Shattered open tibial and fibular fracture, fracture of medial malleolus. Syndesmotic ligaments, however, intact.

b Minimal ORIF and external fixator for the tibia, with primary removal of a devascularized tibial fragment. Secondary autogenous cancellous bone transplant 6 weeks after injury (arrows).

c 1-year result: fracture ideally healed, ankle joint normal.

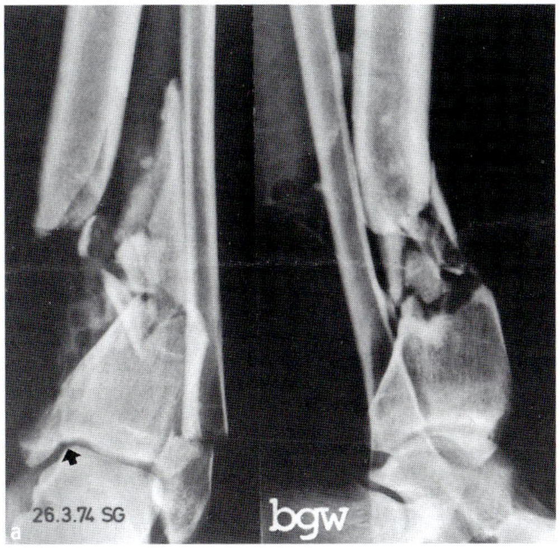

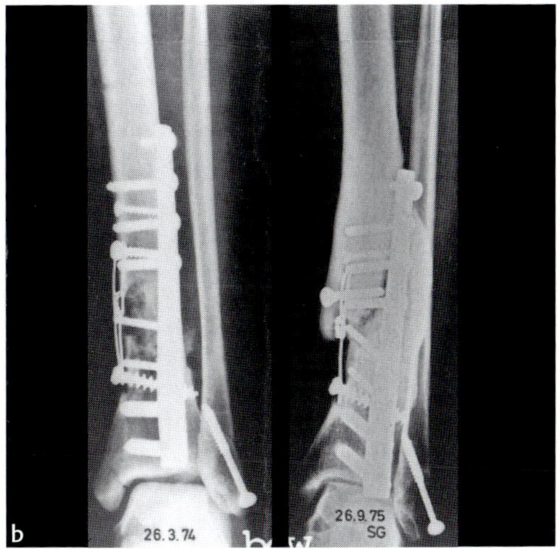

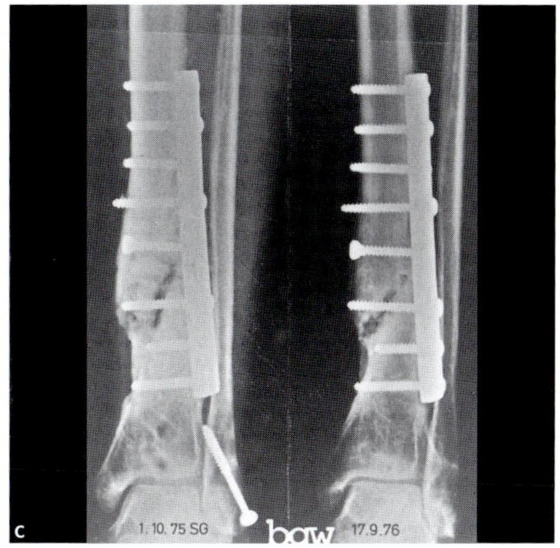

Fig. 3-50a–d According to Fig. 3-46 B.

a Shattered open tibial fracture, fibular fracture buttressing, split fracture of medial malleolus (arrow).

b ORIF and 1 1/2 year later: biologically active nonunion, varus, fibula too long, tibia shortened respectively.

c New plating with lengthening of the tibia in the nonunion and 1 year later.

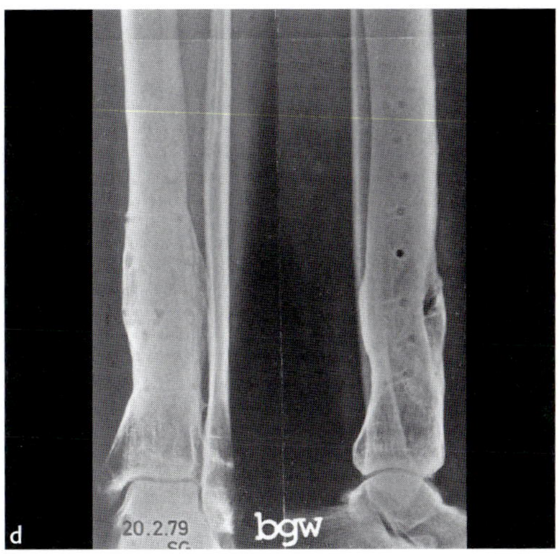

d Late follow-up 5 years after injury: normal leg and ankle joint.

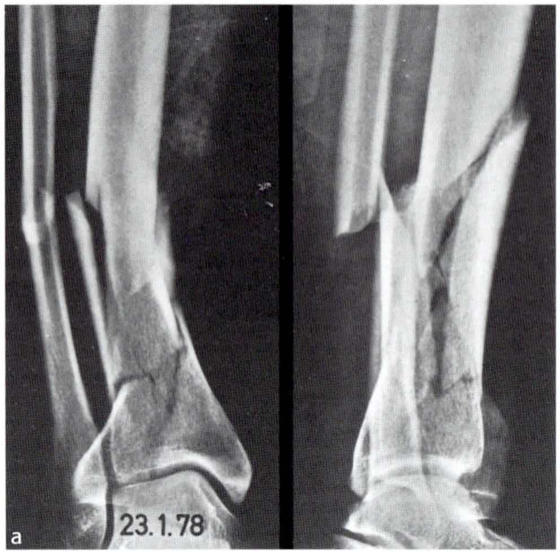

Fig. 3-51a–d According to Fig. 3-46 C.

a Tibial fracture extends into the ankle joint (pilon-like).

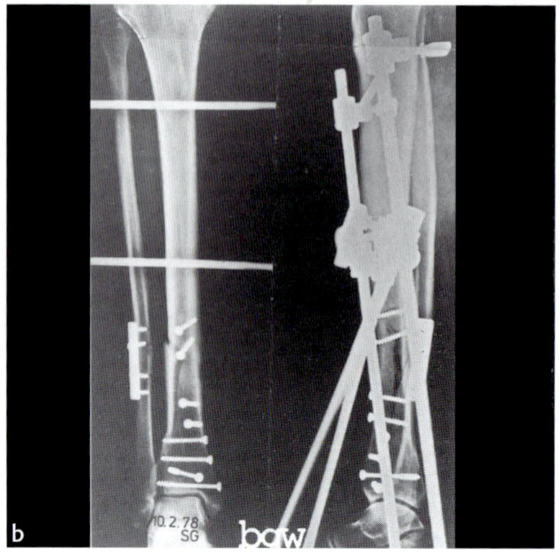

b Plating of the fibula, minimal screw fixation for the tibia, and protective external fixator down to calcaneus and metatarsals.

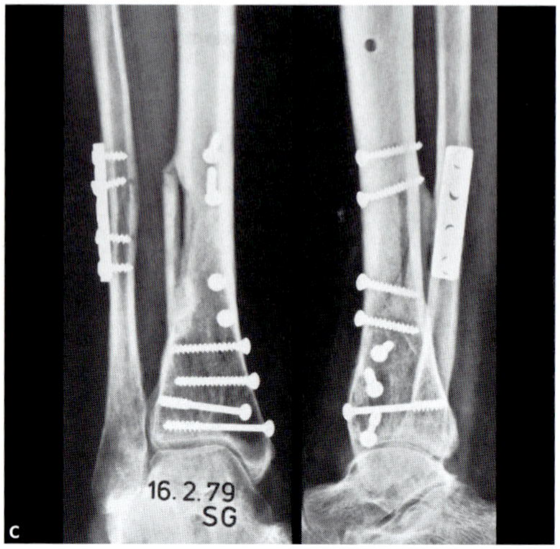

c 1-year result of anatomical 'biological' reconstruction.

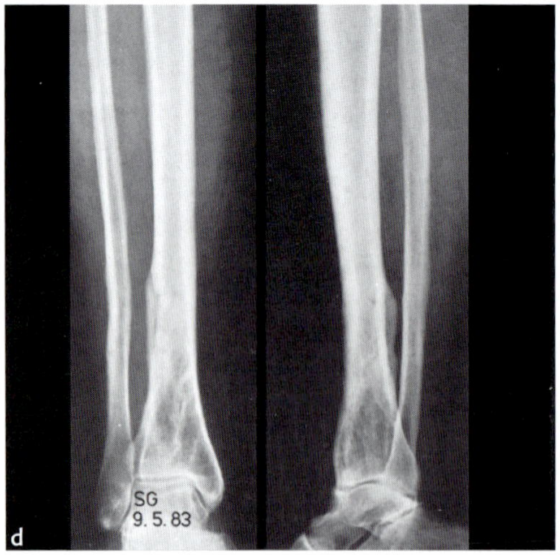

d Follow-up 5 years after injury: back to normal for the leg and the ankle joint.

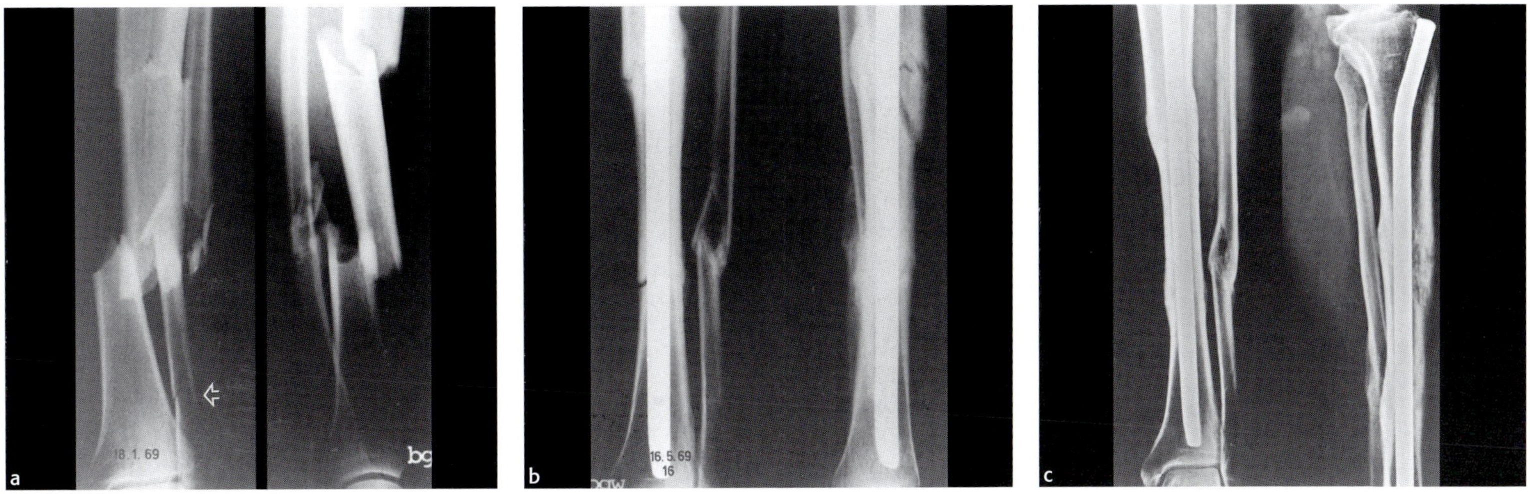

Fig. 3-52a–c According to Fig. 3-46 D.

a Segmental fracture, distal SLIM undisturbed, undisplaced fracture of distal fibula (arrow).

b Focused open reduction through two small anterior incisions, gently reamed nailing. 16 weeks after surgery: 'biological' healing process.

c 1-year result. Ankle joint normal.

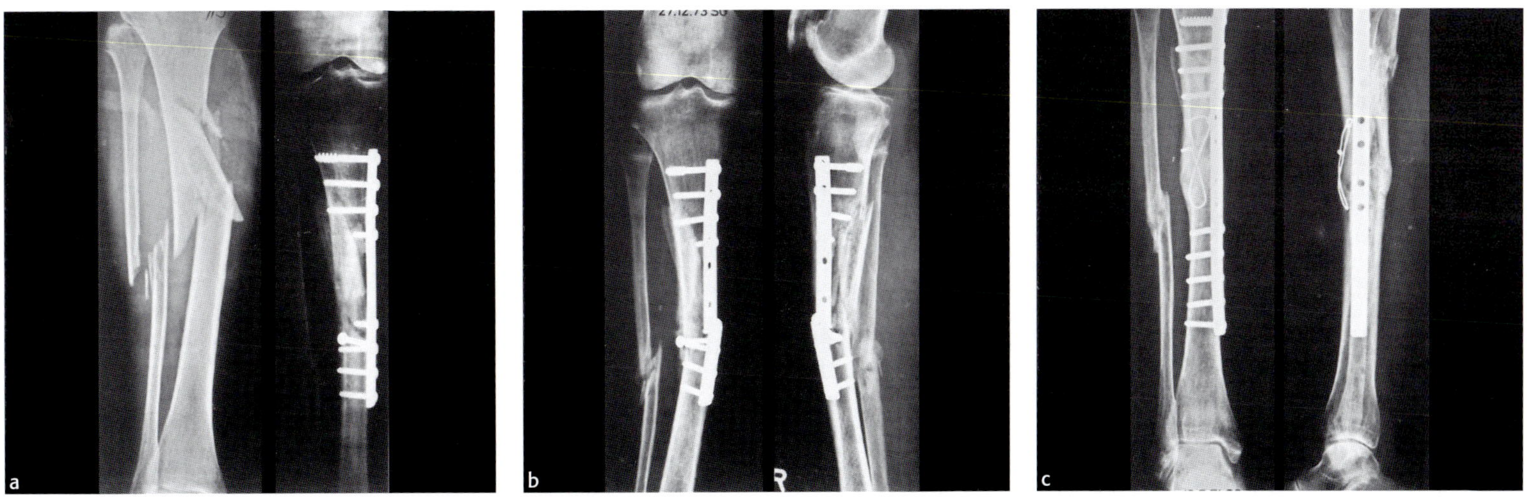

Fig. 3-53a–c According to Fig. 3-46 D.

a Complex open fracture. Distal SLIM undamaged. Bridge plating.

b 3 months after injury: fatigue plate fracture under functional aftercare. Revision plating plus tension-band wiring at that time.

c 8 months after fracture: ideal healing. Note: normal ankle joint.

3.1 Discussion

Fracture anatomy

On standard x-rays, lower leg fractures are easy to describe: undisplaced fissured or displaced, transverse-oblique, spiral, complex. Not evident on x-rays, however, are accompanying damages of SLIM. The state of SLIM and the fibula will determine the function and the fate of the leg and of the ankle joint. The basis for this assessment is the status of the ankle fracture: A B C, with 'harmless' (A), 'serious' (B), or 'very serious' (C).

The various type Fs (fibular fractures) allow prediction of the type or corresponding ruptures of SLIM and the severity of the ankle injury with high certainty. Four of the six type F fractures involve the ankle joint, ie, 66%; 100% when the rare direct blow and fatigue fractures are excluded.

The various type Ts (tibial fractures) also allow prediction of a corresponding SLIM situation and influence on the ankle joint:

- Transverse fractures spare the ankle joint, fractures high or low.
- Low spiral fractures, however, mostly involve the ankle joint the closer to the ankle joint that the tibia is broken.
- High spiral fractures, in contrast, spare distal SLIM and the ankle joint.
- Three of the six type T fractures involve the ankle joint, ie, 50%.

The different types F+T (fibular and tibial fractures) permit the following description:

- Transverse fractures with no or little displacement spare the ankle joint from damage. With marked displacement and the more distal the fracture, the more likely ankle damage is.
- Spiral fractures spare the ankle joint when the fibula fracture is located proximally to the tibial fracture. If, however, the fibular fracture is located further distally from the tibial fracture, then the ankle joint is most likely involved.
- Complex fractures—astonishingly—mostly spare the distal SLIM. The distal tibia, however, may suffer vertical fracturing. The more proximal the fracture area is, the less probable injury traces are down into the ankle joint.
- Six of the twelve type F+T fractures involve the ankle joint, ie, 50%.

Comparison of type F, type T, and type F+T fractures:

Regarding the ankle joint, the type F fractures are the worst ones, ie, 100% involvement. Therefore, these injuries are termed 'ankle fractures'. Less risky for the ankle joint are the isolated type T and the both-bone fractures, type F+T, still with 50% involvement.

The high rate of 50% ankle joint involvement should be kept in mind when treating lower leg fractures.

Fracture treatment in general

Fracture care depends on the surgeon's potential, on the care facilities, and on the patient's expectations. Under this aspect, fracture care—and medical care in general—cannot be the same globally. Even in one country, even in different regions, such as in Switzerland, fracture care is specifically nuanced from trauma facility to trauma facility.

For us in St. Gallen, the following rules have always been valid:

- Suprema lex salus aegroti, primum nil nocere (Hippocrates).
- Strive for restitutio ad integrum (original AO principle).
- Expect the unexpected, ie, "beware of the bear" (Yellowstone Park).

These three main rules imply that fracture care for our patients should be exactly the same as if the surgeons were themselves the patient. What would they wish for themselves?

- Perfect asepsis, ie, sterile enclosure facility.
- A fully trained orthopedic and trauma surgeon, mastering the original AO principles of open reduction and internal fixation, the MINIMAX principle, and Sarmiento's closed treatment [6].

4 Treatment of lower leg fractures

The clinical examples in the chapter on 'Classification of lower leg fractures' demonstrate the following points:

- Lower leg fractures are mostly more than only a fractured tibia. Therefore, different fractures ask for different treatments—conservative or surgical.
- When a **tibial** fracture is **transverse**, either undisplaced or reduced, it has **highest possible intrinsic stability**. With a minimum of additional support, the fracture will heal in spite of progressive weightbearing: In children, a plaster fixation and in adults, a functional brace or an unlocked medullary nail is the right treatment according to MINIMAX.
- When a **tibial** fracture is **spiral**, intrinsic stability is zero. The fragments are shearing or shortening against each other. When the fibula is unbroken—or transversally broken and buttressing, open reduction and internal fixation of the tibia are adequate. When the fibula has no stability, open reduction and internal fixation of the fibula offers additional support, the tibia may be internally fixed by screws and, if needed, with a plate. If the ankle joint is intact, open reduction and internal fixation for the tibia alone is correct.
- In **closed tibial fractures** with severe comminution, a bridging plate or an external fixator offers 'biological' healing conditions. The fibular fracture may be plated first. When the fibula is stabilized, a unilateral external fixator is enough. Fibula and fixator together form a frame with high stability. When the fibula cannot be plated, a bilateral external fixator with frame-configuration is indicated.
- In **open** and **open complex**—often grossly displaced—fractures, the surgeon should consider: The blood supply of the fragments should not be hindered by any type of fixation, in fact it should be to the contrary. Stripped, deperiosted fragments only live for 10–12 weeks from medullary vascular nutrition. It makes no sense to use medullary nails for such critical fractures, even not unreamed; this would be an 'overkill'. Restoration of blood supply to stripped fragments first happens along the medullary cavity only under the following conditions: No occlusion of the bone cavity by a nail, fragments anatomically reduced and minimally fixed with screws or with a small antigliding plate plus an external fixator. Bridging plates are reserved for closed complex fractures. Medullary nails are best used for closed simple midshaft fractures.
- This is not the place to describe the MINIMAX principle (see corresponding chapter). MINIMAX principles must be acquired during training and thereafter. Over time, some kind of clinical instinct develops. Every case is individual, requiring new assessment, decision making, and treatment.
- Open reduction and internal fixation of both leg bones restores a destabilized ankle fork by itself.
- Open reduction and internal fixation of the fibula may be helpful to augment the stability of a fixed tibia.

Conclusions

This chapter on lower leg fracture intends to emphasize the following points:

1. The surgeon should not only analyze the tibial fracture. The whole nature of the leg injury will determine WHAT to treat. Lower leg fractures are mostly more than only a broken tibia.
2. With the 'Classification of lower leg fractures', potential injury of the ankle joint becomes predictable.
3. For ankle fractures type B and C, fibular shortening is typical. For isolated tibial fractures, tibial shortening is typical. In many bone fractures, fibular and tibial shortening are present. In lower leg fractures, the ankle joint needs the same emphasis of treatment as the broken tibia. Therefore, the fibula—unbroken or broken—deserves highest attention.
4. The complexity of lower leg fractures needs a differentiated assessment and surgical treatment. All the reduction and fixation equipment must be disposable and be mastered by the surgeon. Lower leg fracture treatment is much more than only interlocking nailing or plate-bridging of the tibia. In addition, the fibula and SLIM deserve highest attention should restitutio ad integrum be the goal of the fracture care.

5 Bibliography

Blue references indicate links to abstracts of articles online available through Medline (www.nlm.nih.gov).

1. **Müller ME, Nazarian S, Koch P** (1987) *Classification AO des fractures 1, Les os longs.* Berlin Heidelberg New York: Springer-Verlag.
2. **Müller ME, Allgöwer M, Schneider R, et al.** (1991) *Manual of Internal Fixation. Techniques Recommended by the AO Group.* Third Edition. Heidelberg New York: Springer-Verlag.
3. **Rüedi TP, Murphy WM, Colton CL, et al.** (2000) *AO Principles of Fracture Management.* Stuttgart New York: Thieme.
4. **Danis R** (1949) *Théorie et Pratique de l'ostéosynthèse.* Paris: *Masson.*
5. **Le Cœur P** (1938) *La pince malléolaire.* Thèse. Paris: Masson.
6. **Sarmiento A, Latta LL** (1981) *Closed Funtional Treatment of Fractures.* Berlin Heidelberg New York: Springer-Verlag.

4 Open fractures of the lower leg

1 General considerations

The specific high risk of open fractures is infection [1–5].

Closed fractures, treated conservatively with reduction and splintage, do not offer a portal for contamination and infection [4], though dead space, devascularized soft tissues, and bone fragments that might offer an ideal culture medium for bacteria.

Open fractures with their portal of skin disruption are different. Contamination occurs through the portal into the fracture area from the following sources:

- The patients' own skin flora.
- Bacteria, spores, and fungi from the accident scene.
- Airborne [6] or inoculated bacteria from first aid people and those at the emergency department. Their flora may contaminate the open wound directly by manipulation or indirectly from the surrounding air.
- Direct and indirect contamination of the open wound in the conventional operating theater, where real asepsis is absent [6]: Indirect airborne contamination from instruments, implants, the surgeon's hands and direct airborne contamination (see chapter Asepsis).

2 Prevention of contamination

- Wound contamination at the site of the injury is inevitable. Since first aid staff are germ carriers and potential transmitters, they should maximize their avoidance of possible wound contamination. Disinfectants (eg, Betadine) should be used extensively by soaking the patient's clothes and the sterile dressings. Antibiotics should be administrated as soon as possible, at the latest immediately after hospital admission.
- After admission, wound inspection with removal of the primary dressing at the emergency department is strictly forbidden. It should be delayed until after x-ray pictures have been taken, the patient is anesthetized and brought to the operating theater. Here, the risk of further contamination can be minimized to zero by ensuring all the fracture care is under sterile enclosure conditions with a body-exhaust system for all personnel (see chapter Asepsis). In the sterile enclosure, a patient's primary dressing and clothes can be removed for the first time. This unusual sequence of fracture assessment reduces the risk of contamination with dangerous hospital bacteria. However, it requires the surgeon's personal presence—which is generally resisted by surgeons.
- The surgeon, and nobody else before them, is allowed to prepare the patient's injury for treatment. They perform the disinfection, surgery, wound closure, final dressing and the patient's bedding with the assistance of the whole surgical team, using the same body-exhaust system to prevent wound contamination (Fig. 4-1).

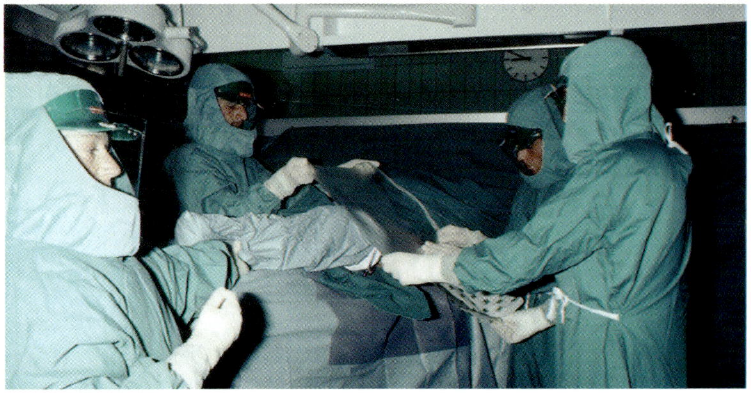

Fig. 4-1 Surgery in sterile enclosure with body-exhaust system.

- The general fracture treatment includes debridement of devitalized tissues, fragment fixation, occlusion of dead spaces and suction wound drainage. Wound closure is aimed for, whenever possible. The wound closure possibilities vary from minimal trimming, skin-defattening, primary skin-splitting coverage, and flap-shifting, to Picot-flap moving around the lower leg. Primary vascularized skin-flap coverage has not been done in our institutions in over 40 years, other than occasionally for infected nonunions.
- Postoperative wound control is also performed under sterile enclosure conditions until the vital barrier against contamination has been rebuilt. Antibiotics are administered during that period, but for no longer than 8–10 days (Fig. 4-2a–c).
  When primary wound closure is impossible, the open wound may be protected from further contamination on the ward with a local enclosure of the limb.

3 Fixation techniques

Fixation techniques in closed lower leg fractures focus on restoring the normal anatomy of the tibia and fibula with special attention to the ankle joint. Both here, and also for open fractures, the treatment strives to attain 'back to normal' status (see chapter Classification of lower leg fractures).

MINIMAX fixation techniques [7] are valid for both closed and open fractures. In open fractures, however, the soft tissue damage requires additional attention, especially the skin lesion over the tibia in open lower leg fractures. 'Biology' has highest priority [5, 7–9].

Most open fractures are high energy injuries [1–3]. Therefore, open lower leg fractures ask for refined MINIMAX-fixation techniques, all of which are already biological fixations [8]:

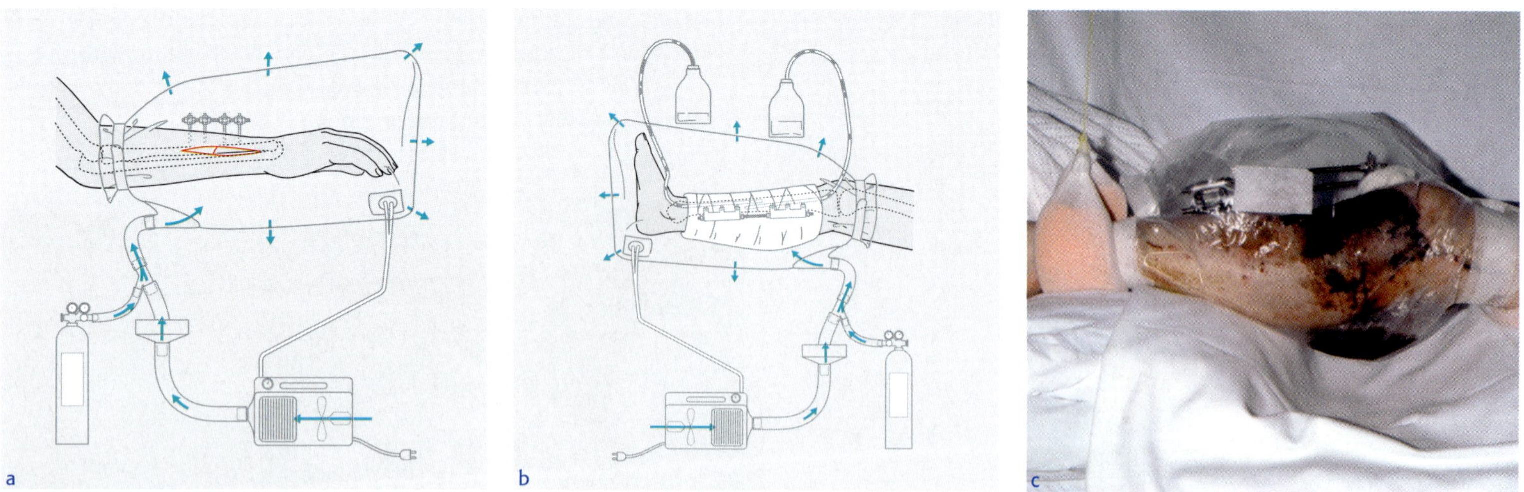

Fig. 4-2a–c Sterile enclosure air bag.
a Sterile air from high efficiency particle absorption filter and oxygen are inflated.
b The same for a lower leg.
c Clinical case.

MINIMAX fixations for open fractures of the lower leg

1. Non-standard fixations with standard plates.
2. Intramedullary nail fixations with limited indication.
3. External fixations, to be permanently in place for the entire fracture healing period [5].
4. Minimal local internal fracture fixations that need mechanical protection with an external fixator (ExFix) [5].
5. Plate fixation of the fibula for indirect reduction of the tibia fracture and as stability augmentation of ExFix [5].
6. Primary removal of devitalized fragments and secondary autogenous bone defect compensation.
7. Secondary change to another fixation type.
8. Skin-lesion management.

These eight treatments can be used individually or more often combined according to the given circumstances. Endless injury variations within the AO classification of open fractures grade I II [1], III [2, 3] need customized treatment for every case.

Our surgery relies on the original standard AO implants [1, 8]. The problem is not the implants, as they can meet all surgical demands. The problem and the challenge is the skilful application of screws, plates, nails, external fixators, and soft-tissue management.

On one hand, the following cases demonstrate the severity and complexity of open lower leg fractures, but on the other hand they also demonstrate the chance for good healing results.

4 Cases—open lower leg fractures and their MINIMAX treatment

A MAXIMAL healing result with MINIMAL surgical insult is the goal of treatment [7].

Open fractures have already suffered the trauma of considerable insult to the bone and soft tissues. Bone fragments are more or less disconnected from the soft-tissue envelope and therefore separated from blood perfusion. Periosteal blood supply under such circumstances is interrupted, and the remaining blood supply to the main fragments arrives at the most along the medullary canal. Reduction maneuver and fixation must take this vascular deficit into account and should favor revascularization. Treatment must not increase the pre-existing traumatic vascular insult. The soft tissue damage does not permit the same open reduction and internal fixation techniques that are useful in closed fractures. After debridement of the site, the amount and the pattern of fixation devices must be applied in such a way that additional tissue violation and vascular insult are avoided.

4.1 Non-standard plate fixations with standard plates

The standard plate site for open reduction and internal fixation of closed tibia fractures is the medial tibia flat surface, which is curved and twisted distally and which is covered by nothing other than the skin. Skin slough has brought tibia plating into disfavor. Interlocking nailing and subcutaneous bridge plating are now preferred for both closed fracture nailing as well as for open fractures [3].

In open fractures, plating of the medial aspect of tibia is out of the question. However, the other two surfaces of the tibia may lend themselves to plate fixation, as a plate may be well covered by vascularized soft tissue and by the muscle envelope.

Comment

Non-standard plating interferes less with the blood supply of fragments than intramedullary nailing does. From that standpoint, plating is a biological fixation according to the MINIMAX principle [5, 7, 9].

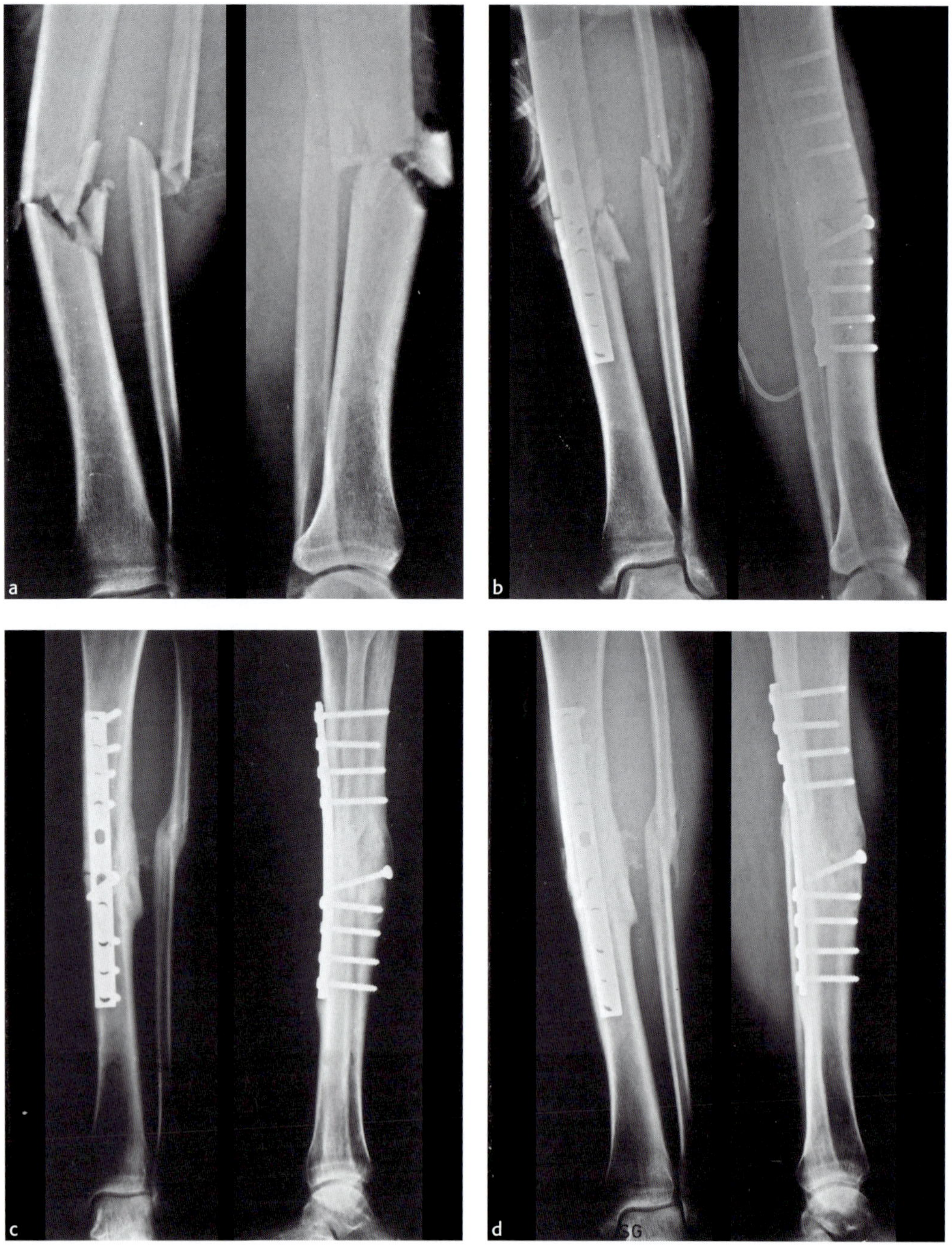

Fig. 4-3a–d Grade II (30-year-old patient).

a Skin disruption and contusion medially. Plate fixation through the open wound to the posterior tibial surface. The plate is protected, covered by sound soleus muscle.

b The plate on the posterior tibia surface.

c Healing process 54 weeks later.

d Late result 2 years after fracture.

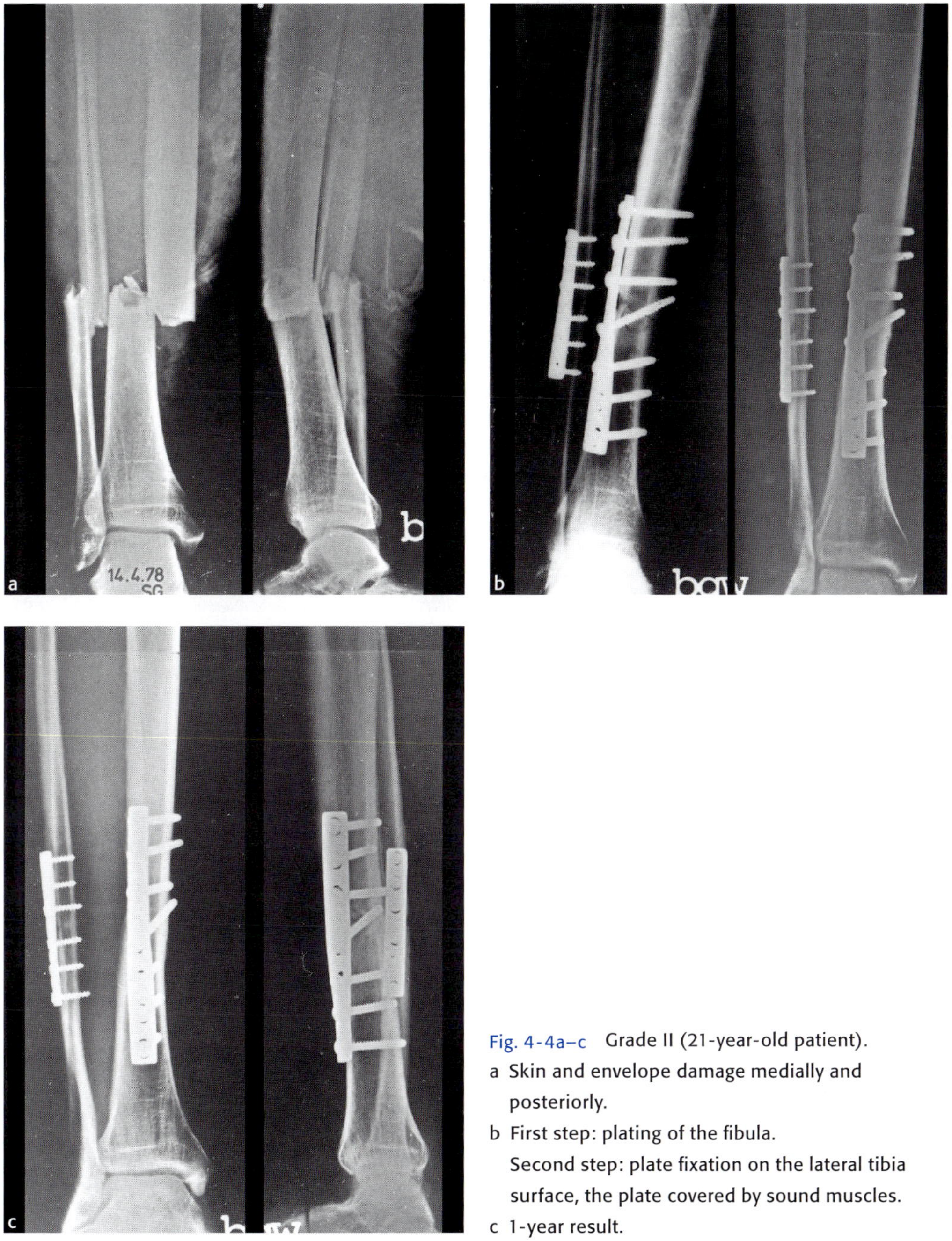

Fig. 4-4a–c Grade II (21-year-old patient).

a Skin and envelope damage medially and posteriorly.

b First step: plating of the fibula.
Second step: plate fixation on the lateral tibia surface, the plate covered by sound muscles.

c 1-year result.

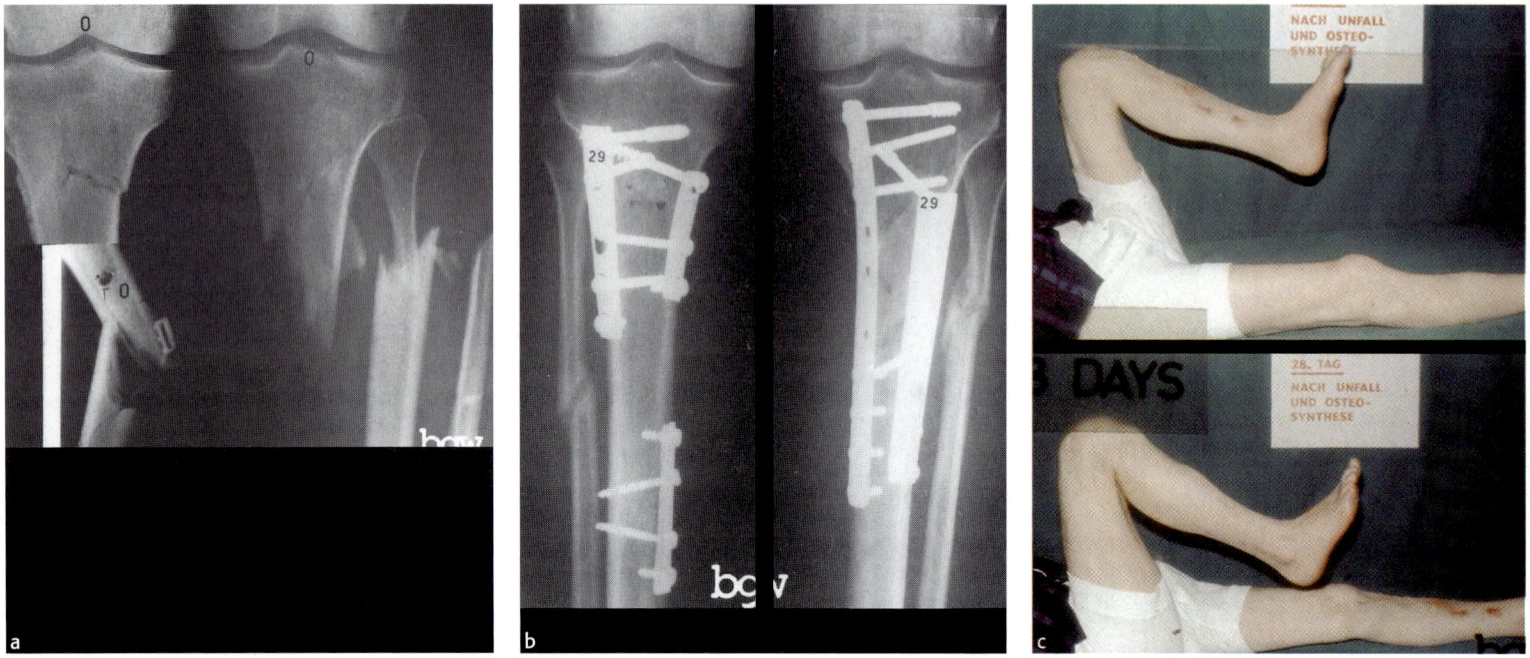

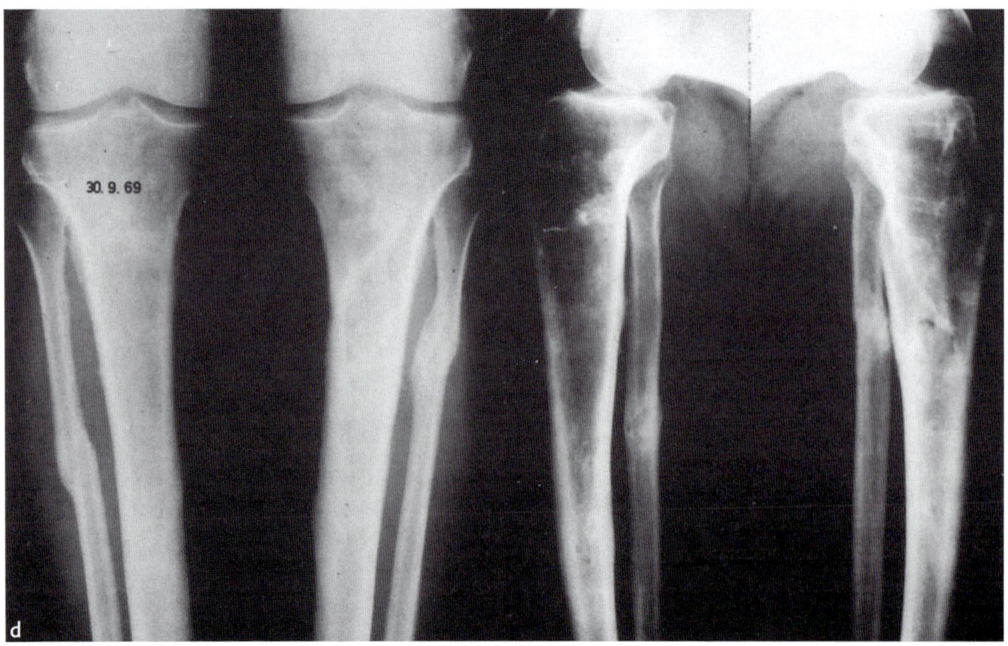

Fig. 4-5a–d Grade II (62-year-old patient).

a Right leg: segmental fracture. Left leg: gross displacement of fracture.

b 29 weeks after plating on both sides with contoured semitubular plates, all of them protected by well-vascularized muscle.

c The function 28 days after open reduction and internal fixation.

d 3 years after injury, 1 year after metal removal. Full restoration.

4.2 Intramedullary nail fixations with limited indication

The ideal indication for intramedullary nailing is the undisplaced or slightly displaced closed midshaft fracture of the tibia. In these fractures, the periosteal blood supply is not seriously disturbed and the surgery-related insult to the intramedullary blood distribution is well tolerated. These fractures heal rapidly by periosteal callus formation.

In open fractures, Grade II III in which the soft-tissue envelope and therefore the periosteal blood supply is damaged, medullary nailing would cause 'overkill' of bone-blood perfusion. Nailing under such circumstances is not biological at all.

Grade I open fractures without significant envelope-stripping, however, are, from the point of view of blood supply, similar to closed and non-displaced tibia fractures. They may also be stabilized with intramedulary nailing.

Comment

Intramedullary nailing in open tibial fractures is successful as long as the periosteal blood supply of the tibial fragments has not been destroyed. However, when one or both fragments are separated from the soft-tissue envelope and also when the endosteal blood circulation is insulted by the nail, callus fixation may fail. Under adverse vascular focal conditions, medullary nailing should be avoided in favor of stabilization with an external fixator.

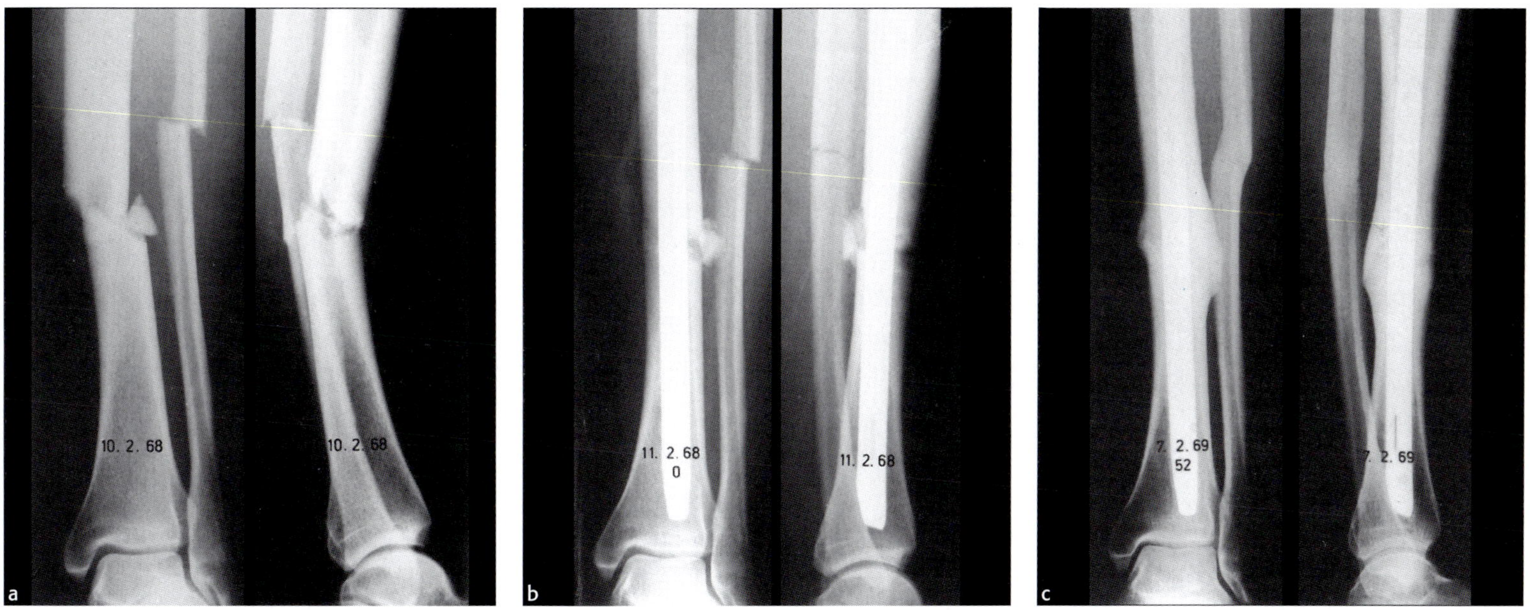

Fig. 4-6a–c Grade I (47-year-old patient).
a Grade I injury, extensive skin degloving over distal fragment.
b Closed nailing and primary wound closure.
c 1 year later: Sound periosteal fracture healing, more voluminous callus mass laterally than medially, as to be expected.

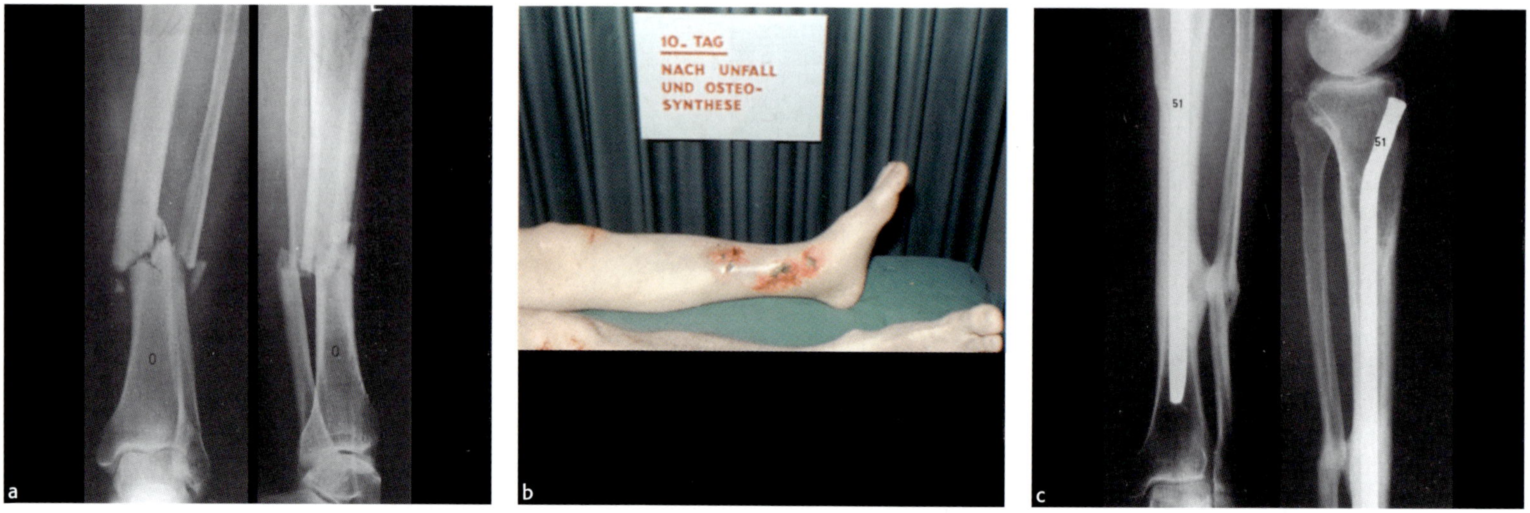

Fig. 4-7a–c Grade I (53-year-old patient).

a Grade I injury with serious skin contusion proximal to medial malleolus.

b 10 days after open reduction and internal fixation with nail.

c 51-week result. Massive callus mass laterally at the site of lesser degloving by the original injury.

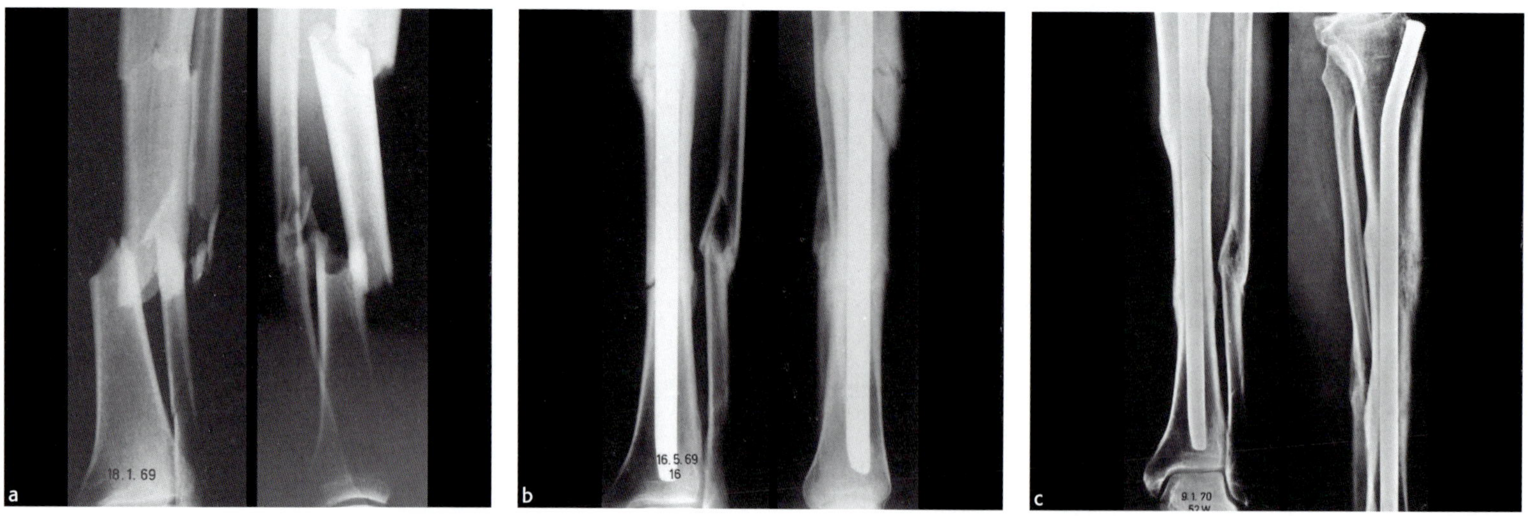

Fig. 4-8a–c Grade II (patient's identification lost).

a Grade II segmental fracture with heavy skin contusion, considerable displacement of the distal fracture.

b 16 weeks after closed reduction proximally, open reduction through the skin disruption distally and nailing. Note: poor callus production at the distal site with degloving of the fragments.

c 52 weeks after fractures: uneventful periosteal fracture healing.

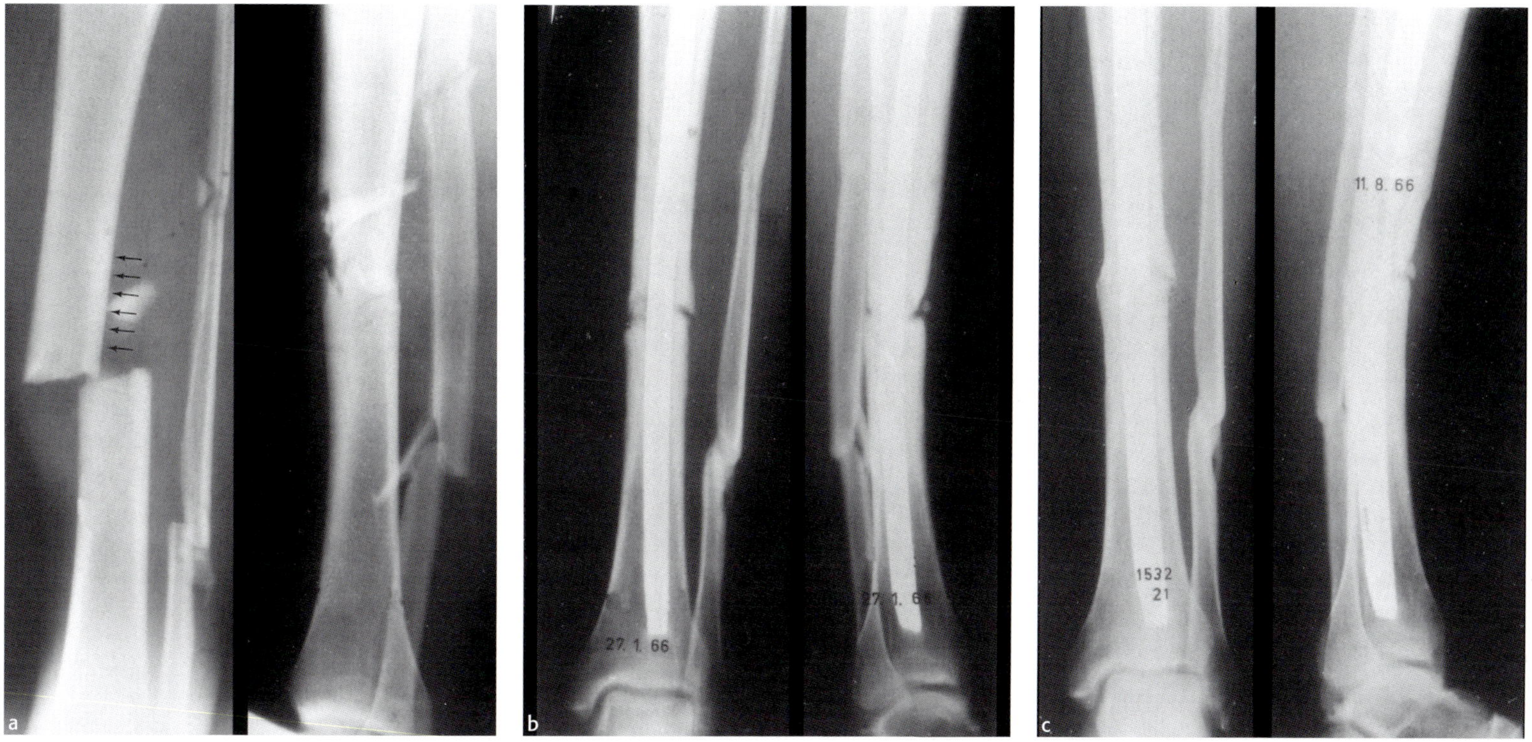

Fig. 4-9a–c Grade II (30-year-old patient).

a Grade II fracture. Extensive envelope stripping from the proximal fragment medially and from the interosseous membrane (arrows).

b 37 weeks after open reduction through the skin disruption and unreamed nailing: poor periosteal callus formation, nonunion. Therefore, closed renailing with a thicker nail.

c 16 months after fracture: the fracture is uniting only with difficulty, with only a small amount of periosteal fixation callus. The blood supply of the fragments was doubly impaired, by the degloving and by the medullary nailing.

4.3 External fixator to be permanently in place for the entire fracture healing period

The general policy for open fractures is that the external fixator is a preliminary fixation. It is removed at the time of wound healing, when the threat of infection is gone, and it is replaced by another fixation of a nail, plate, or a brace.

Our concept is different: The external fixator should offer fixation for the entire healing period. Our arguments in favor of that policy are as follows: The external fixator, ie, Steinmann pins or Schanz screws hardly interfere with the intramedullary blood circulation or with the periosteal blood supply. Stability of reduced and locally fixed fragments favors their healing and secondary operations for failed bone healing are seldom necessary. Minimal open reduction, internal fixation, and fixation with the external fixator is therefore the greatest biological stabilization possible [5, 7, 8]. This is our treatment of choice for grade II and III injuries—it simultaneously benefits the soft-tissue healing process and the fracture healing.

Comment

The external fixator preserves the blood supply of fragments to the maximum [5]. A wide range indication is available for open fractures as well as for complex closed fractures.

Our refinements to the original threaded-rod external fixator [5] makes it superior to other systems in several ways. Its main advantage is the high stability due to the fixed right-angle clamps on threaded rods and on rods that may be bent to accommodate axial adjustment. To understand the threaded-rod external fixator, see our monograph "The external fixator" [5].

Practically all requirements of an external fixator can be satisfied with the Synthes external fixator, with its few elements on one hand and trained skill on the other.

What can be done with the threaded-rod external fixator?

1. Hold fragments.
2. Hold and compress fragments.
3. Neutralize internal fixations.
4. Distract fragments, lengthening.
5. Approximate fragments, shortening.
6. Angulate fragments, axial correction.
7. Stretch soft tissues.

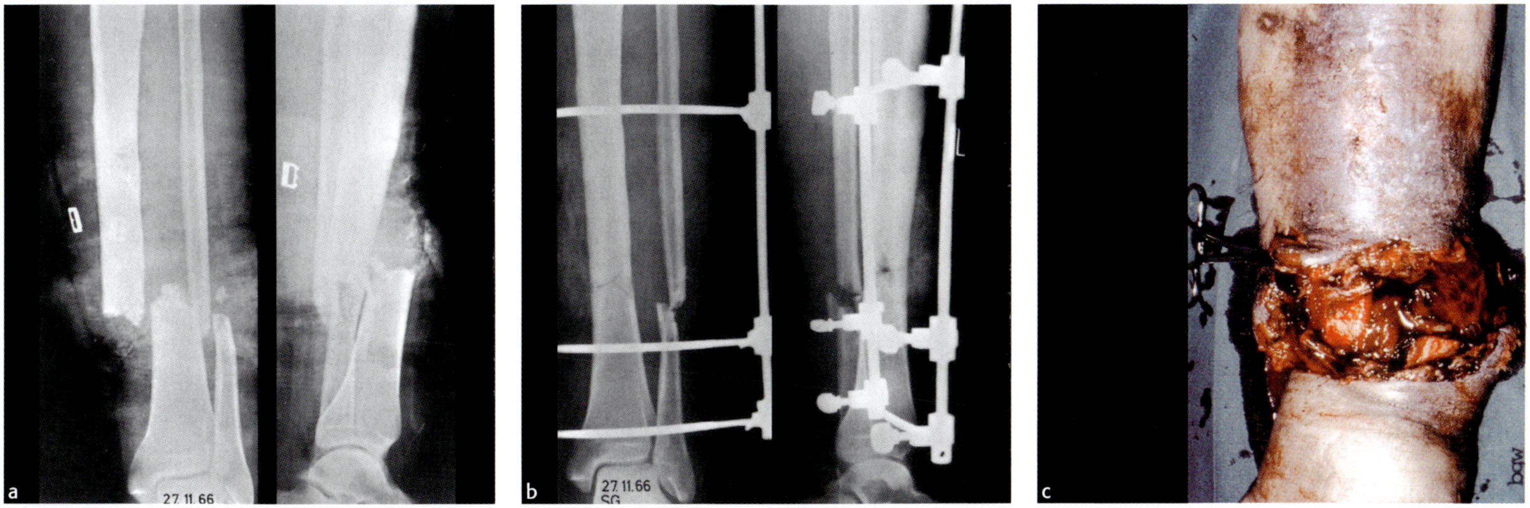

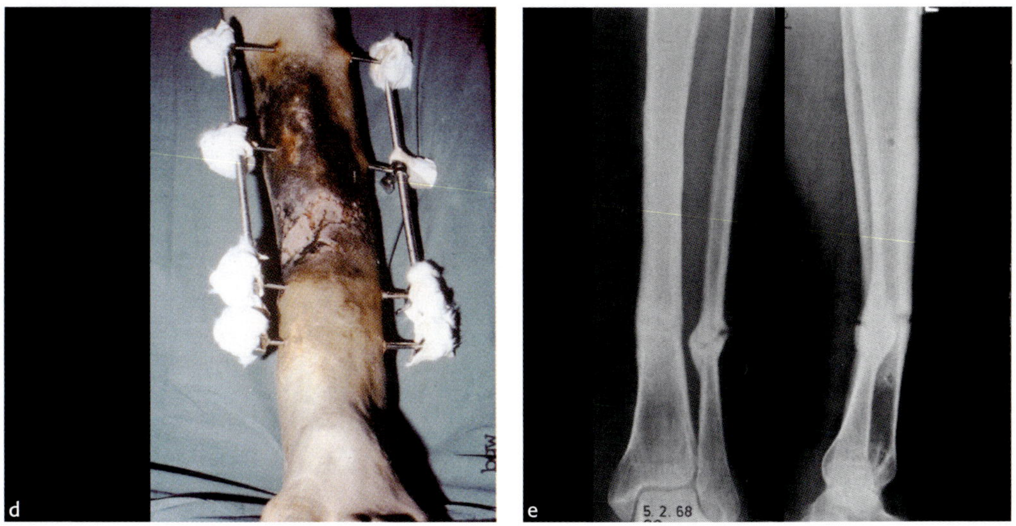

Fig. 4-10a–e Grade III (32-year-old patient).

a Grade III fracture through a chronic leg ulcer with gross displacement. Tibia and fibula are in normal relation to each other, ie, the soft-tissue envelope of both fragments is not seriously disturbed over a long distance.

b The fracture is anatomically reduced through the ulceration and stabilized with a prestrained compression fixator frame.

c Skin ulcer and fracture.

d 5 weeks later, 2 weeks after split skin grafting on granulations.

e 14 months after fracture: fracture of the tibia is healed by periosteal and endosteal callus. The fibula is almost completely united and the chronic leg ulcer is also healed.

4.4 Minimal local internal fixations that need mechanical protection with an external fixator

With minimal open reduction and internal fixation, restoration of the fragment perfusion along the intramedullary route is encouraged and the closure of the soft-tissue envelope is favored. To stabilize the minimal local internal fixation, an external fixator is applied that is stable enough to allow early-immediate increasing function, continuous passive motion plus continuous active function (CPM plus CAF).

Comment

Frame or unilateral external fixator allows functional treatment of anatomically and biologically reduced and fixed open grade I and III tibial fractures. Fracture healing occurs mainly by endosteal callus formation due to corresponding restoration of the blood supply of the fracture area along the medullary canal.

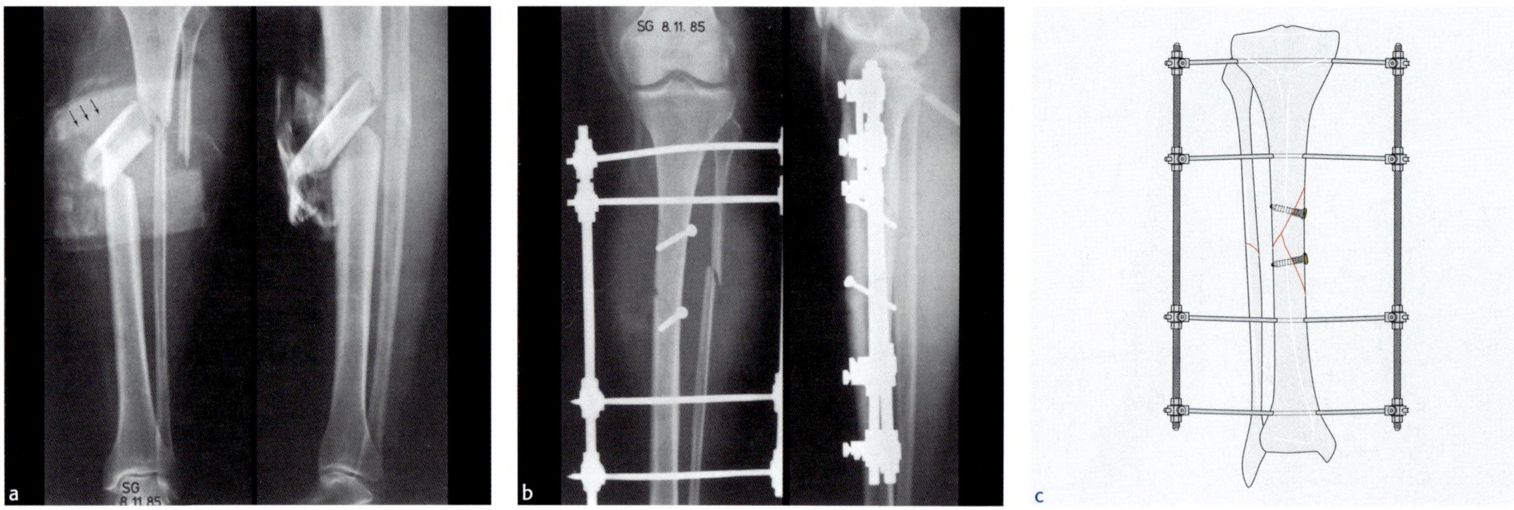

Fig. 4-11a–f Grade III (59-year-old patient).

a X-rays with primary dressing (arrows), outside sterile enclosure not removed.

b Minimal waterproof open reduction and internal fixation with two lag screws. The principle of the holding frame: the proximal and distal pair of Steinmann pins are prestrained against each other to provide undisplaceable stability with the bone. Such stability is very much in favor to prevent pin-track infection.

c Waterproof internal fixation and prestrained external fixator frame.

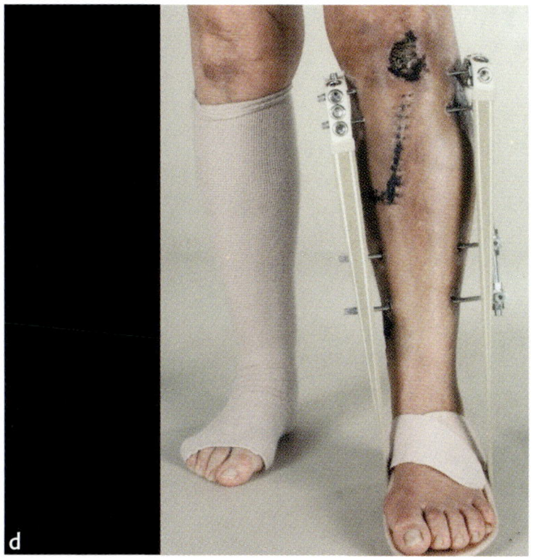

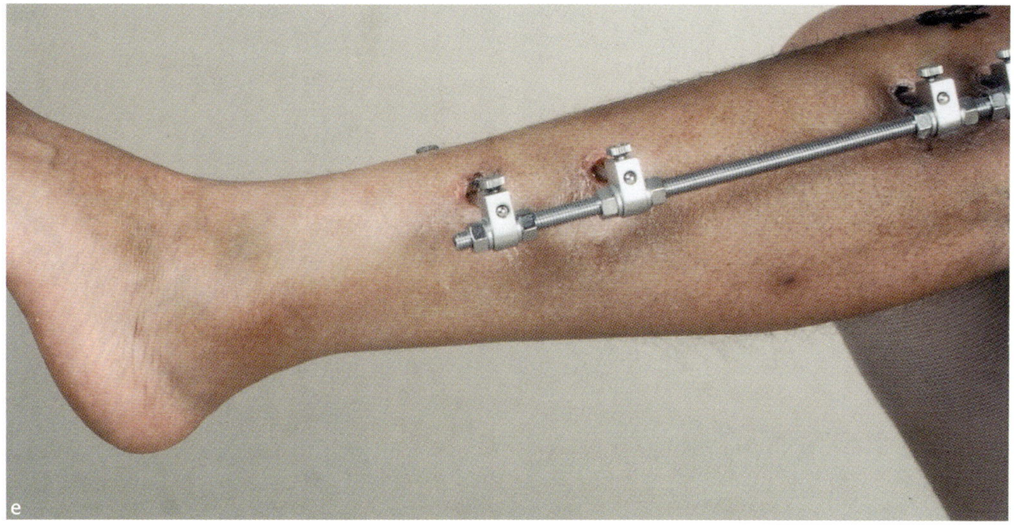

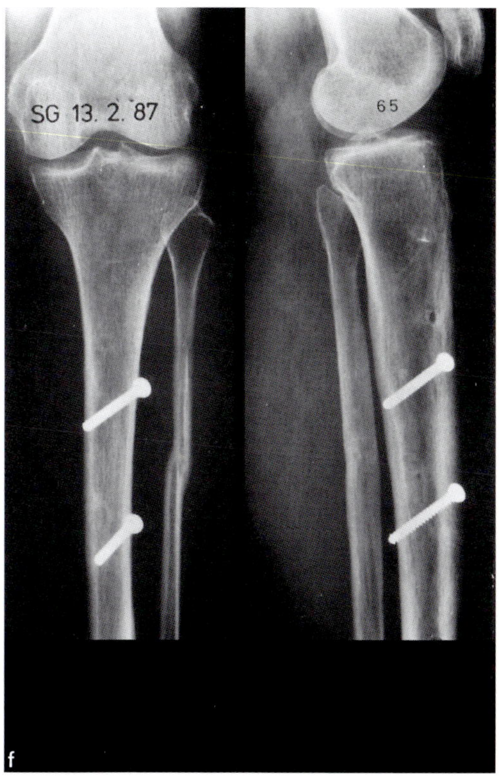

Fig. 4-11a–f cont.

de Early function. Plantar support against equinus. Sound wound healing after primary local-limited rotation skin flap.

f 65 weeks after injury: back to normal.

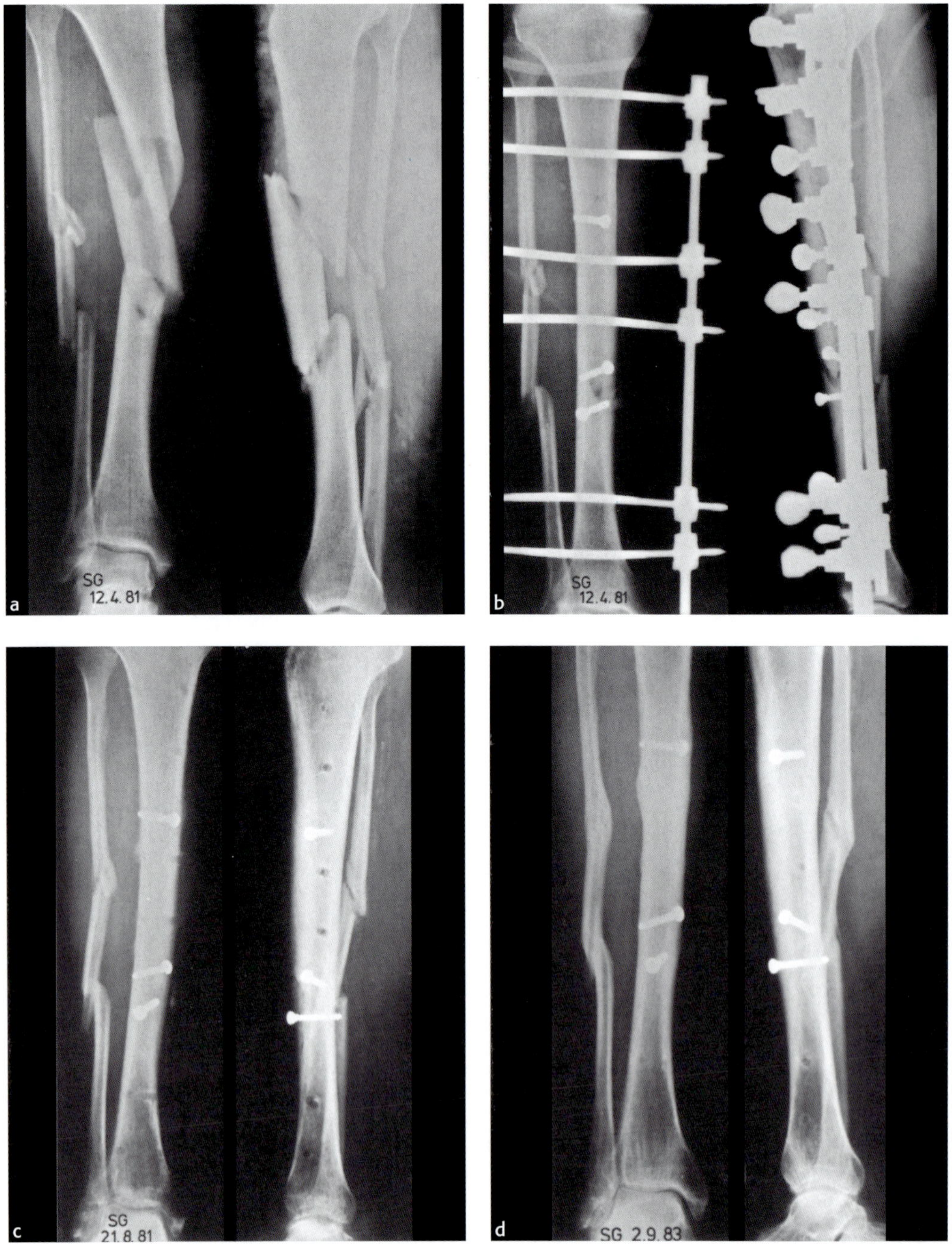

Fig. 4-12a–d Grade II (53-year-old patient).

a Segmental fracture, skin disruption, skin contusion.

b Waterproof internal fixation with lag screws and protective prestrained external fixator frame.

c 4 months after injury, immediately after fixator removal. A removable functional brace is given for another 4 months.

d Late follow-up 2 years 5 months after injury: full recovery.

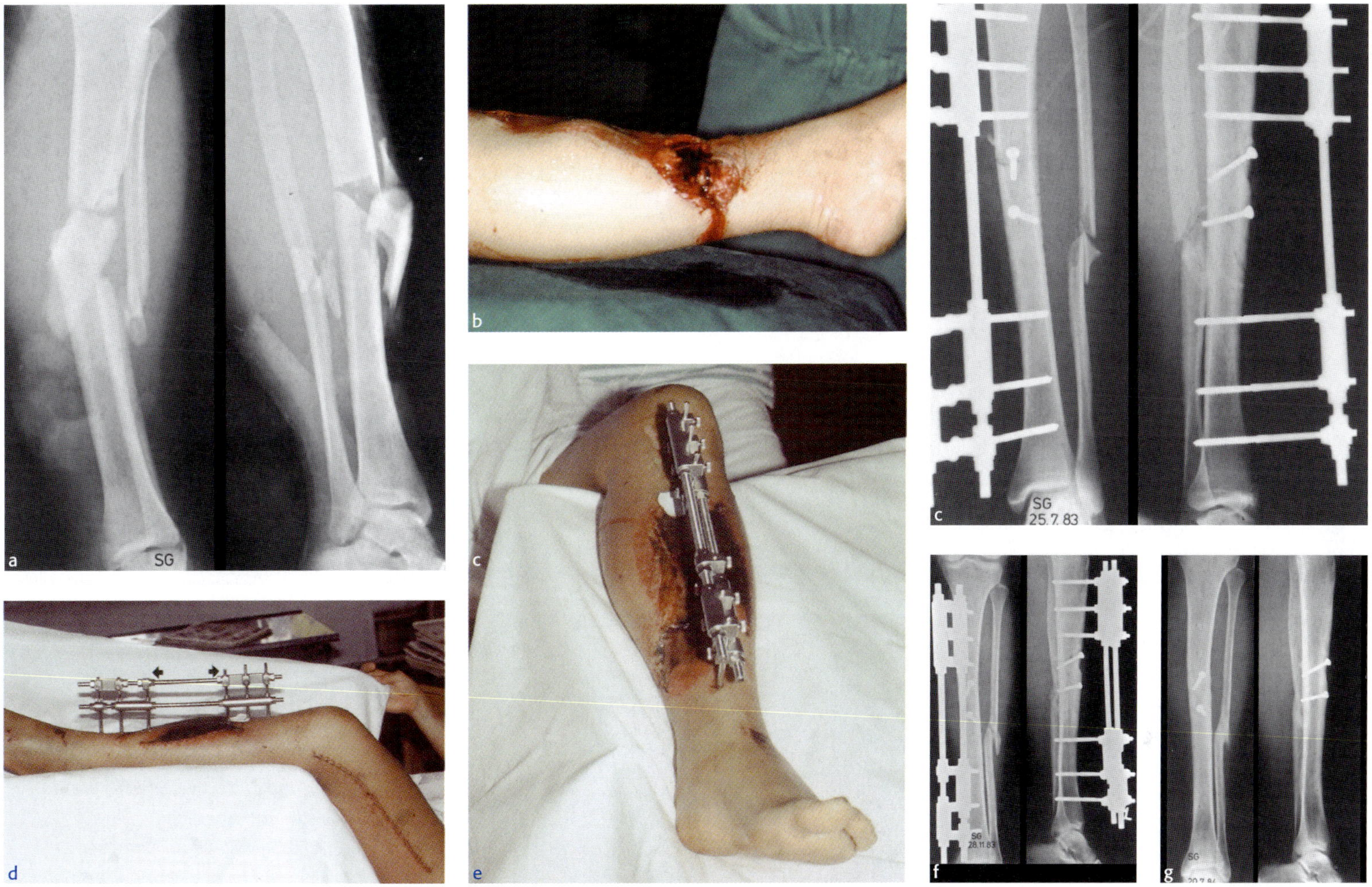

Fig. 4-13a–g Grade III (16-year-old patient).

a Complex fracture.

b The skin lesion: rupture, contusion, degloving.

c Minimal open reduction and internal fixation with protective unilateral external fixator. Note: three screws per main fragment, two threaded rods prestrained against each other to prevent deformation of the construction.

d 3 weeks after the fracture: clinical aspect. Sound wound healing, dry skin necrosis over the tibia. Note: prestrain by distraction (arrows).

e Note: one rod on one side, one rod on the other side of the Schanz screws with the effect of a frame, ie, of maximal stability against varus-valgus.

f 4 months after injury: endosteal fracture healing.

g The 1-year result: back to normal.

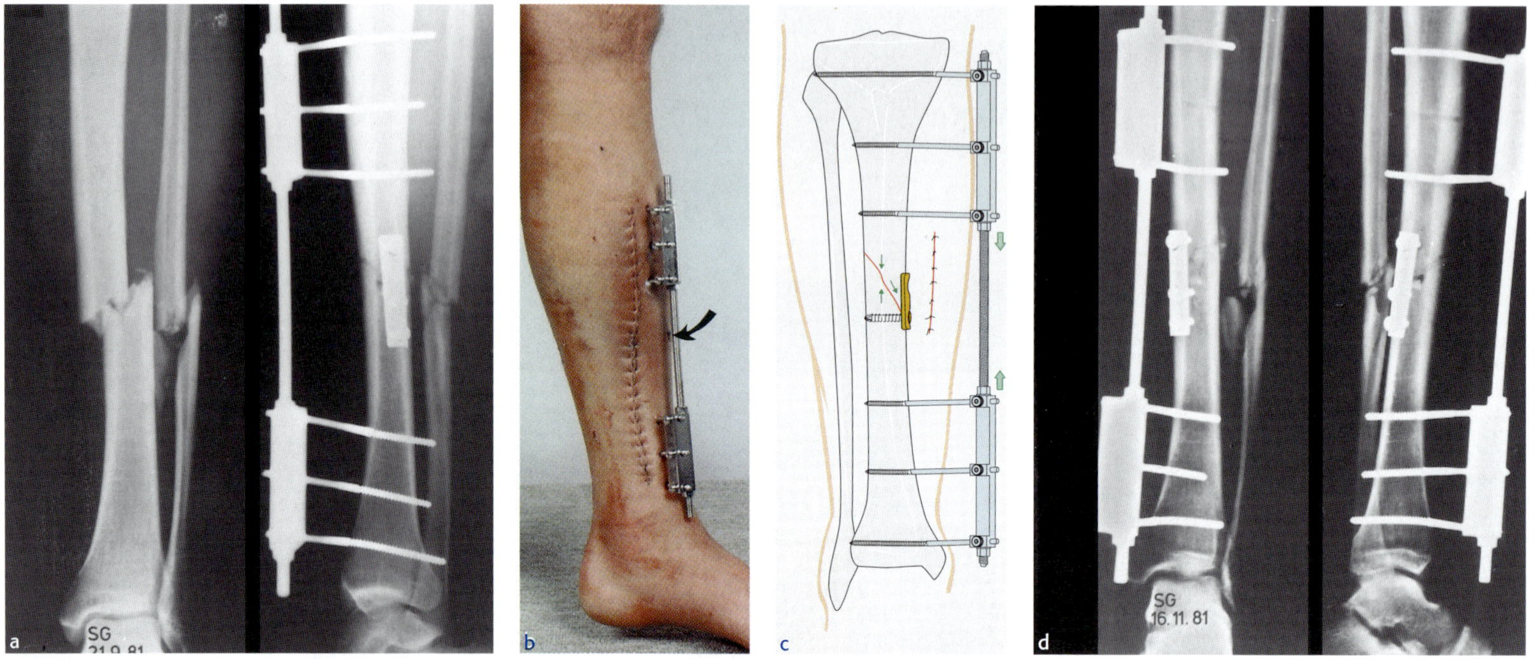

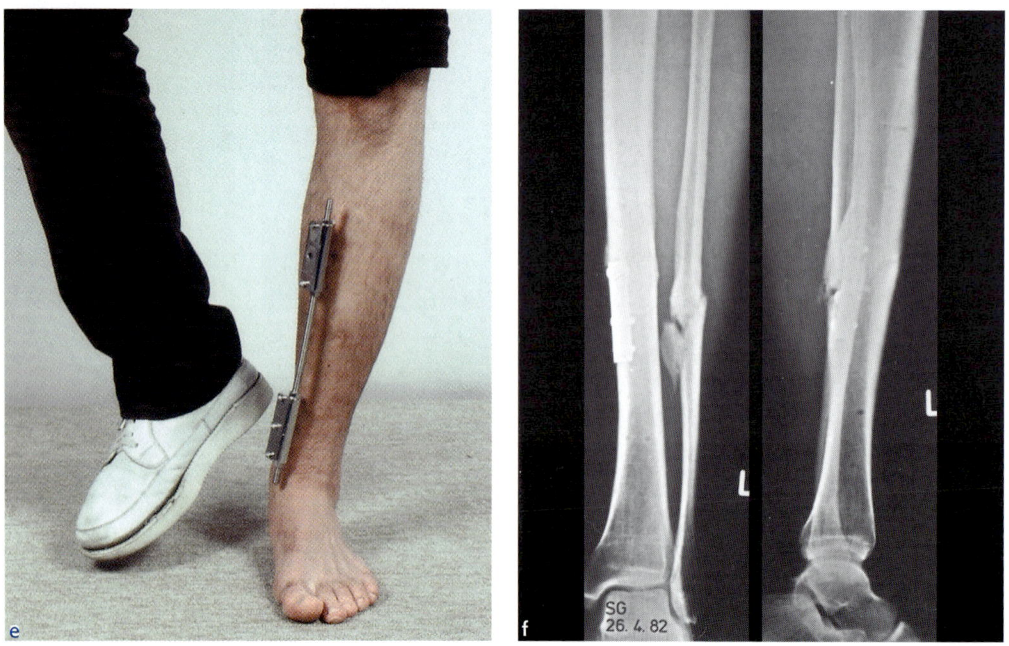

Fig. 4-14a–f Grade I (22-year-old patient).

a Open reduction and internal fixation with semitubular antigliding plate on the medial-posterior tibial crest.
Unilateral one-rod protective external fixator.

b Clinical aspect 8 days after injury. Skin perforation by the proximal tibia fragment left open (arrow). The long skin incision served for the removal of an extended degloving hematoma and for open reduction and internal fixation.

c The mechanics of the fixation: antigliding plate allowing axial loading of the oblique fracture. The unilateral fixator exerts permanent axial compression (arrows).

d 2 months after fracture.

e Full weightbearing at 2 months. The external fixator is removed at 10 weeks.

f 7 months after the accident: full restoration.

4.5 Plate fixation of the fibula for indirect reduction of the tibial fracture and as a stability augmentation of the external fixator

First plate fixation of the fibula makes reduction of the tibia fracture easy. The stabilized fibula and a unilateral external fixator form a stable frame so that a reduced tibia fracture can be left free from open reduction and internal fixation.

Comment

The plating of the fractured fibula may spare the tibial fracture from direct fixation when the reduction results in intrinsic stability. An unilateral external fixator with the plated fibula forms a stable frame, and functional aftercare is possible. An autogenous bone graft may accelerate the bony union.

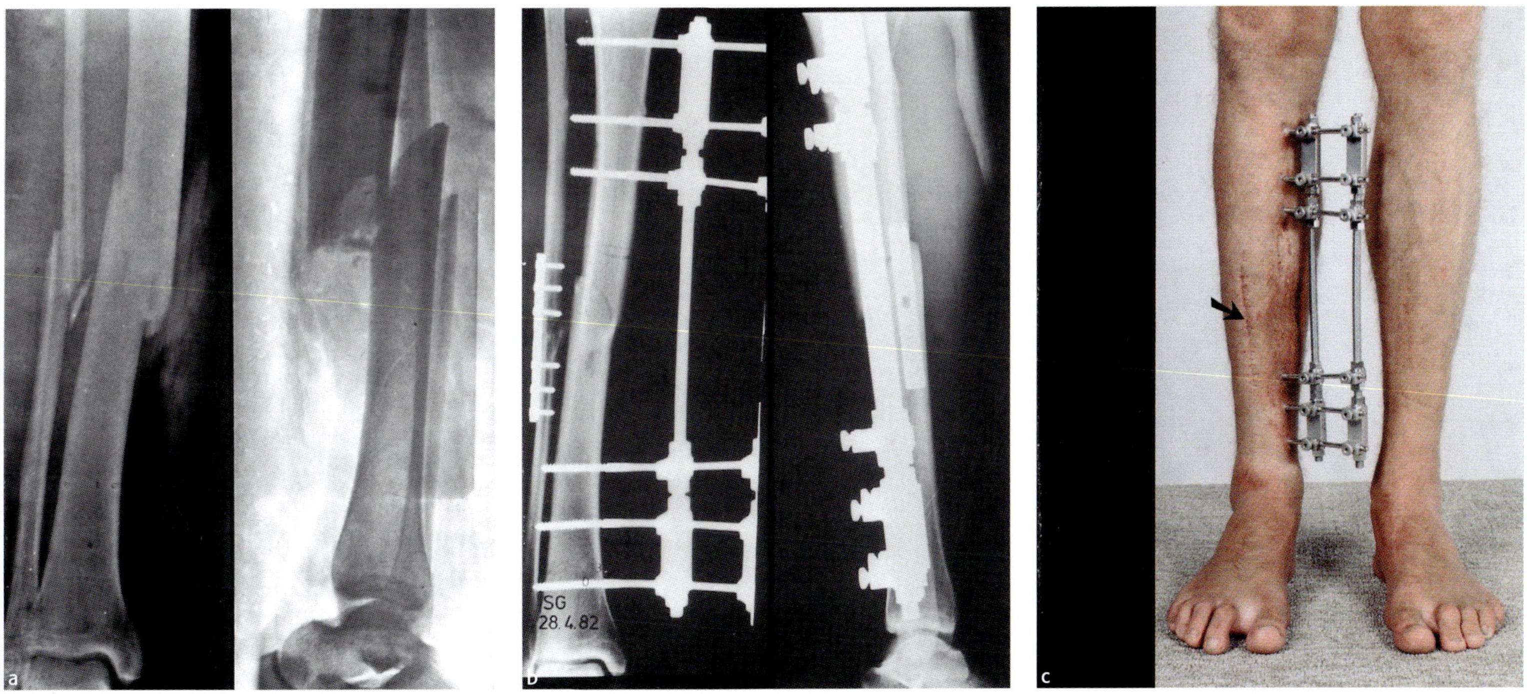

Fig. 4-15a–f Grade III (25-year-old patient).
a The fracture with serious soft-tissue injury.

b Stabilizing frame with plated fibula and unilateral external fixator. Tibial fracture reduced through open wound, but not internally fixed. At 4 weeks, autogenous cancellous bone graft to accelerate fracture healing.

c 2 months from injury: patient is weightbearing. Anterior scar from bone grafting (arrow).

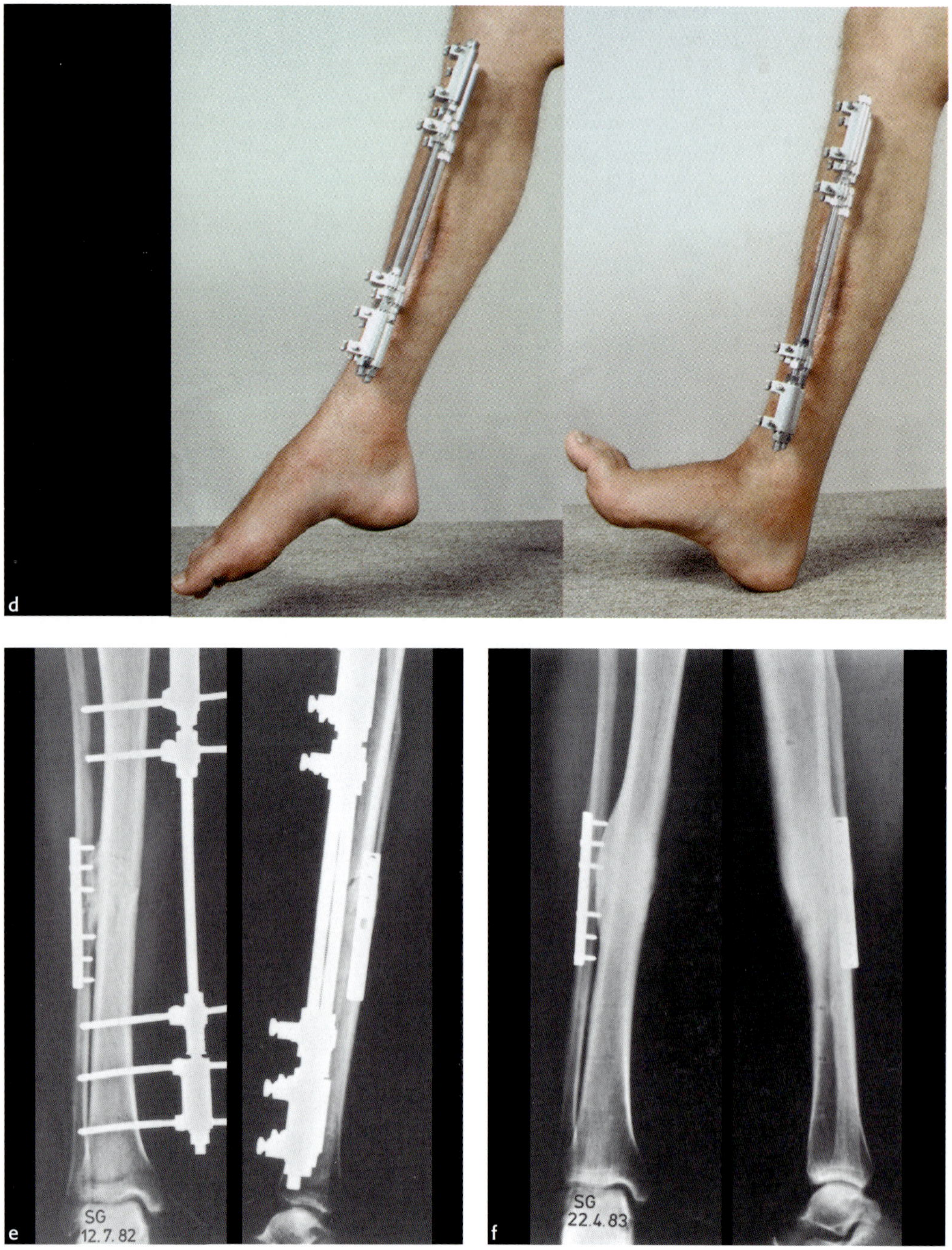

Fig. 4-15a–f cont.

d Function of the foot at that stage.

e The x-ray at 2 months, when the external fixator is removed and a functional brace is applied for 6 weeks.

f Final result 1 year after the accident: sound healing of the tibial fracture by endosteal and periosteal callus and by the graft.

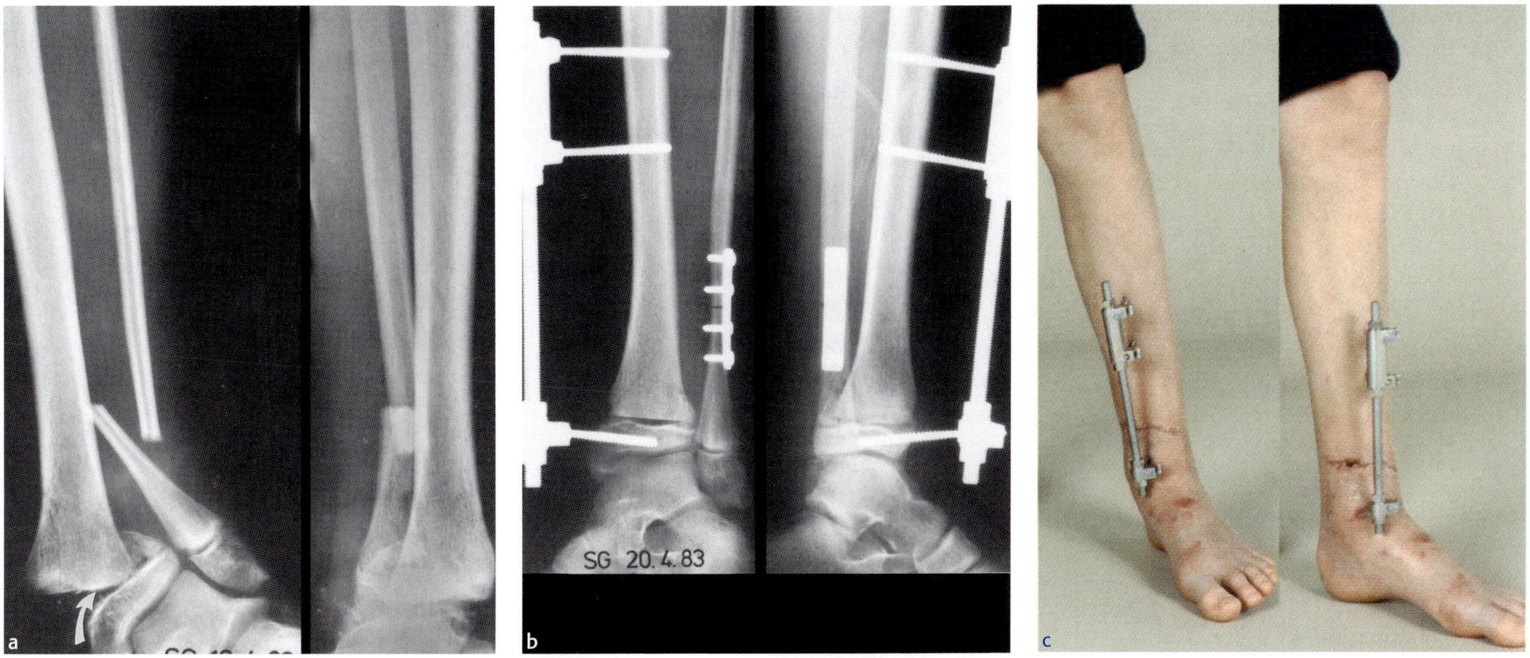

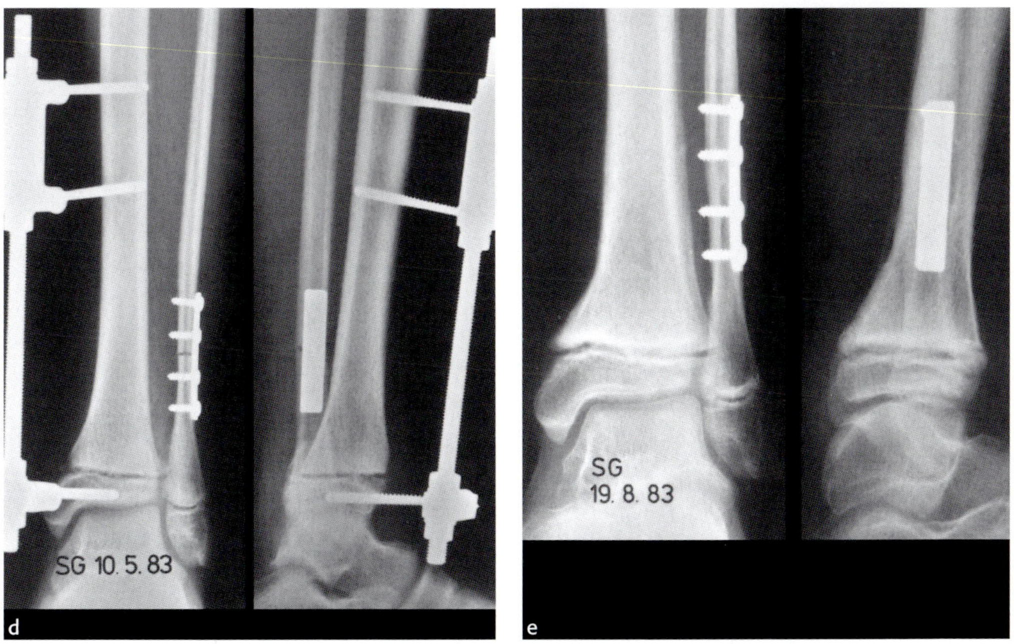

Fig. 4-16a–e Grade II (12-year-old patient).

a Gross displacement, periosteal stripping from the proximal tibia fragment on the medial side, skin rupture and partial degloving. Perichondrium and periosteum are entrapped into the lysis (arrow).

b Open reduction and internal fixation of the fibula by plating. Open reduction of tibial fracture, replacement of entrapped periosteum. Unilateral medial external fixator, bridging the growth plate.

c The clinical aspect 3 weeks after injury. Healing of the skin lesions.

d X-ray at 3 weeks, when the external fixator is removed and replaced by a lower leg walking brace for 4 weeks.

e Undisturbed healing at 4 months, no growth disturbance from the growth plate is seen, as expected.

4.6 Primary removal of devitalized fragments and secondary autogenous bone defect compensation

The x-ray and the first local assessment of the fracture allow us to recognize devitalized fragments. In closed, non-contaminated fractures, they may be incorporated into open reduction and internal fixation. Not so in contaminated open fractures: Fragments deprived of blood supply must be considered necrotic and contaminated, and at risk of becoming infected sequesters. For that reason, they are better primarily removed and replaced secondarily at a later stage. The best time for defect compensation with autogenous grafting is then, when aseptic wound healing has occurred. That stage may vary between 3 and 12 weeks after injury. Grafting is safest performed along a safe route, separate from the initial skin lesion.

Autogenous grafts are harvested from the iliac crest: blocks, slivers, sticks, flakes, and small pieces [5, 10].

Comment

In open fractures, which all are contaminated, loose, and devascularized fragments are potentially infected sequesters. They are better removed primarily. The remaining bone defect is compensated for as soon as wound healing is achieved, 3–12 weeks after injury. The best possible material is autogenous bone from the patient's own ilium.

Should bone healing after external fixator fail, a secondary better fixation with an external fixator follows. This process does not interfere with the blood supply at the fracture site, which would be the case with an intramedullary nail or a plate.

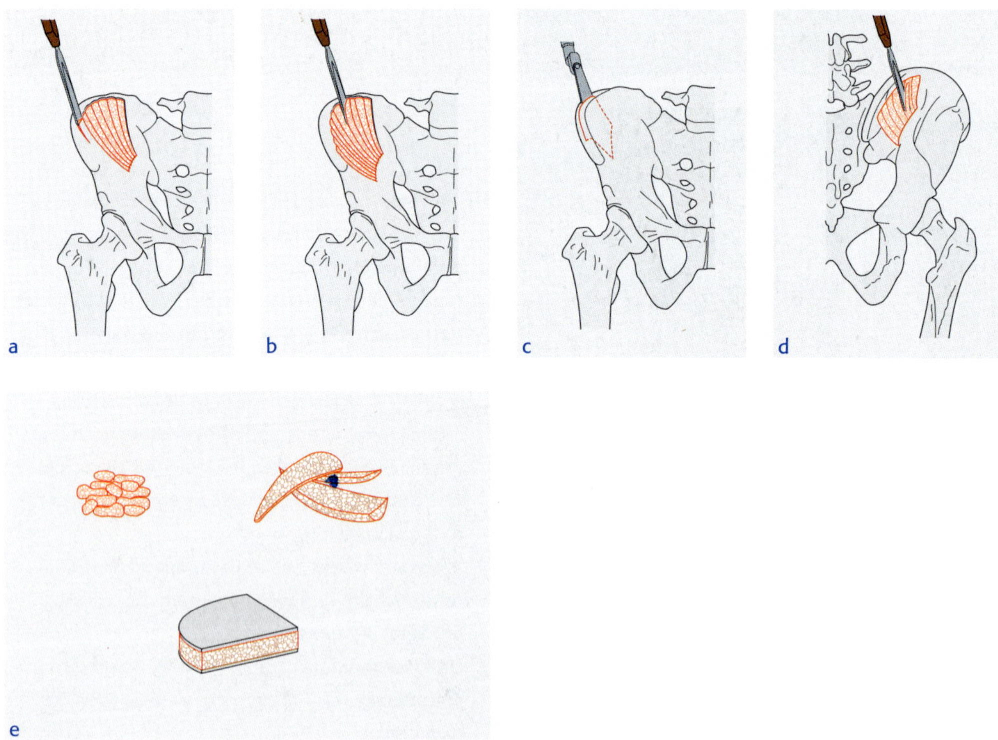

Fig. 4-17a–e Harvesting of autogenous grafts from the ilium.

ab Grafts are removed with graft chisels of various configurations from the inner wall of the iliac wing.

c Corticocancellous blocks are removed with the oscillating saw.

d Occasionally (for lumbosacral fusion, certain nonunions) the grafts are removed from the lateral wall of the posterior ilium.

e Different grafts are harvested according the given requirements.

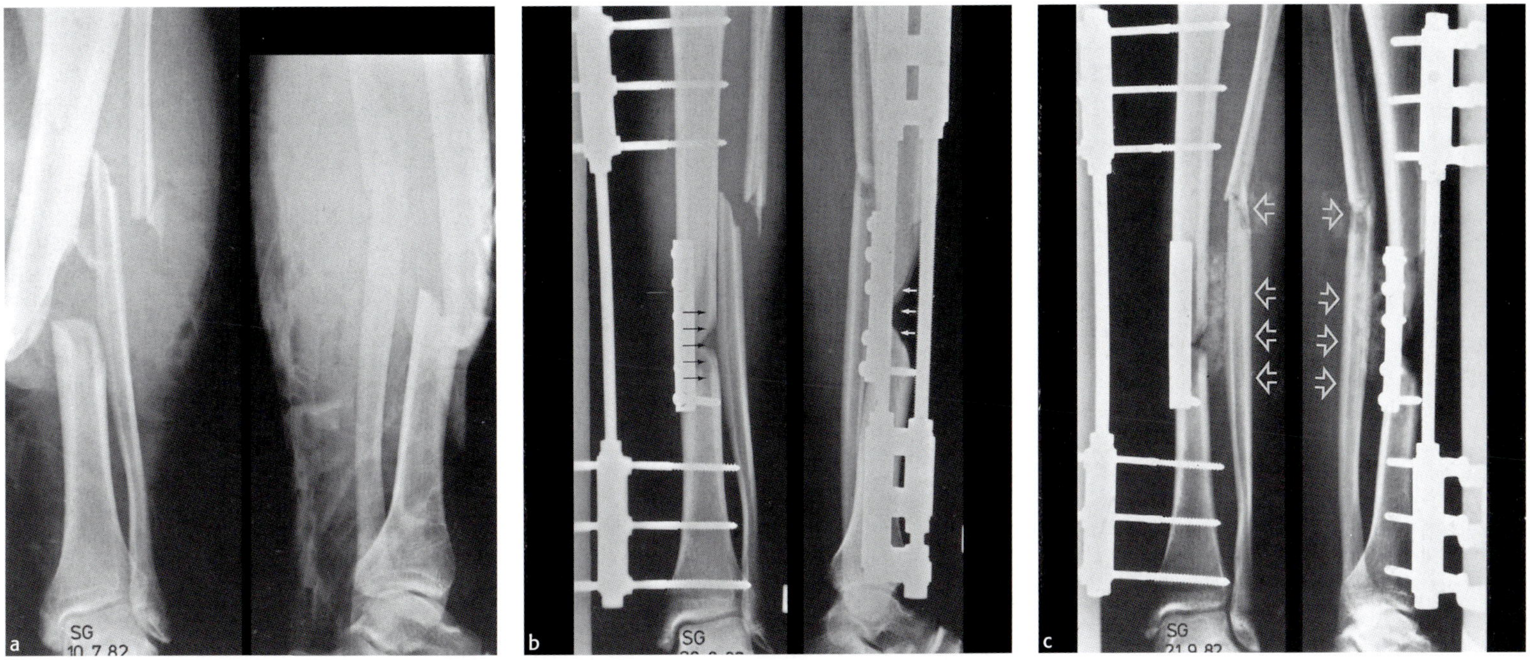

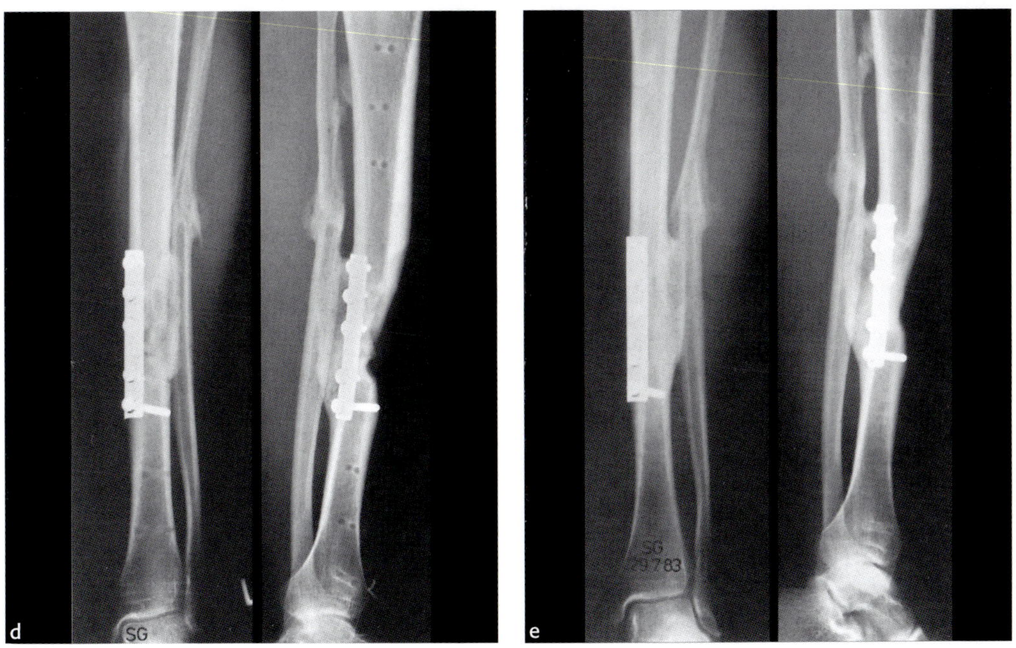

Fig. 4-18a–e Grade III (18-year-old patient).

a The fracture: one fragment is missing, was lost on the road. Open reduction and application of an external fixator are performed.

b 5 weeks later: wound is healed and grafting is performed the next day to compensate the defect (arrows).

c Harmon approach: incision over the fibula, approach posterior along the interosseous membrane to the defect of the tibia. The displaced fibular fracture is reduced from the same approach, application of grafts (arrows).

de 8-month and 1-year follow-up: sound healing of the fracture and remodelling of the bone grafts.

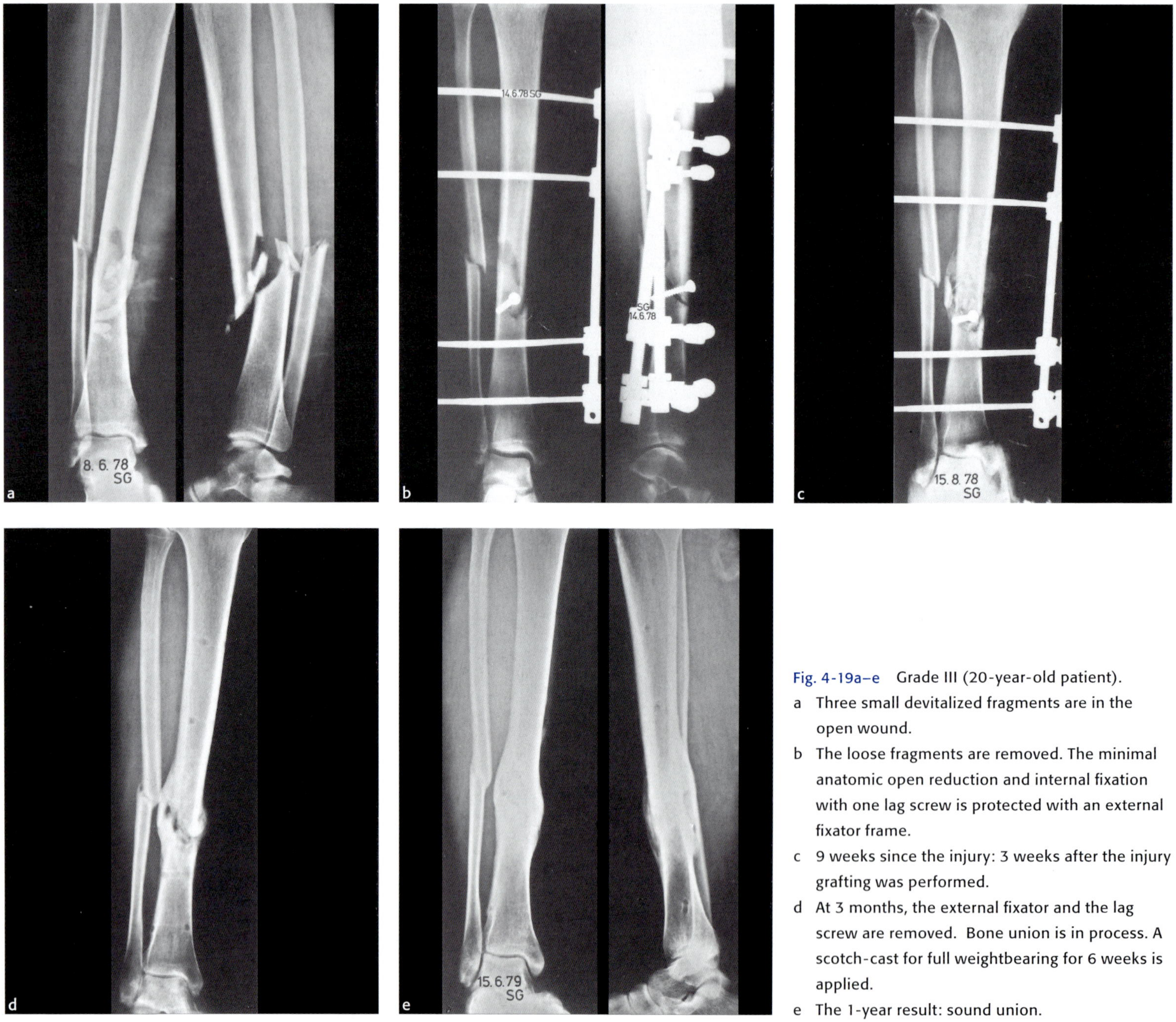

Fig. 4-19a–e Grade III (20-year-old patient).

a Three small devitalized fragments are in the open wound.

b The loose fragments are removed. The minimal anatomic open reduction and internal fixation with one lag screw is protected with an external fixator frame.

c 9 weeks since the injury: 3 weeks after the injury grafting was performed.

d At 3 months, the external fixator and the lag screw are removed. Bone union is in process. A scotch-cast for full weightbearing for 6 weeks is applied.

e The 1-year result: sound union.

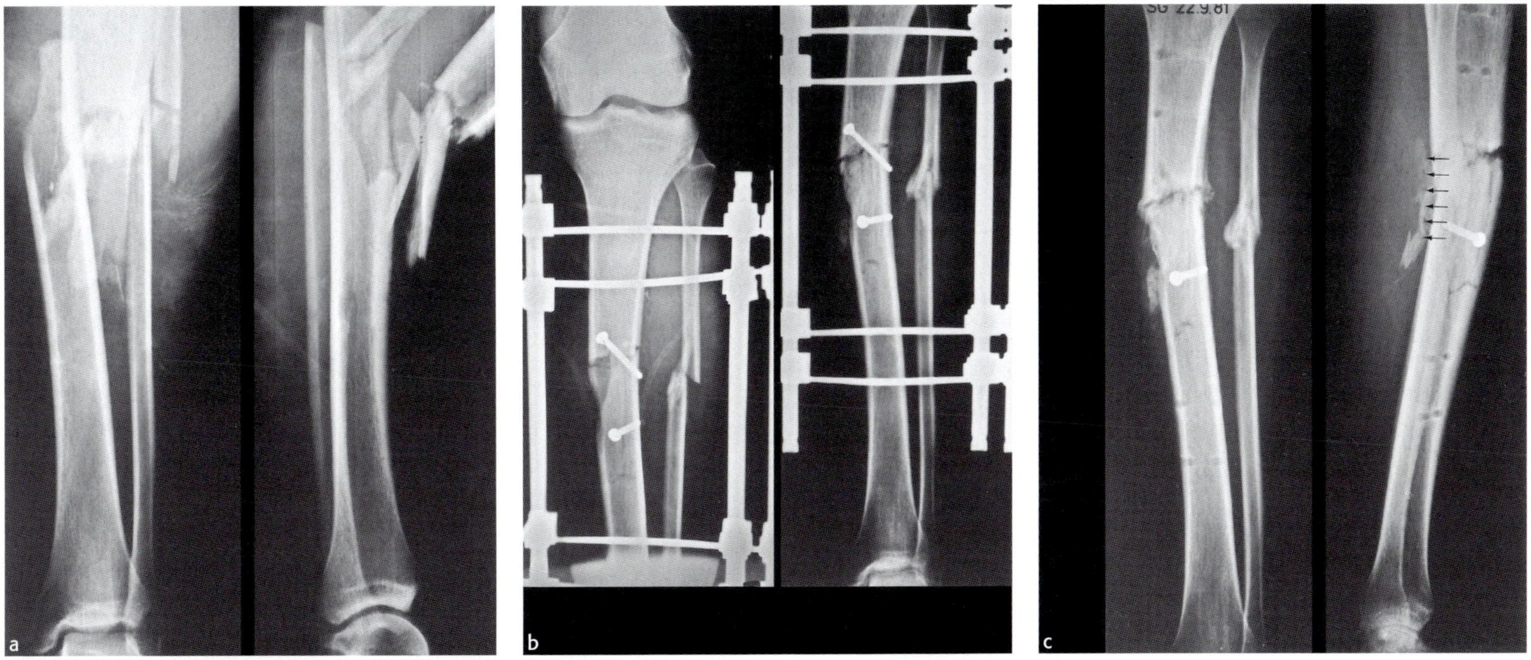

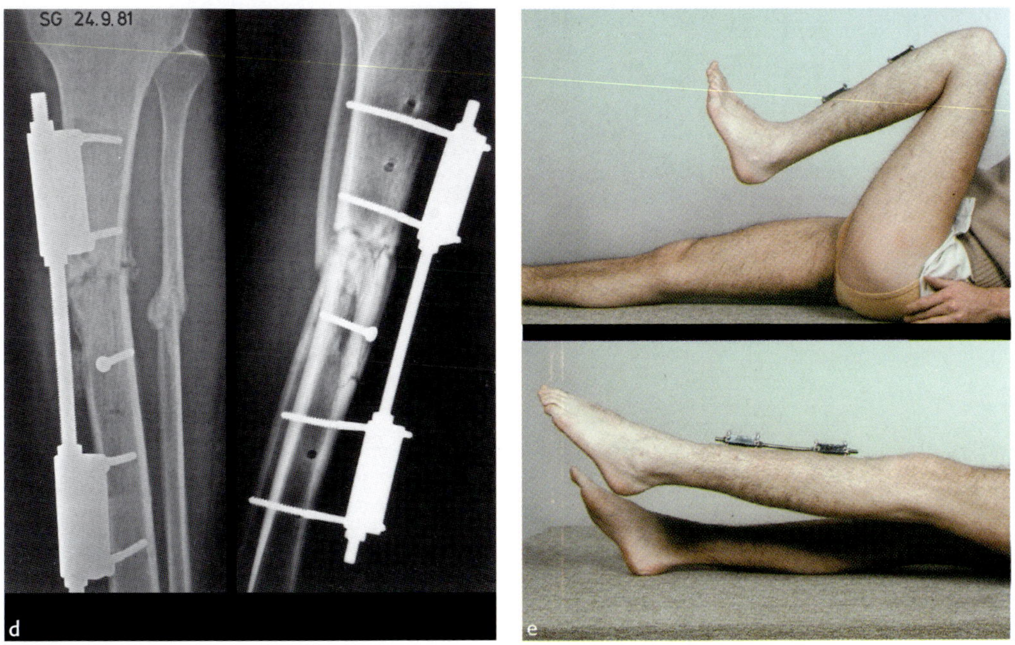

Fig. 4-20a–h Grade III (21-year-old patient).

- a Extensive stripping of distal fragment several devitalized and loose fragments.
- b The loose fragments are removed, not fully successful minimal focal fixation, protecting external fixator.
- c 3 months later: the wound is healed. A biologically active nonunion with local osteoporosis develops. External fixator and screw are removed. For bone stimulation, decortication of the posterior tibial surface (arrows) is performed.
- d Treatment of the nonunion: with unilateral tension band compression external fixator. A virtual frame fixation together with the healed fibula is created.
- e The clinical aspect 6 months after the accident: normal joint functions.

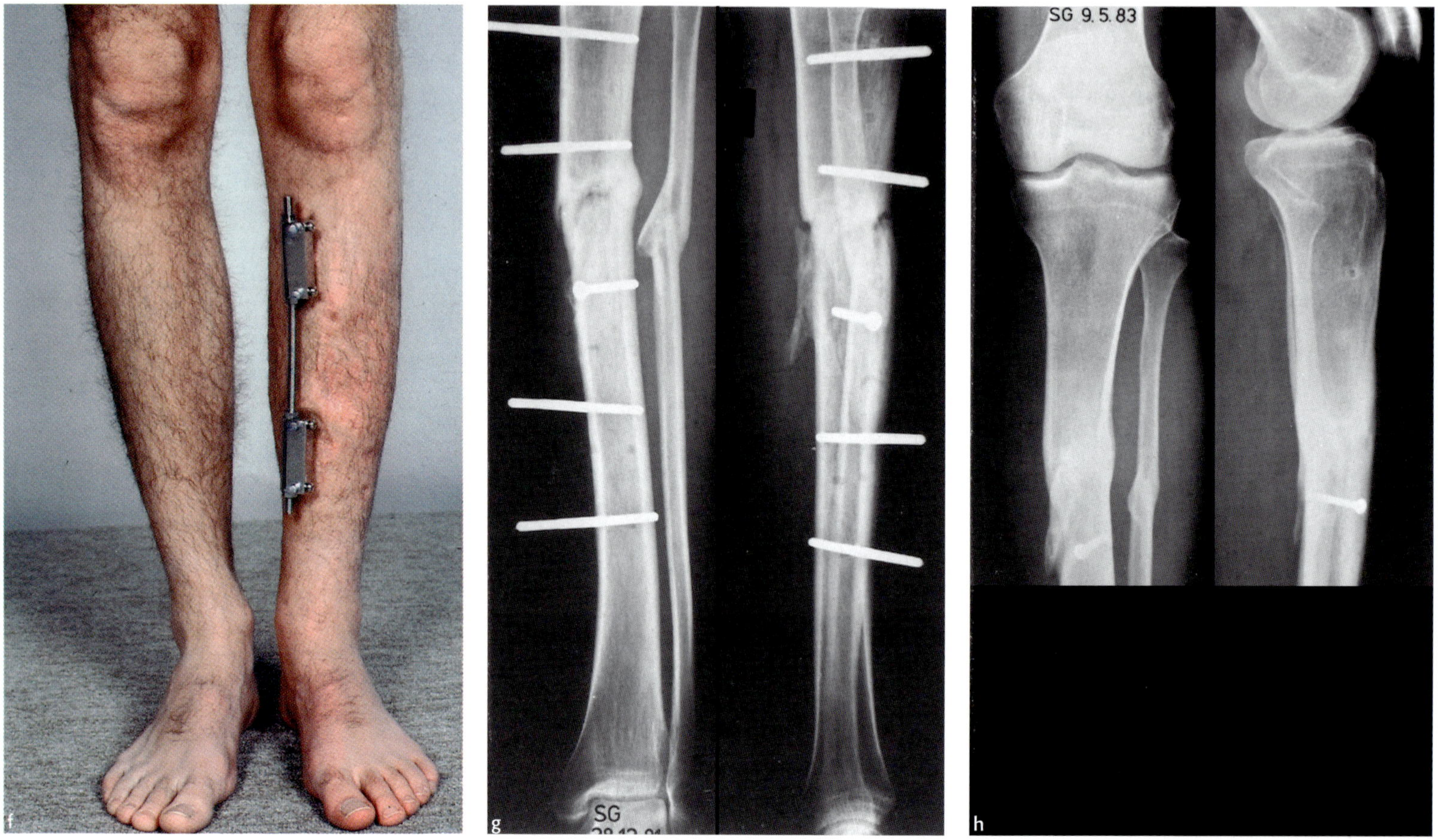

Fig. 4-20a–h cont.

f Full weightbearing at this stage.

g Bone healing allows removal of the external fixator 6 months after the fracture.

h 2 years after the injury: full recovery.

4.7 Secondary change to another fixation type

The primary fixation may fail and, thus, require secondary measures.

The most promising secondary measure depends mainly on the 'biology' at the fracture site: refixation with the same fixation type, with external fixator (see Fig. 4-20), or with another fixation and with bone healing stimulation by bone grafting or decortication shingling [5, 10].

Comment

With failure of fixation and fracture healing, secondary measures to accelerate the healing process should not be delayed. Refixation with the same or with another fixation technique and bone healing stimulation with autogenous grafting or decortication shingling are indicated. In the worst injuries, after careful assessment and attempts to save the limb, primary amputation can spare the patient a long and disappointing treatment period.

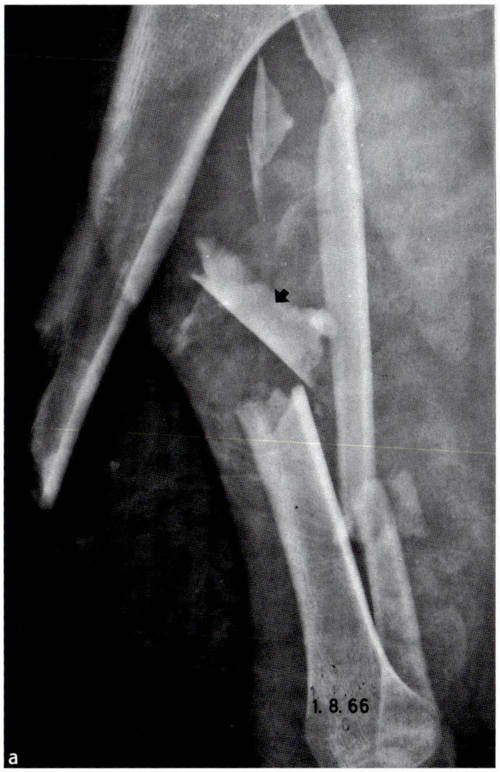

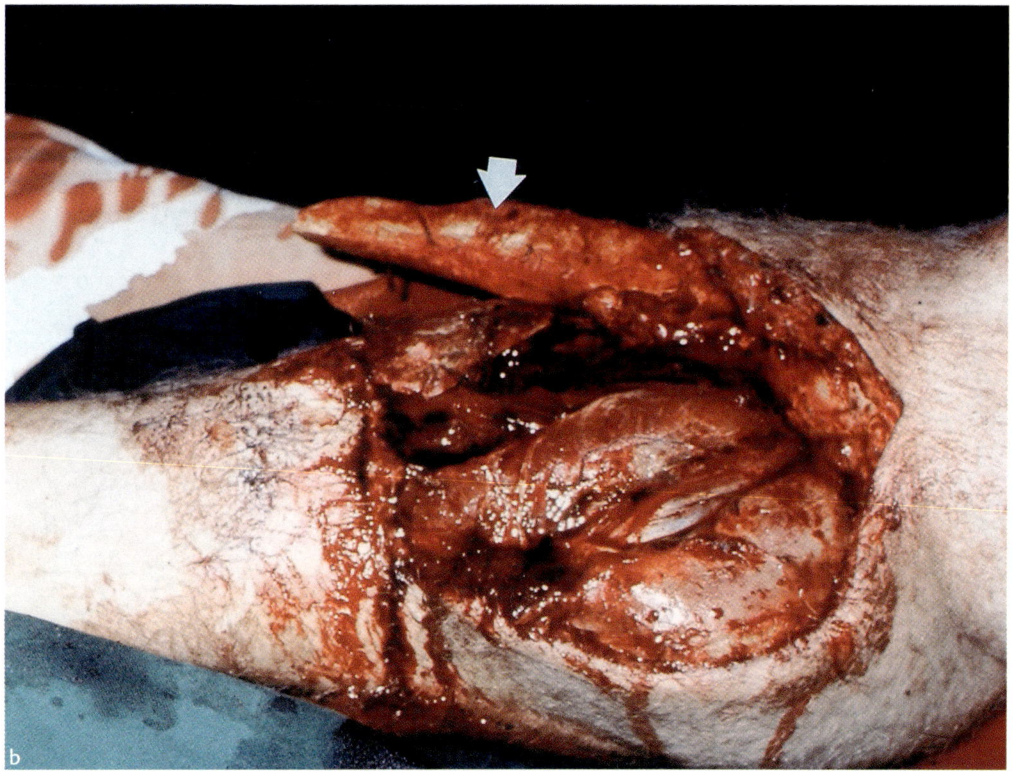

Fig. 4-21a–g Grade III (20-year-old patient).

a Extreme fragment stripping. The third anterolateral fragment, however, is still attached to the extensor muscles (arrow).

b The clinical aspect. The proximal main fragment is largely degloved (arrow).

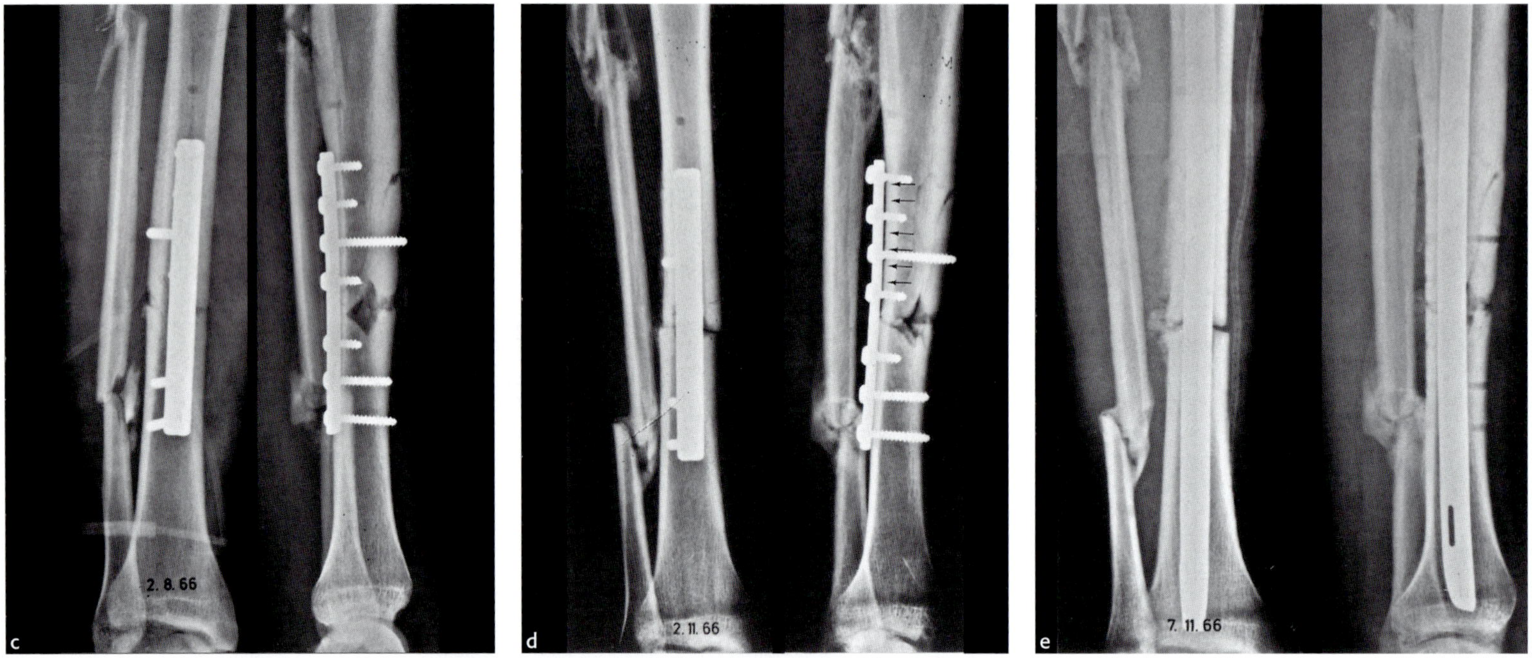

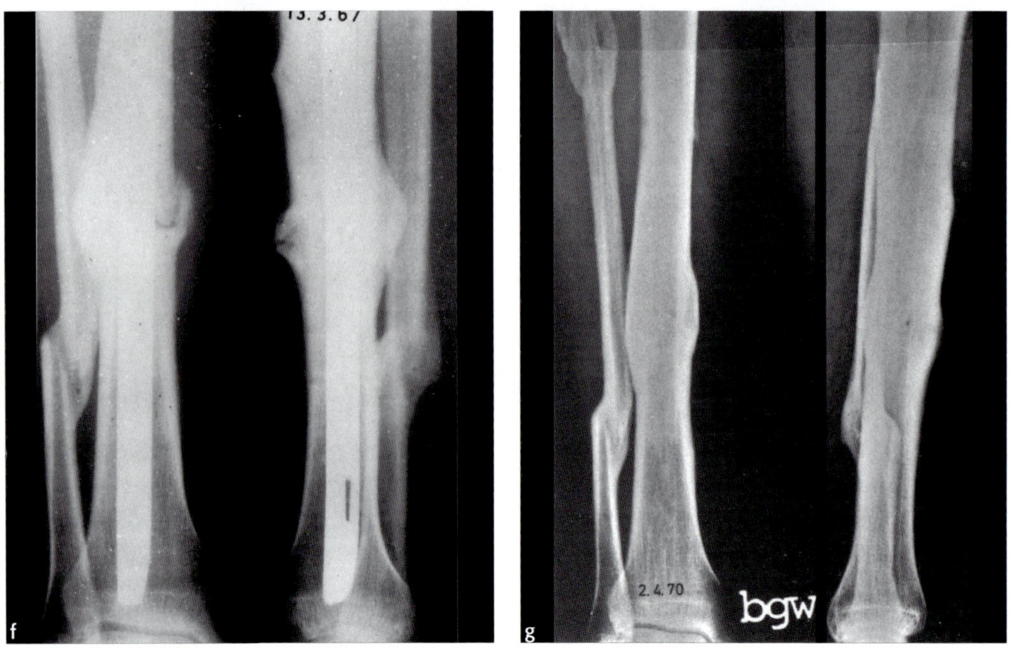

Fig. 4-21a–g cont.

c X-ray of next day: a narrow 4.5 mm plate was applied through the open wound to the posterior tibial surface. Two small loose fragments were removed.

d 5 months after the accident: plate has loosened (arrows). The nonunion asks for a fatigue resistant 'elastic' secondary stabilization and for stimulation.

e Removal of the plate and medullary nailing with gentle reaming. Application of autogenous cancellous bone grafts to the posterior plane of the tibia, where the plate was seated.

f 7 months after the accident, 4 months after nailing and bone grafting: intensive periosteal fixation.

g Late follow-up at 4 years: full recovery. The nail was removed 2 years after injury.

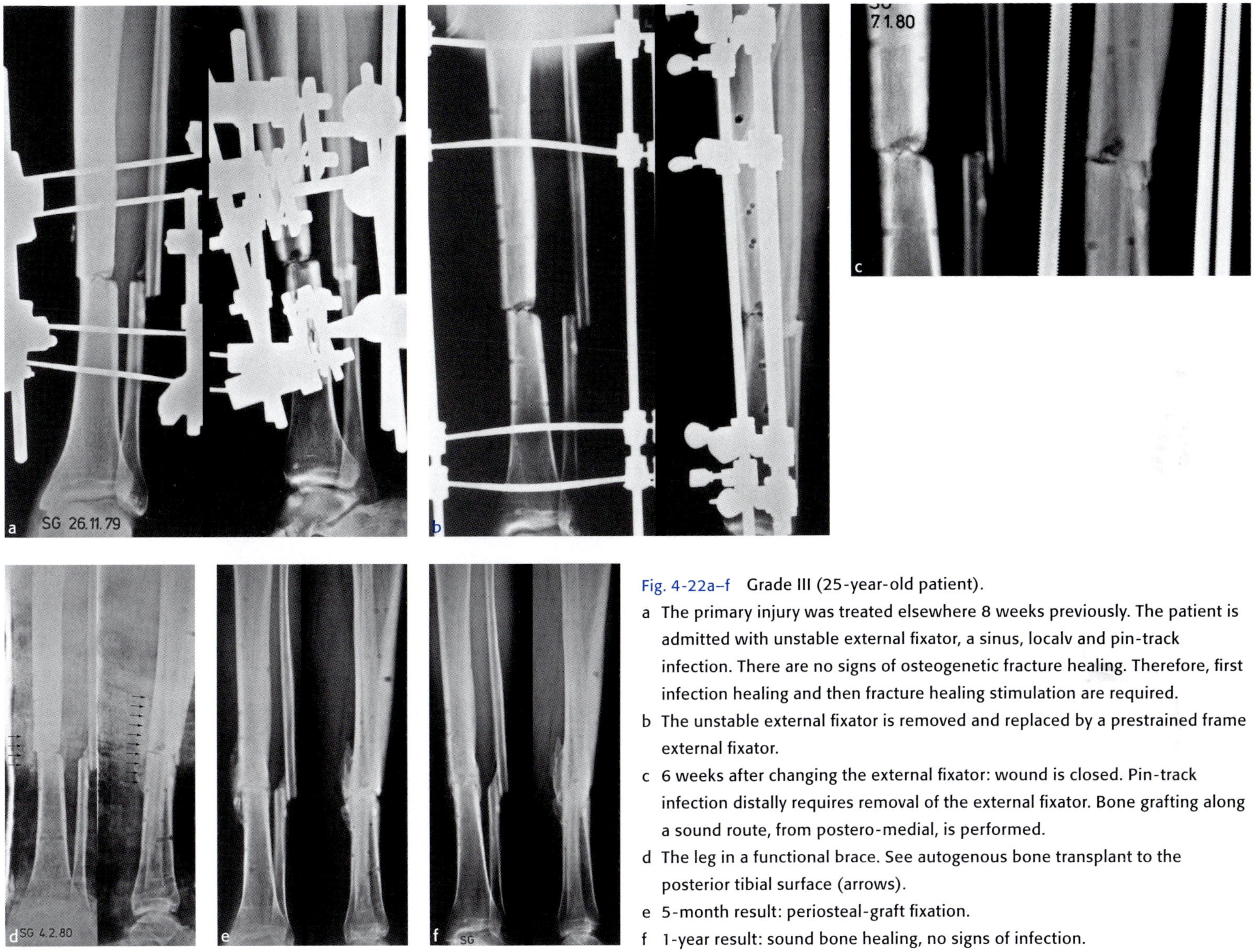

Fig. 4-22a–f Grade III (25-year-old patient).

a The primary injury was treated elsewhere 8 weeks previously. The patient is admitted with unstable external fixator, a sinus, localv and pin-track infection. There are no signs of osteogenetic fracture healing. Therefore, first infection healing and then fracture healing stimulation are required.

b The unstable external fixator is removed and replaced by a prestrained frame external fixator.

c 6 weeks after changing the external fixator: wound is closed. Pin-track infection distally requires removal of the external fixator. Bone grafting along a sound route, from postero-medial, is performed.

d The leg in a functional brace. See autogenous bone transplant to the posterior tibial surface (arrows).

e 5-month result: periosteal-graft fixation.

f 1-year result: sound bone healing, no signs of infection.

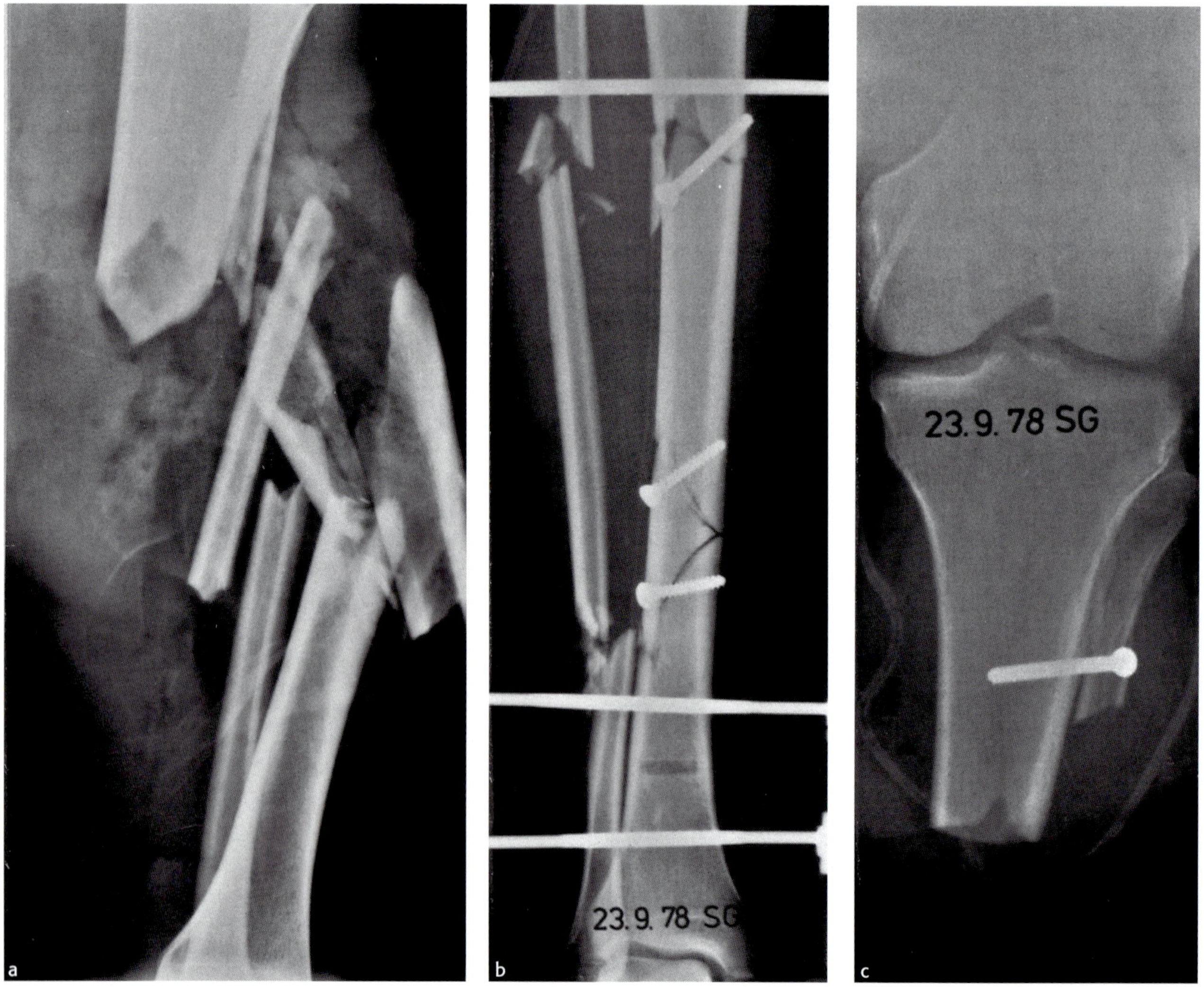

Fig. 4-23a–c Grade IV (32-year-old patient).

a Run over by a truck injury, damage to nerves and vessels.

b Reconstruction attempt and new assessment regarding blood supply to the periphery: the high risk of infection of the crushed tissues rules out vascular and neural reconstruction.

c The consequence: primary amputation.

4.8 Skin lesion management

In open lower leg fractures, the skin is more or less violated and it determines the type of fracture fixation. As a rule, the skin quantity is not decreased, however its quality. The skin lesion shows the following patterns:

Skin lesion patterns

1. Perforation from inside by a fragment without further damage of importance or with degloving, ie, with subcutaneous dead space.
2. Perforation from outside by an object, without or with foreign material displaced into the wound.
3. More or less extended contusion and disruption of the skin with degloving of the adjacent skin from the fascia cruris, often with foreign body pollution.

The skin healing depends on the intracutaneous blood flow and on the blood supply of the skin arriving through the fascia cruris.

Measures that favor skin healing

1. Meticulous debridement, closure of dead space with suction drainage.
2. Prevention of extensive secondary swelling of the limb: by elevation-bedding, multiple skin incisions, compartment fascia splitting.
3. Defattening of degloved skin to full-thickness skin graft, eventual resection of underlaying fascia to allow revascularization from muscle.
4. Localized limited rotation flap.
5. Removal of nectrotic skin, granulation cultivation of the defect area, and secondary coverage with split-mesh skin grafts or Reverdin patch skin grafts.
6. Prolonged care of necrotic skin and waiting for spontaneous, shedding and closure by concentric epidermic migration.
7. Picot-mobilization of the skin around the lower leg.

Comment

Serious skin coverage problems in open lower leg fractures can be managed with local measures. The situation requires patience and compliance. Contemporary vascularized skin transplantation may be superior although I do not have personal experience. 'Conservative' skin problem management may need to be recalled as it was helpful for our patients.

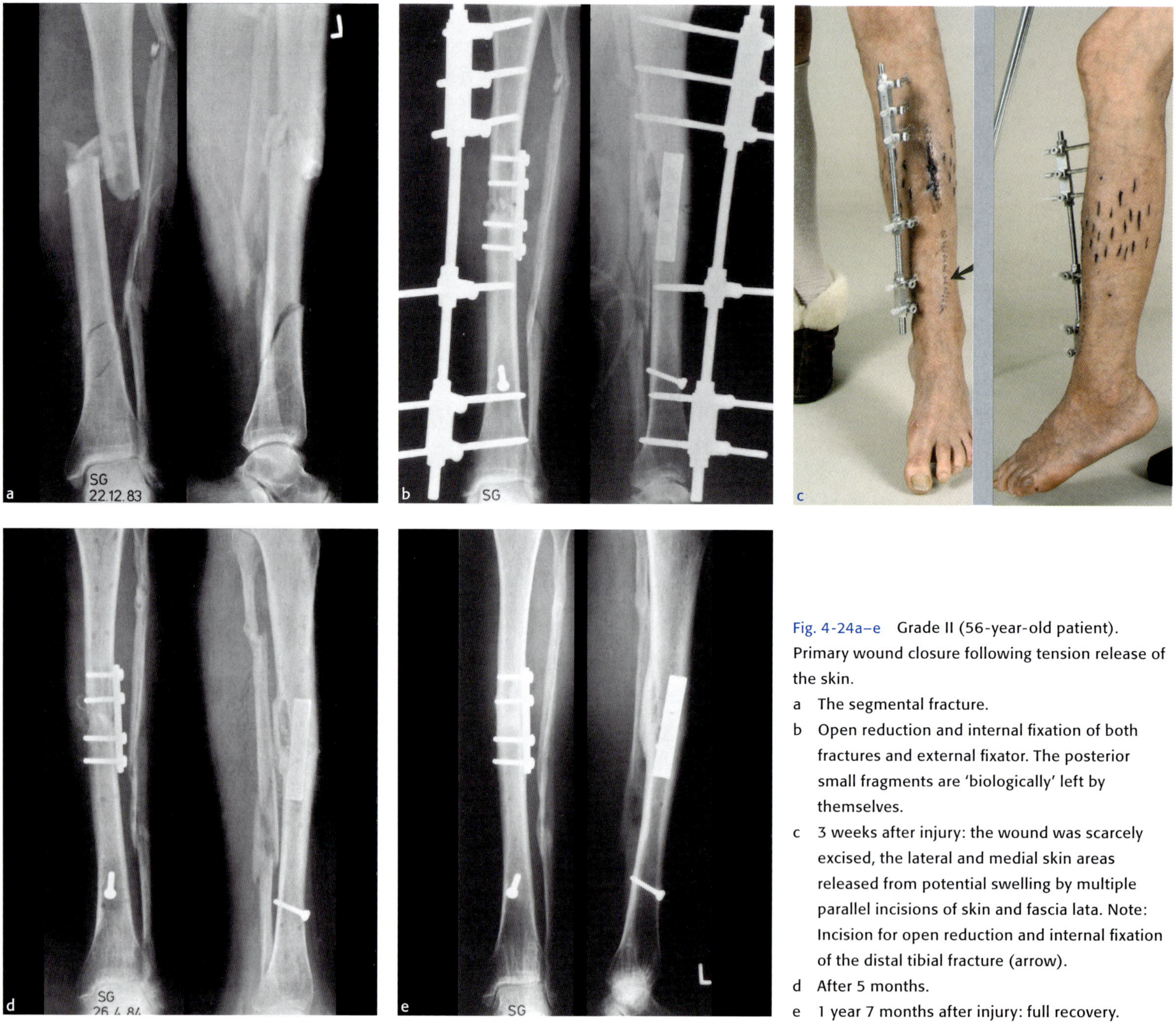

Fig. 4-24a–e Grade II (56-year-old patient). Primary wound closure following tension release of the skin.

a The segmental fracture.

b Open reduction and internal fixation of both fractures and external fixator. The posterior small fragments are 'biologically' left by themselves.

c 3 weeks after injury: the wound was scarcely excised, the lateral and medial skin areas released from potential swelling by multiple parallel incisions of skin and fascia lata. Note: Incision for open reduction and internal fixation of the distal tibial fracture (arrow).

d After 5 months.

e 1 year 7 months after injury: full recovery.

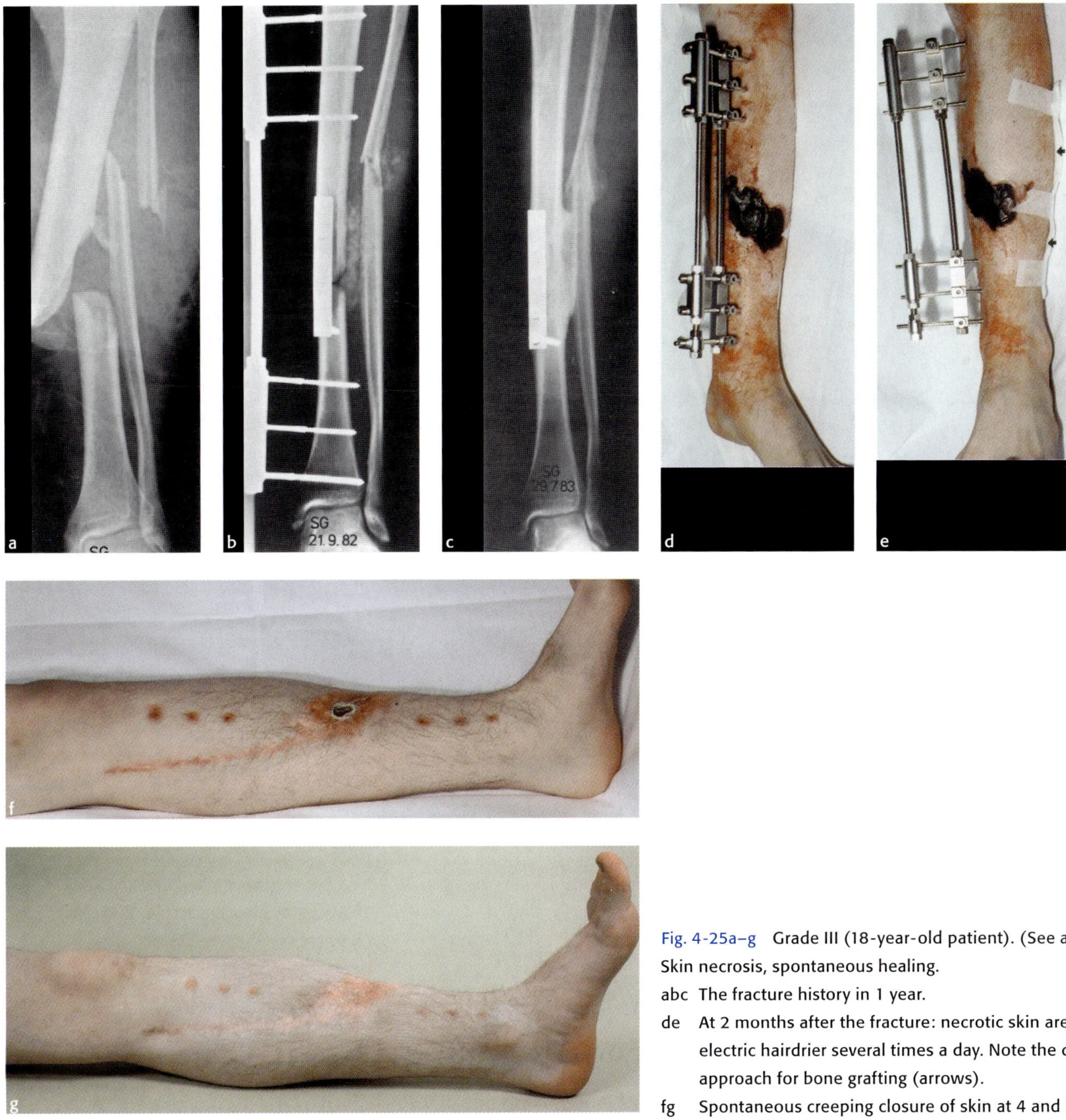

Fig. 4-25a–g Grade III (18-year-old patient). (See also Fig. 4-18.)
Skin necrosis, spontaneous healing.

abc The fracture history in 1 year.

de At 2 months after the fracture: necrotic skin area is kept dry with an electric hairdrier several times a day. Note the dressing from the Harmon approach for bone grafting (arrows).

fg Spontaneous creeping closure of skin at 4 and 5 months.

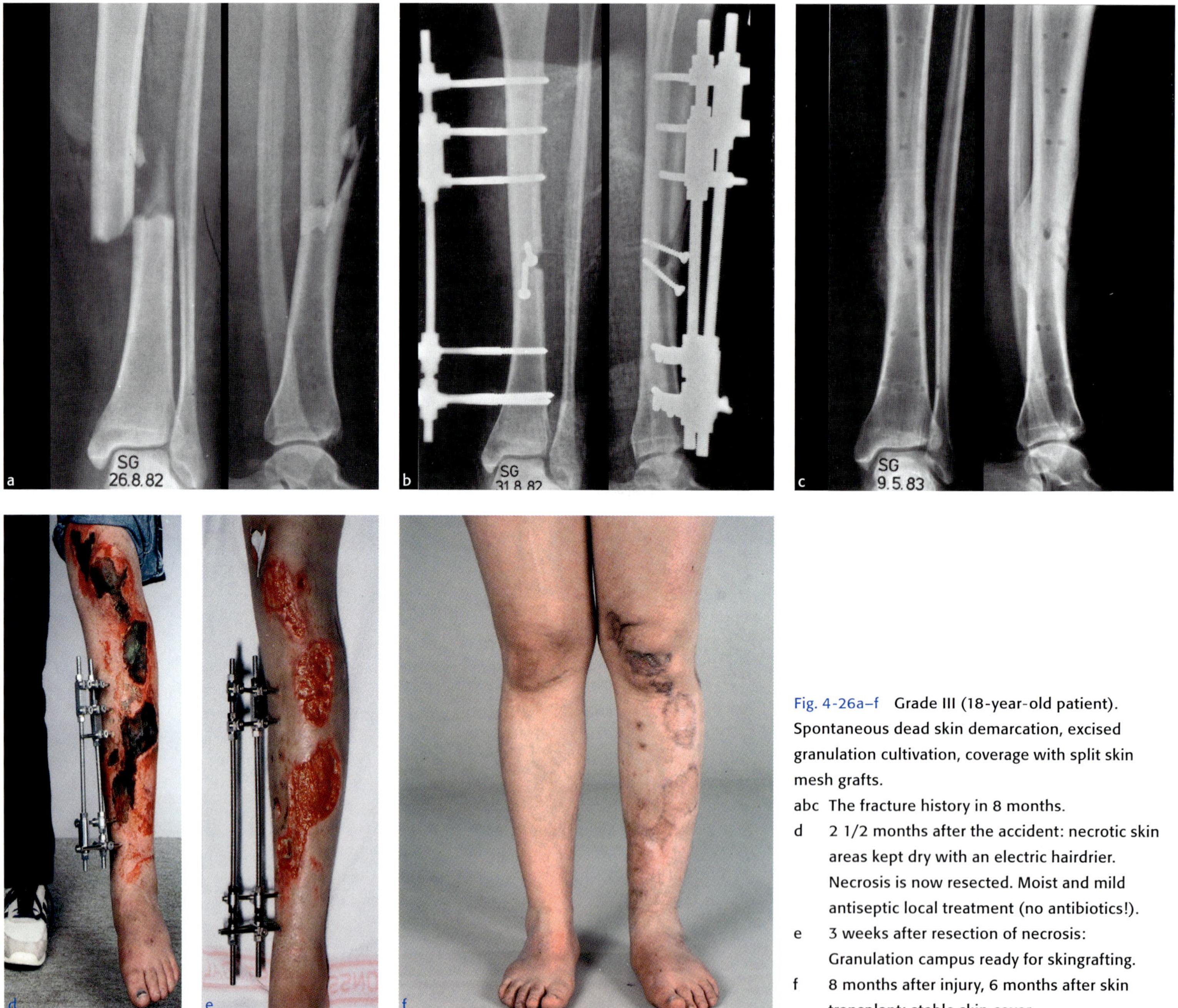

Fig. 4-26a–f Grade III (18-year-old patient). Spontaneous dead skin demarcation, excised granulation cultivation, coverage with split skin mesh grafts.

abc The fracture history in 8 months.

d 2 1/2 months after the accident: necrotic skin areas kept dry with an electric hairdrier. Necrosis is now resected. Moist and mild antiseptic local treatment (no antibiotics!).

e 3 weeks after resection of necrosis: Granulation campus ready for skingrafting.

f 8 months after injury, 6 months after skin transplant: stable skin cover.

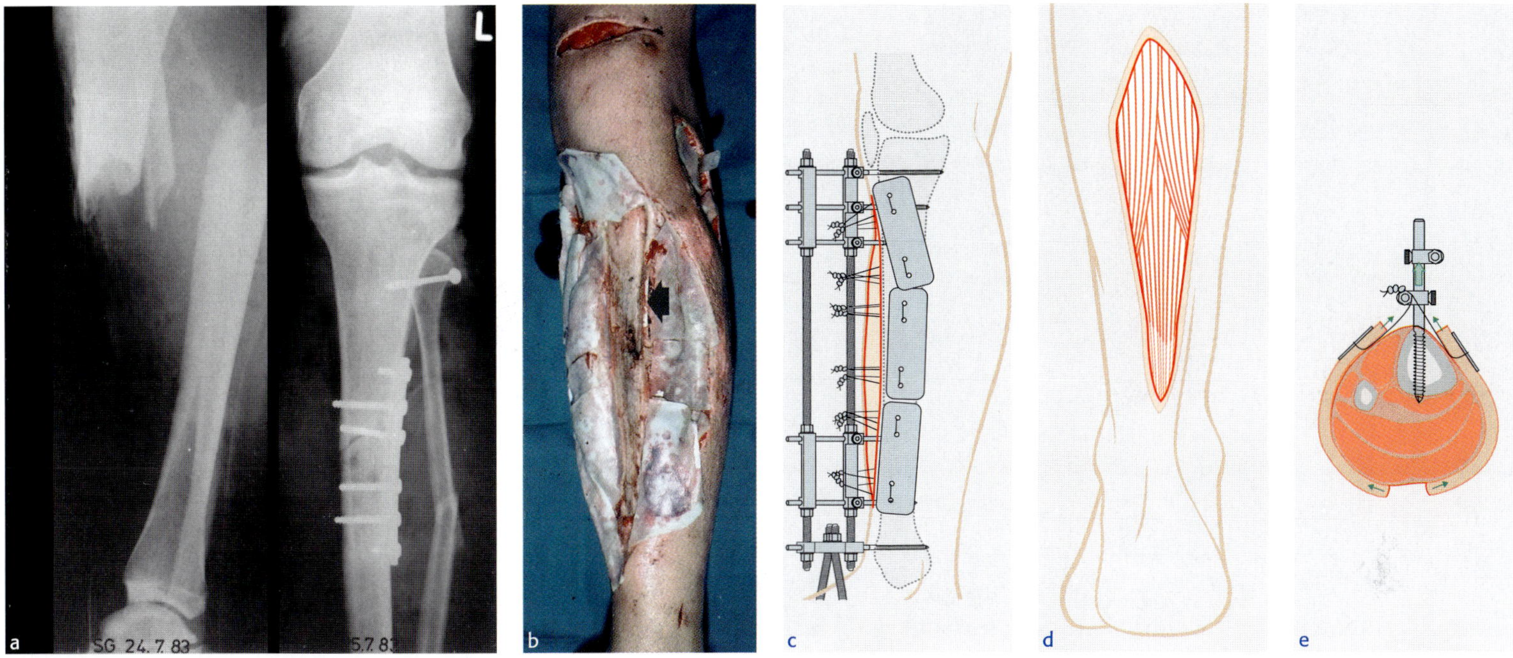

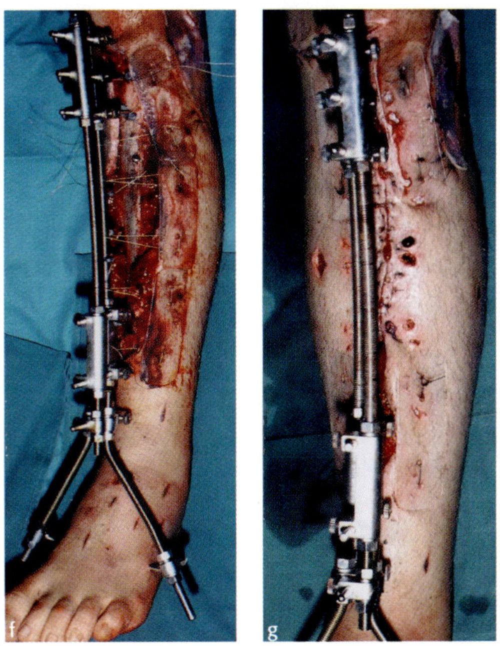

Fig. 4-27a–m Grade III (22-year-old patient). 'Motorized' Picot skin flaps.

a Injury and primary treatment in another hospital.

b Admission at 8 days: tibial and lateral plate (arrow) lie open in the infected wound.

c The plate is removed and replaced by a single lag screw. Protective fixation with an anterior external fixator. The two lips of the wound are tied to one of the two threaded rods with steel wires.

d The skin over the calf is largely split open. Split skin grafting follows when flap transport is made.

e Cross-section view: one rod is used as a spindle onto which the steel cables are wound forward by twisting by daily 2 mm increments.

fg In 2 weeks, the flaps have migrated to achieve contact. The necrotic tibial surface was scarcely shingled away. The gap of the skin on the rear of the calf was closed with split-skin mesh. 3 weeks after start of flap migration.

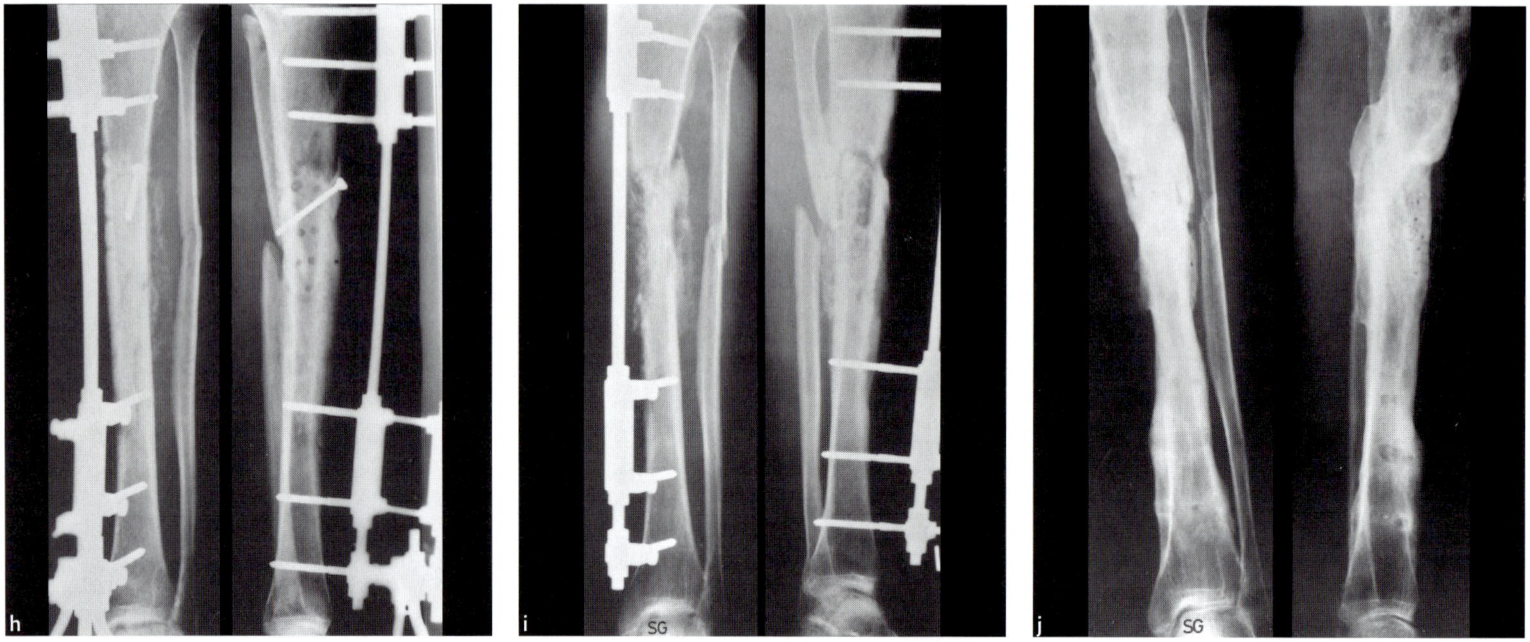

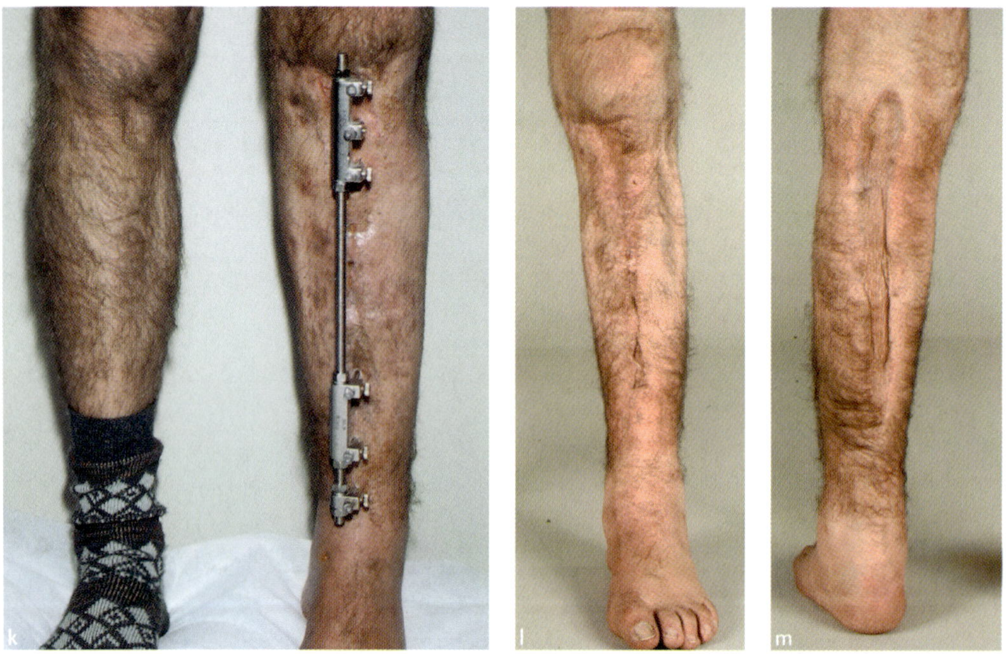

Fig. 4-27a–m cont.

hij The history of fracture healing: 2 months (h), 6 months (i) and 2 years 3 months (j) after the leg saving treatment.

k 6 months after accident.

lm 1 year after accident: no sign of infection. Good function of the leg, but with cosmetic impairment.

5 Summary

The assessment of the biological conditions of bone and soft tissues is of central importance to open fractures of the lower leg. Covering the medial tibial aspect with only skin is unique. With that in mind, subcutaneous plates are unsuitable. Plate fixations may occasionally be helpful when placed on the lateral or on the posterior aspect of the tibia, where the metal is safely covered by well-vascularized muscle tissue.

Nailing is suitable in open tibial midshaft fractures (grade I), where the fracture is transverse or short oblique, with only a small amount of soft tissue damage, ie, when the periosteal blood supply to the main fragments is maintained.

The external fixator is the fixation device of choice for most grade II and III fractures, since it does not disturb either the periosteal or the intramedallury blood circulation.

Restoration of the blood supply to the main fragments and to the fracture site is favored by minimal open reduction and internal fixation. The intramedullary blood circulation across the fracture zone is restored best when the fracture is reduced end to end. However, such anatomical 'waterproof' reduction needs protective stability with the help of the external fixator.

In case of bone fragment loss, autogenous bone grafting after wound healing will prevent delayed and nonunion.

The skin injury can be managed in most cases locally without vascularized skin transplant procedures. Such sophisticated surgery is, for us, indicated in infected nonunions, where the local wound healing capacity is exhausted.

It must be stressed that the demonstrated fixations with external fixators are strictly linked to the original threaded-rod fixator, which has been refined over the years with regard to its elements, but especially to its application technique. These problems can be studied in the monograph "The external fixator" [5], published in English and German in 1985. The chapter "External fixation" in the "AO Principles of Fracture Management" [3] is particularly relevant. One of the advantages is said to be: "External fixation requires less experience and surgical skill than standard open reduction and internal fixation".

However, we cannot confirm such a statement. The refined application of MINIMAX is very difficult as is the general fracture care philosophy that we have practised in St. Gallen since the mid 60s. The techniques described ask for intensive surgical training, considerably more than only workshop experience.

Understanding of fracture biology, clean room facilities with a body-exhaust system and surgical skill vary from place to place. There will never be globalized fracture care.

This chapter on open lower leg fractures is exemplary for the St. Gallen concept of fracture care, a concept that has been maintained by most of those who have ever worked in our institution. Many of them have become teachers in Switzerland, Europe, and overseas—they continue to cultivate our principles: Biological fracture treatment as included in our MINIMAX principles.

6 Bibliography

Blue references indicate links to abstracts of articles online available through Medline (www.nlm.nih.gov).

1. **Müller ME, Allgöwer M, Willenegger H** (1963) *Technik der operativen Frakturenbehandlung.* Berlin Göttingen Heidelberg: Springer-Verlag.
2. **Müller ME, Allgöwer M, Schneider R, et al.** (1991) *Manual of Internal Fixation.* Berlin, Heidelberg, New York: Springer-Verlag.
3. **Rüedi TP, Murphy WM, Colton CL, et al.** (2000) *AO Principles of Fracture Management.* Stuttgart New York: Thieme.
4. **Sarmiento A, Latta LL** (1981) *Closed functional treatment of fractures.* Berlin Heidelberg New York: Springer-Verlag.
5. **Weber BG, Magerl F** (1985) *The external fixator.* Berlin Heidelberg New York Tokyo: Springer-Verlag.
6. **Weber BG** (1984) Reinraumtechnik in der orthopädischen Chirurgie. In: Draenert K, Rütt A, editors. *Erfahrungen mit dem operativen Gelenkersatz.* München: Art and Science: 117–123.
7. **Weber BG** (2000) MINIMAX-Prinzip für Osteosynthesen beim Erwachsenen. In: Dubs L, editor. *Orthopädie an der Schwelle.* Bern Göttingen Toronto Seattle: Huber: 19–133.
8. **Brunner ChF, Weber BG** (1982) *Special Techniques in Internal Fixation.* Berlin Heidelberg New York: Springer-Verlag.
9. **Weber BG, Brunner Ch, Freuler F** (1980) *Treatment of Fractures in Children and Adolescents.* Berlin Heidelberg New York: Springer-Verlag.
10. **Weber BG** (1976) *Pseudarthrosis.* Bern Stuttgart Wien: Huber.

5 Trauma of the ankle joint and of its neighborhood

1 Introduction

The AO classification as well as open reduction and internal fixation [1–3] of the common ankle joint fractures [4–6] have enjoyed worldwide acceptance since the sixties. Some finer points are reported here again.

The following suggestions may be used by those who are familiar with standard ankle joint repair surgery:

Finer points

Open reduction and internal fixation (ORIF):

- Ankle joint fracture type B
- The posterior lip fragment of the tibia
- Medial malleolus avulsion fragment

Consequences

- The short fibula
- The long fibula
- The fibulotibial synostosis
- Secondary and primary ankle joint fusion
- Secondary clubfoot following Salter III/IV fracture of the medial malleolus (excision of epiphyseal fusion)

Achilles tendon

- Acute rupture and repair
- Achilles tendon defect reconstruction
- S. T. Hansen muscle transfer
- Foot flexor stretching with an external fixator

Acute and recurrent ankle sprain

- Diagnosis of acute or chronic ankle sprain
- Treatment of acute rupture of fibular collateral ligaments
- Treatment of recurrent ankle sprain

2 Open reduction and internal fixation (ORIF)

2.1 Type B fibular fracture

The original AO plate fixation method [1–3] with the plate on the lateral surface of the fibula has four inconveniences:

- The plate lies under the vulnerable skin.
- The most distal screws may penetrate into the joint.
- Poor screw hold in the relative soft lateral malleolus leads to screw pull back.
- Secondary displacement as result of poor fixation.

To avoid these problems, the following open reduction and internal fixation has been in use for 30 years for type B fibular fractures (Fig. 5-1a–d).

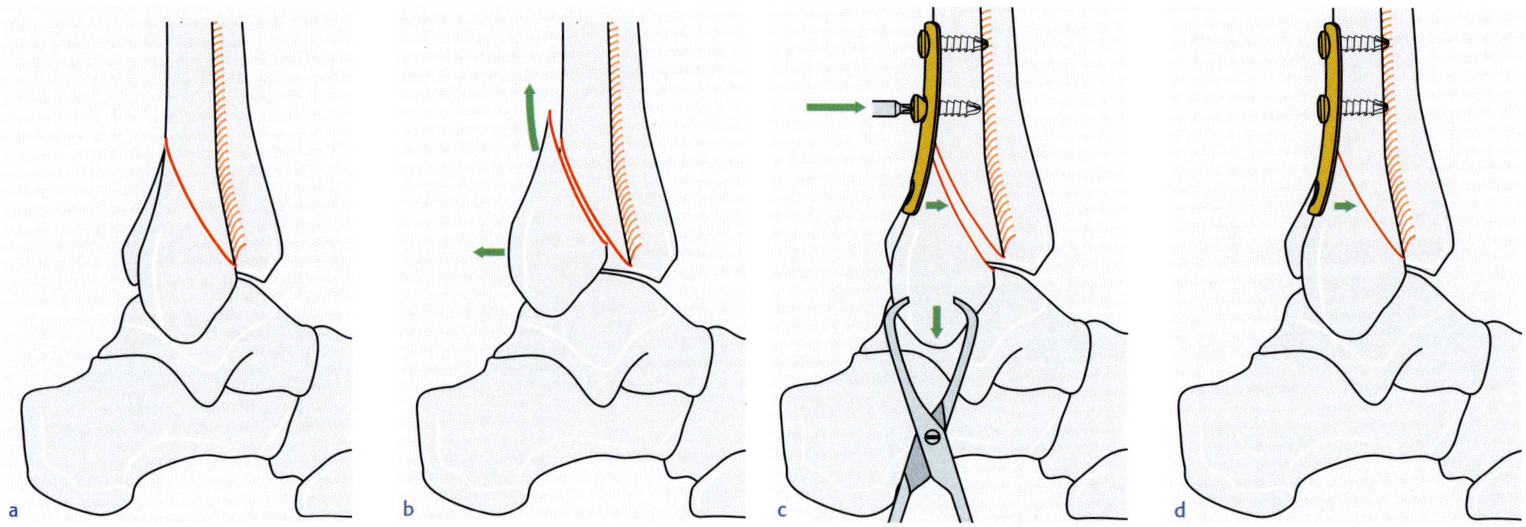

Fig. 5-1a–d Antigliding plate on the posterior or posterolateral aspect of the distal fibula [7–9].
The fibula is exposed from the lateral side, the peroneal tendons are elevated from the fibula. Their anchorage distally is left intact to prevent dislocation of the two tendons.

a Type B fracture immediately before the occurrence (future fracture outlined).
b The malleolus displaces backwards and upwards and rotates externally. The distal peroneal tendons are already separated from the proximal fibula fragment by the trauma.
c A one-third tubular plate with 3–5 holes is selected and not contoured. The most distal screwhole in the proximal fragment is drilled first and the plate is fastened halfway. The uncontoured plate is 'overbent', and when tightening the screw, the plate automatically pushes the distal fragment back to its original place. The fragment is reduced, the distal fragment may be adjusted to 'waterproof' position with the help of a towel clamp.
d The rest of the screws are inserted. An additional compression screw may be set across the fracture plane to add stability (arrow). The antigliding plate acts opposite to the deformity according to the MINIMAX principle. The plate does not disturb the skin over the lateral malleolus, or the gliding of the peroneal tendons.

2.2 Posterior lip fragment of the tibia in the absence of a fracture of the medial malleolus

With open reduction and internal fixation of a fractured fibula type B or C, a posterior lip fragment is at least partially reduced. A small shell-like fragment is left by itself. A fragment of 1/4 or larger size of the tibial surface, however, requires 'waterproof' reduction and fixation [6].

When the medial malleolus is broken, waterproof reduction is easily performed by widening its fracture gap. Inspection of the tibial joint surface allows reduction under sight control through the fracture gap. Preliminary fixation with a K-wire is followed by a lag screw, inserted from the front of the distal tibia. After which the broken medial malleolus is screwed back to its place [6]. This procedure cannot be performed when the medial malleolus is unbroken, not even when a ruptured deltoid ligament is present instead of a fracture. A second para-achillar incision approach would be needed. The following optimal approach is preferred (Fig. 5-2a–c).

The surgical sequence is inverted here compared to the standard repair of the ankle joint, which starts with the fractured fibula. But not here! A similar approach can be used in type C fibular fractures: The distal fragment is displaced by external rotation, offering visual control of the lip fragment in the fibular notch.

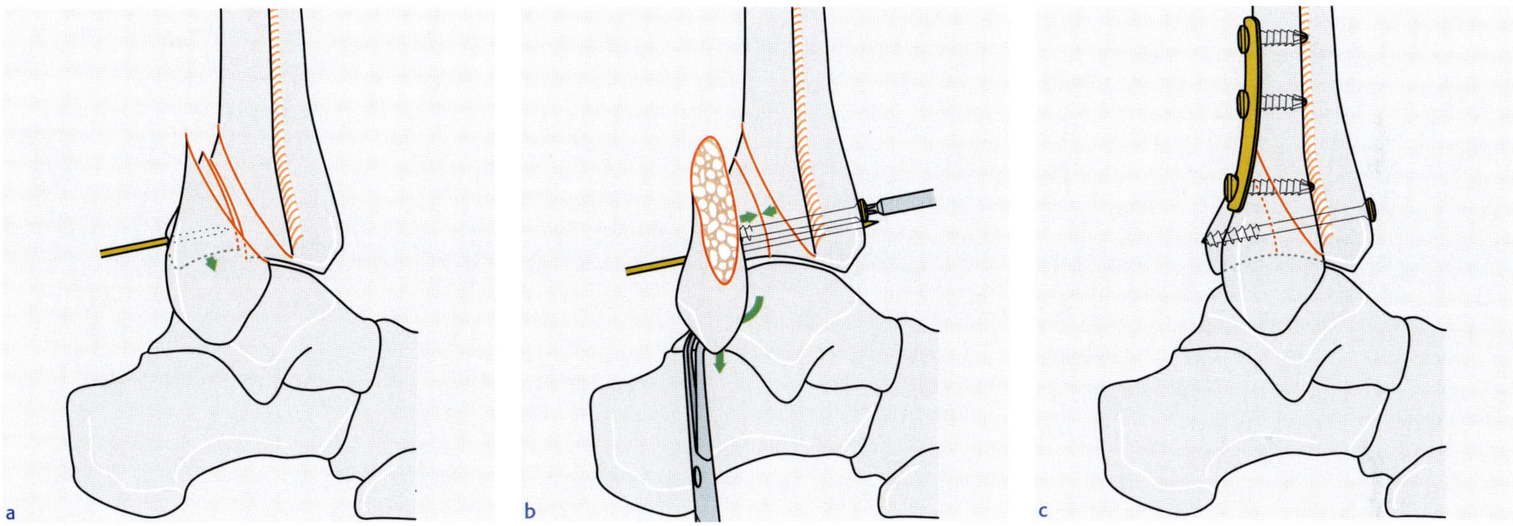

Fig. 5-2a–c Reduction of the posterior lip fragment of the tibia through the type B fibular fracture [8].

a The broken malleolus is overdisplaced with a small spreader. The lip fracture becomes visible in the fibular notch. With a K-wire, inserted from behind the fibula, the lip fragment is manipulated into place and fixed.

b With a lag screw, inserted from the front of the distal tibia, the lip fragment is rigidly fixed.

c Only now does the fibula undergo open reduction and internal fixation.

2.3 Medial malleolus avulsion fragment

The small avulsion fragment of the medial malleolus, when pinned or screwed, risks being redisplaced because the fixation device cannot be inserted at a right angle to the fracture plane. Instead of compression/ fixation, shear ends up with lateral redisplacement (Fig. 5-3a–f).

The sequence of ordinary open reduction and internal fixation is also irregular here: only after medial malleolus fixation is the fibula fracture reduced and fixed.

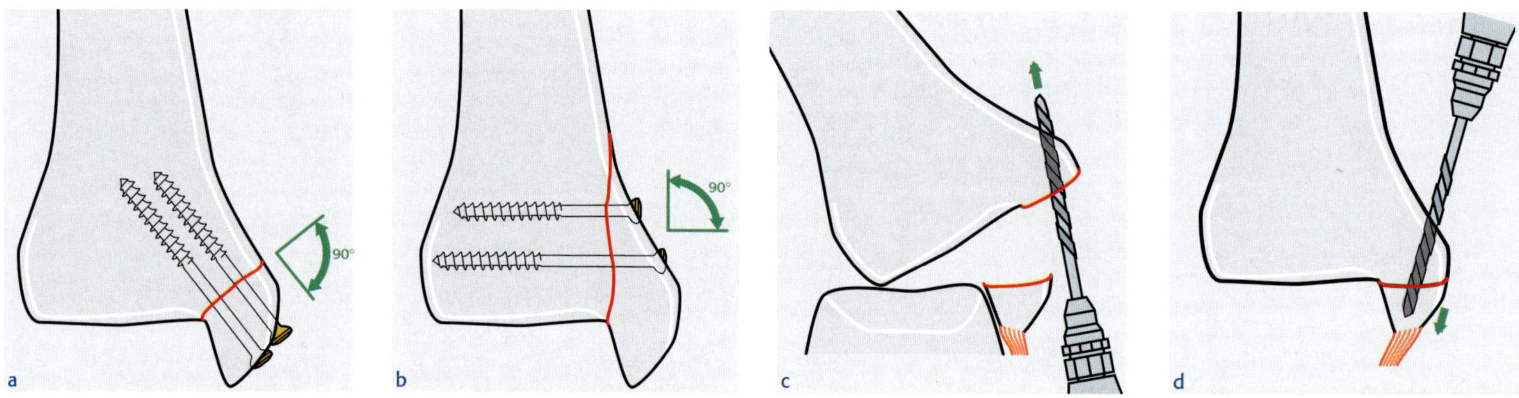

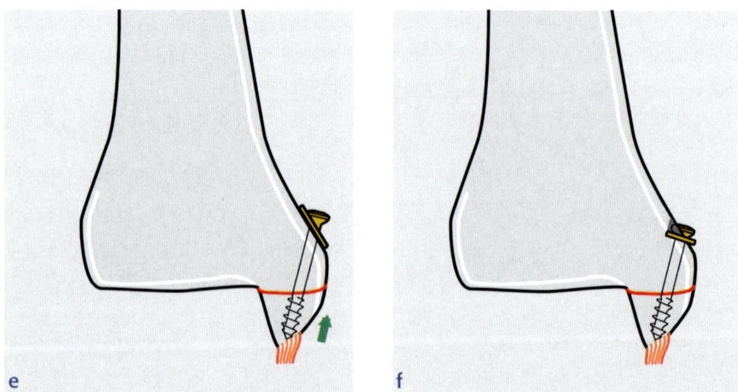

Fig. 5-3a–f Retrograde lag screw fixation of the avulsed medial malleolus [8].

ab Typical fractures of the medial malleolus to be treated with anterograde screw fixation, perpendicular to the fracture plane.

c Retrograde fixation technique.
First step: avulsed small fragment, unsuitable for anterograde fixation, foot is subluxated laterally and a 3.5 mm gliding hole is drilled upwards.

d Second step: reduction of the tip fragment with a towel clamp. Downward drilling of a threaded hole, tabbing, insertion of a 3.5 mm lag screw.

ef Washer is not necessary, flat on the cortex or lodged in a small chisel slot.

Clinical examples are described in Fig. 5-4–5-8:

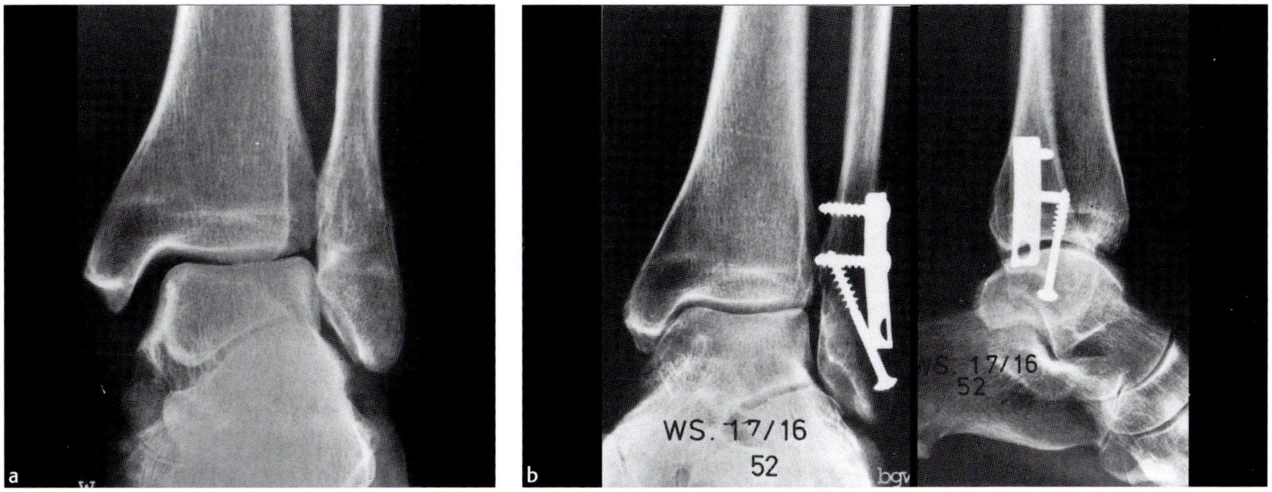

Fig. 5-4a–b

a Type B fibular fracture with rupture of the deltoid ligament.

b 52 weeks later, after open reduction and internal fixation as well as ligament suture.

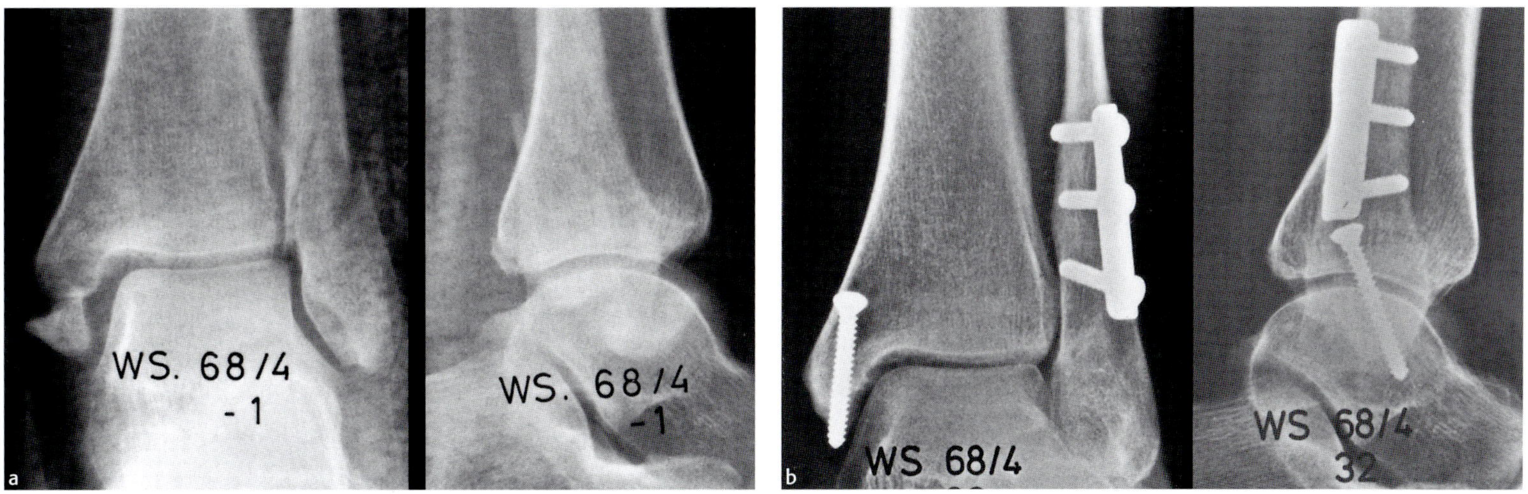

Fig. 5-5a–b

a Avulsion fracture of the tip of the medial malleolus.

b 32 weeks after open reduction and internal fixation.

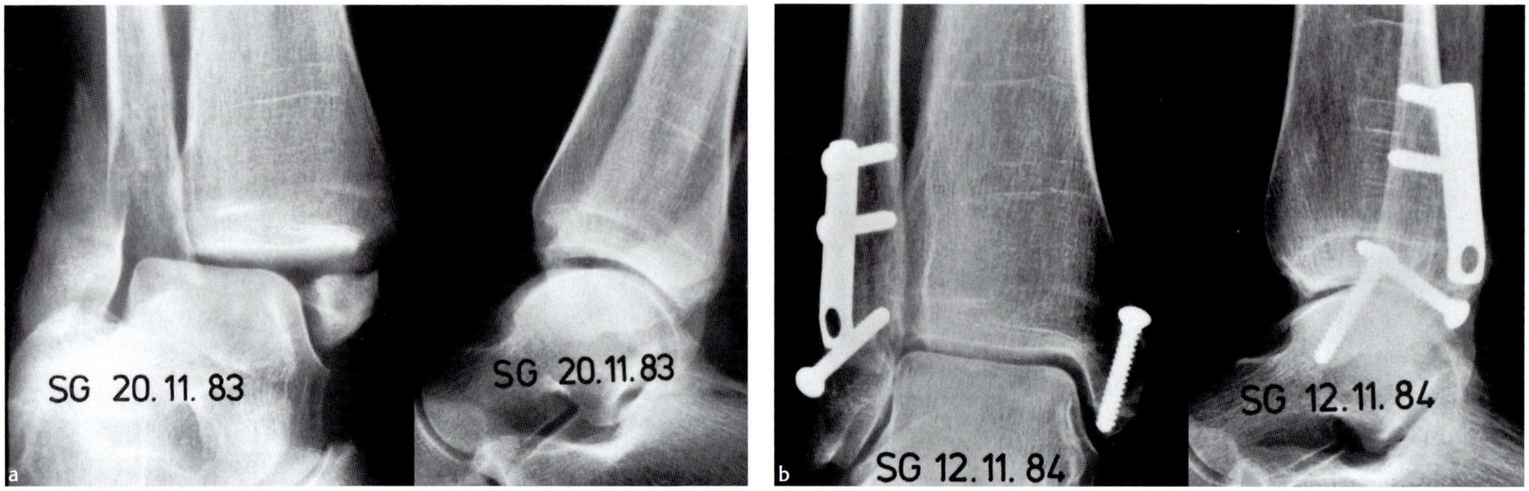

Fig. 5-6a–b

a Avulsion fracture of tip of medial malleolus.

b 1 year after open reduction and internal fixation.

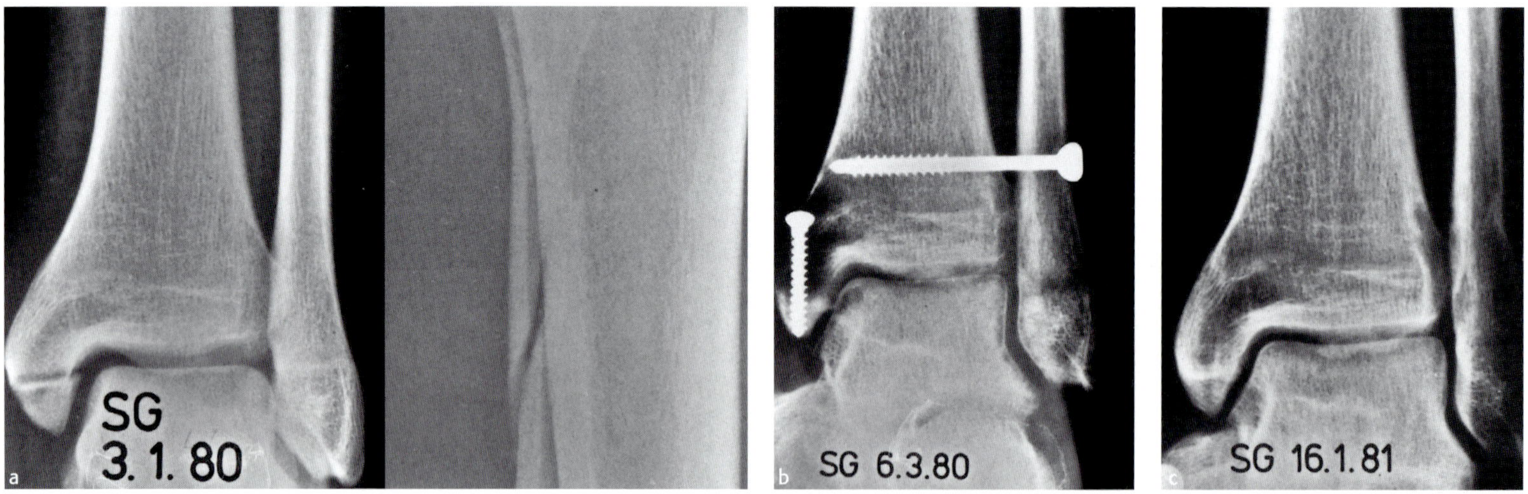

Fig. 5-7a–c

a Type C fibular fracture plus avulsion fracture of the tip of the medial malleolus.

b 3 months after open reduction and internal fixation and positioning screw for the syndesmosis and interosseous membrane.

c 1 year after open reduction and internal fixation, 10 months after screw removal.

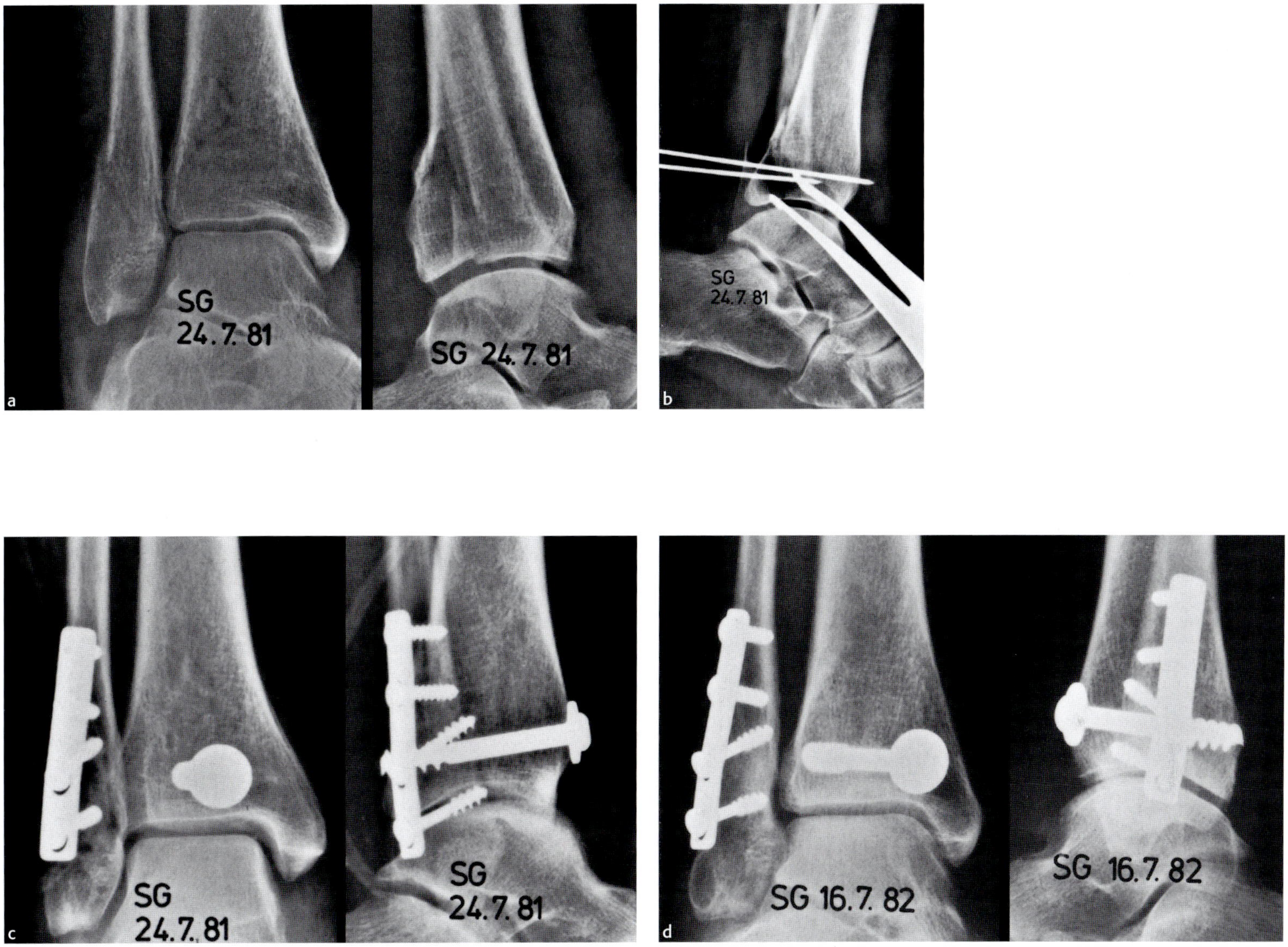

Fig. 5-8a–d

a Type B fracture of fibula, big posterior lip fracture of tibia, no lesion medially.

b Pinning reduction 'through' the fibular fracture.

c Immediately after open reduction and internal fixation.

d 1 year after open reduction and internal fixation.

3 Consequences

3.1 The short fibula

Type B and C fractures risk healing with shortening, and with lateral and external-rotation displacement of the distal fibula [6] (Fig. 5-9a–b).

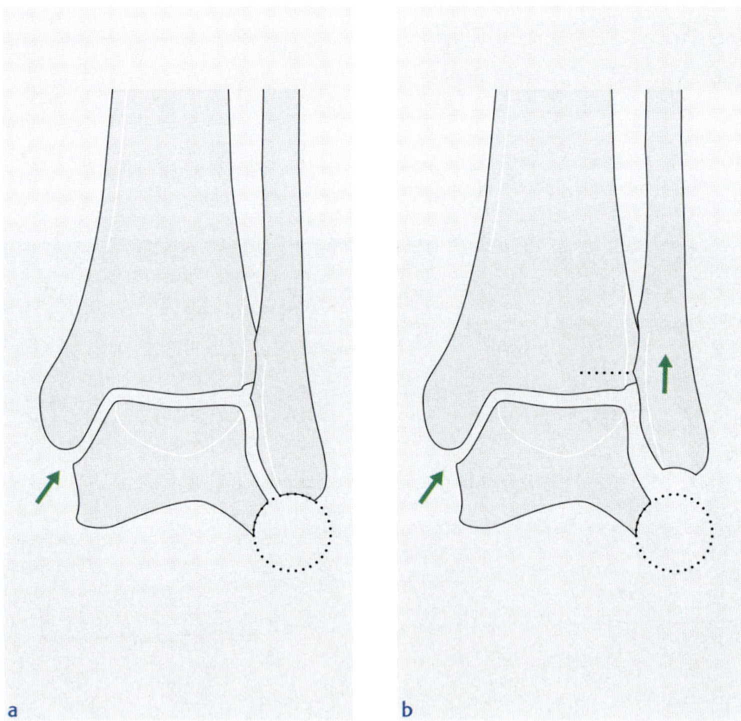

Fig. 5-9a–b The normal and the short fibula on the x-ray [6, 10].

a Normal x-ray of ankle joint: Regular joint space, unbroken subchondral line, fitting of a virtual ball against fibula and talus.

b X-ray of short fibula: Break in the subchondral line, misfit of the virtual ball, widening of the joint space medially (arrows).

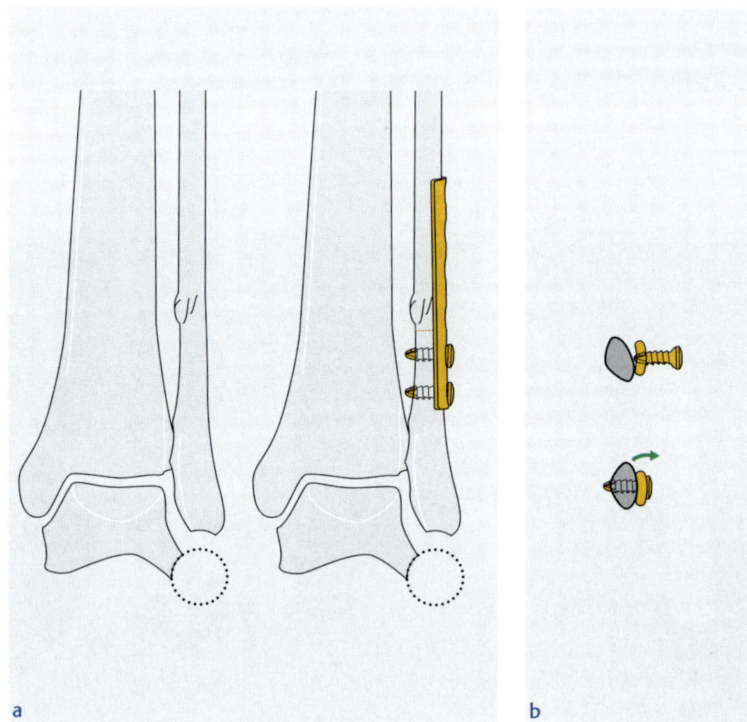

Fig. 5-10a–e Technique of fibular lengthening [6, 10, 11]—malposition of the short fibula is corrected as follows.

a Plate fixed to the distal fragment.

b Anticipation of medial rotation to be performed after osteotomy.

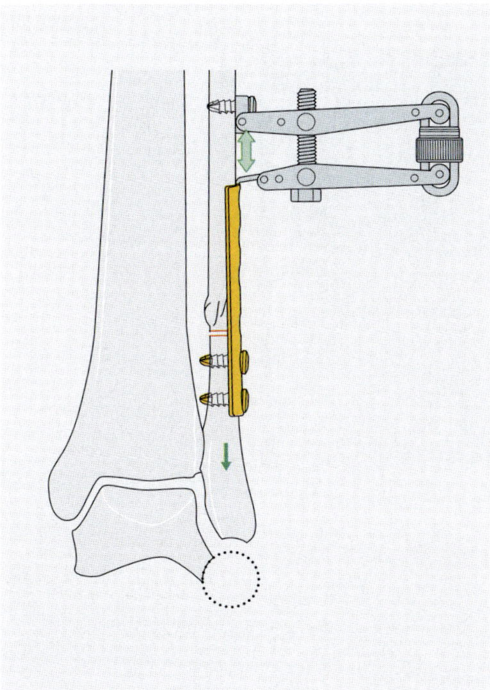

c

c Lengthening with a distraction device.

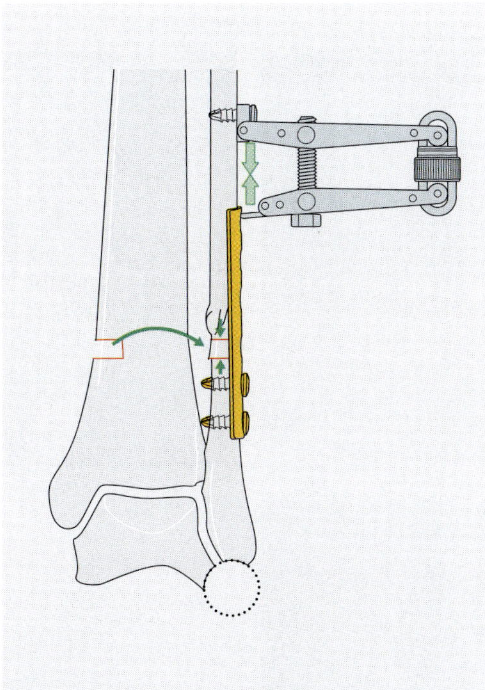

d

d Locking of a corticocancellous bone graft with the converted device for compression. The graft is harvested from the tibia, proximal to the medial malleolous.

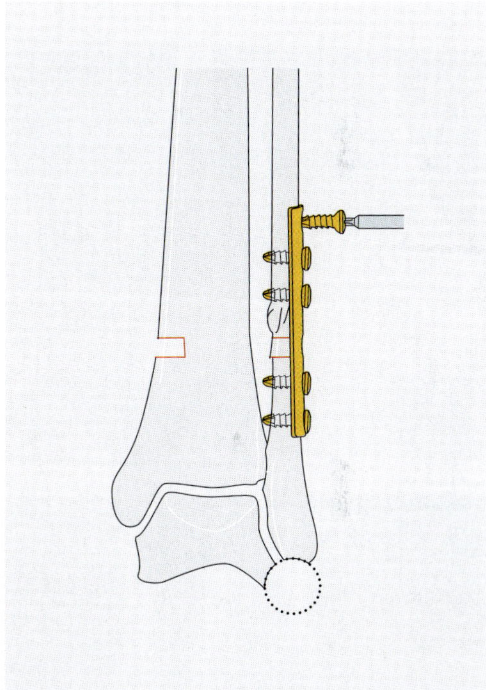

e

e Restoration of the joint with fibular lengthening.

Clinical examples described in Fig. 5-11–5-13:

If syndesmotic ligament repair is not performed, the ankle fork will remain stable since scar tissue develops during the 10-week scotch-cast bracing and continuous active function (CAF), ie, with weightbearing.

The widened joint space medially and the syndesmotic notch always need to be assessed for interposed scar tissue. If present, it must be removed before reconstruction.

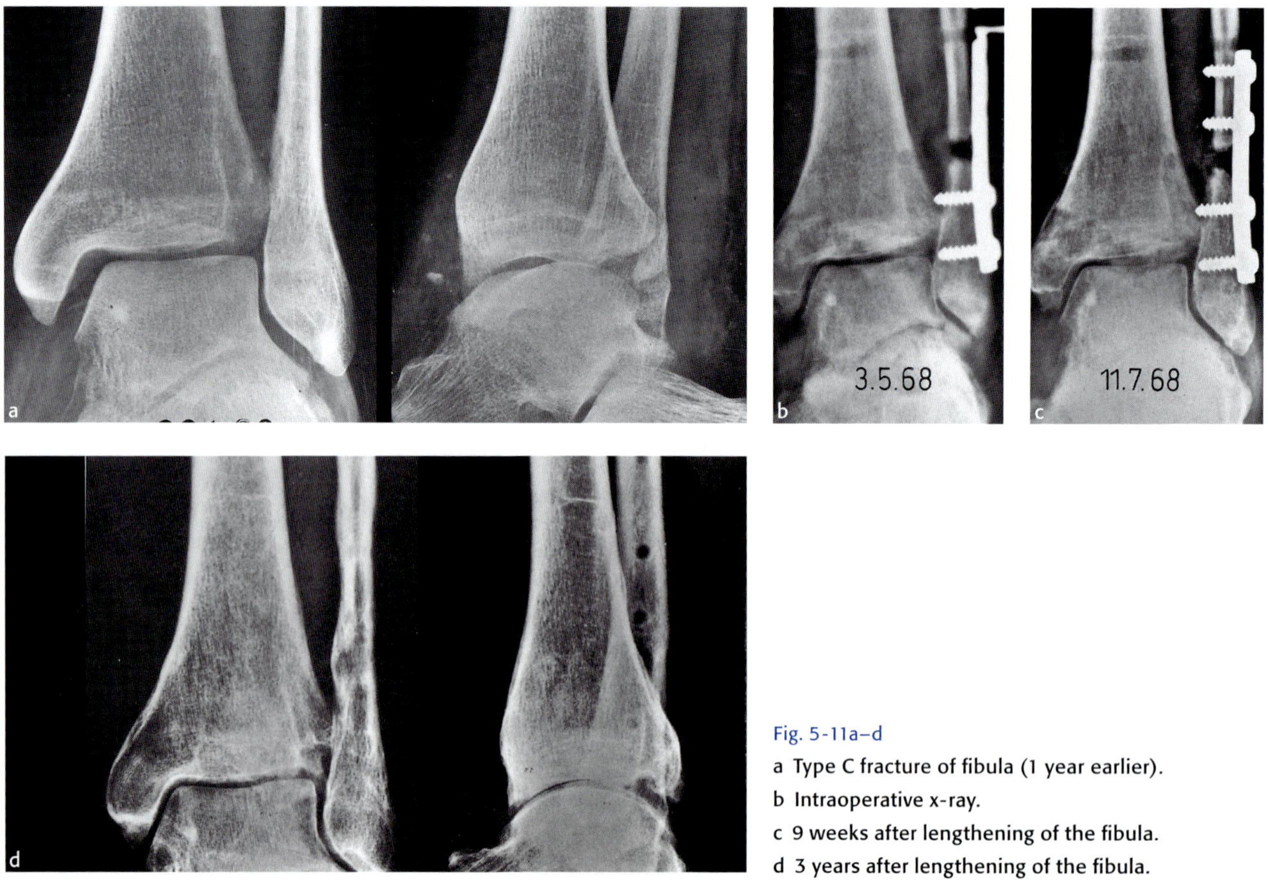

Fig. 5-11a–d

a Type C fracture of fibula (1 year earlier).

b Intraoperative x-ray.

c 9 weeks after lengthening of the fibula.

d 3 years after lengthening of the fibula.

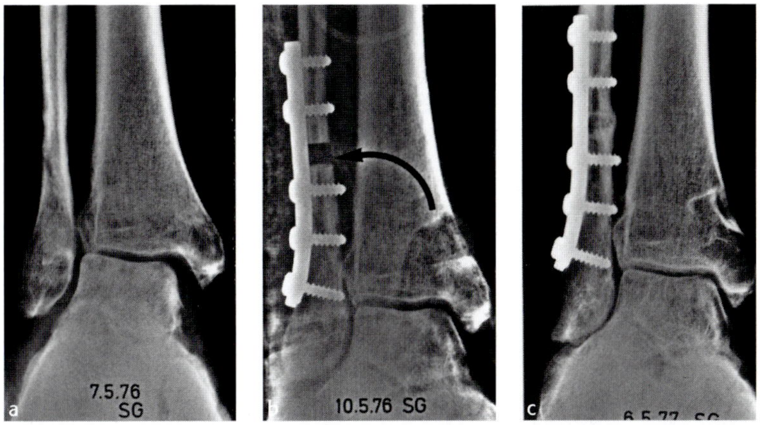

Fig. 5-12a–c

a 1 1/2 year after low type C fracture.

b Postoperative view after lengthening of fibula (arrow).

c 1 year after reconstruction.

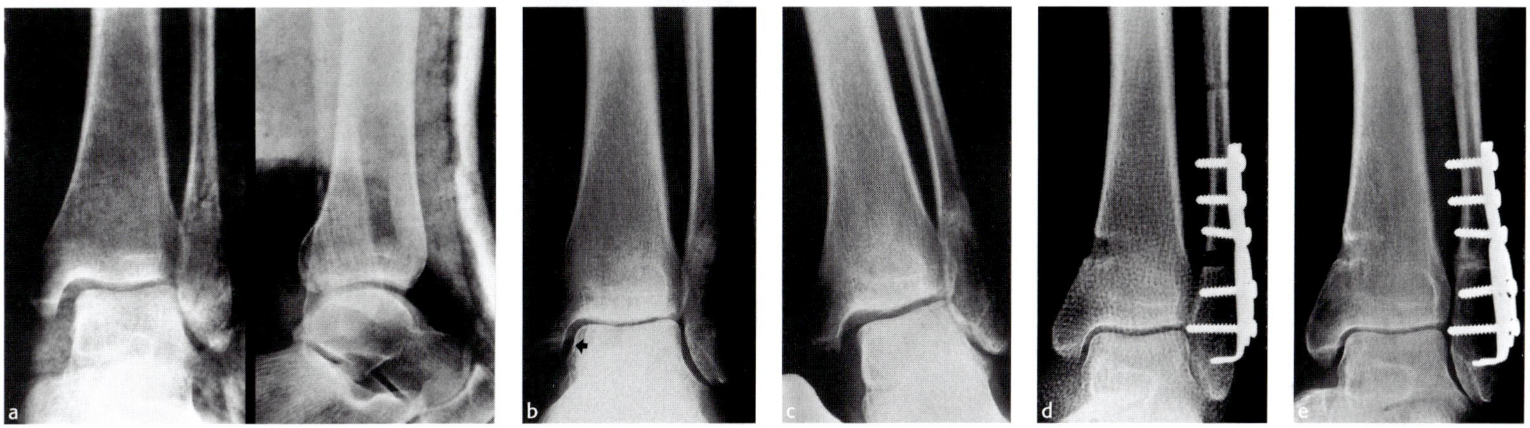

Fig. 5-13a–e

a The fresh type B fracture in a brace.

b 3 months later: widened joint space medially (arrow).

c Stressed x-ray in pronation: shortening of the fibula is evident.

d 2 months after lengthening of the fibula.

e 8 months after reconstruction. Note: Two one-third tubular plates superimposed and 10° twisted were used to fit the thin fibula.

3.2 The overlong fibula

In lower leg fractures where the fibula stays unbroken, the tibial fracture may heal with shortening, resulting in the fibula being relatively too long. The joint is incongruent, dorsiflection of the foot is hindered, the joint is at risk of osteoarthritis. A distal tibial fracture may also heal in slight varus with minimal or no fibula shortening, causing malalignment of the ankle joint (see chapter Lower leg fractures with and without involvement of the ankle joint and the consequences for fracture treatment).

The three options to restore ankle joint anatomy are: fibula shortening, tibia lengthening, or supramalleolar osteotomy (Fig. 5-14a–c).

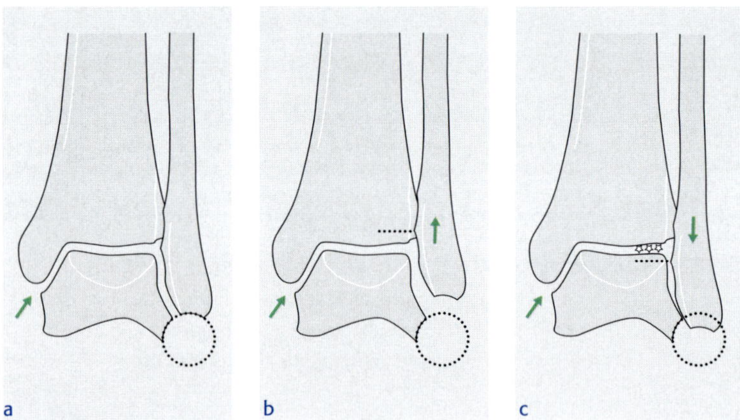

Fig. 5-14a–c

The normal, the short, and the overlong fibula.

a Normal.

b Short fibula.

c Overlong fibula. The joint space may be widened (starlets).

Fibular shortening

Fibula shortening is performed when the pilon of the tibia is spared in the original injury, ie, when a tibial shaft fracture has healed with shortening. The technique is identical to fibula lengthening, but with resection of a slice of the fibula shaft (Fig. 5-15a–c).

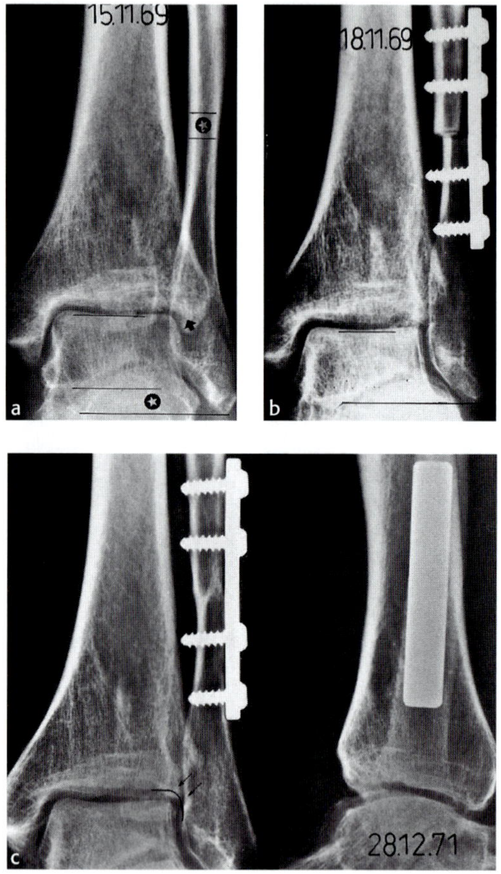

Fig. 5-15a–c

a The overlong fibula. Preoperative planning: size of shortening (starlets) and a reactive spur to be removed (arrow).

b Revision clearing of the fibular notch. Resection of the spur. Shortening osteotomy and compression plating of the fibula.

c 2 years after reconstruction: normal radiology of joint space and of subchondral joint line (arrows).

Tibial lengthening [6]

Where the original fracture of the tibia had run through the pilon with both shortening and malposition resulting from crush impaction, lengthening and realignment of the distal tibia are indicated (Fig. 5-16a–c).

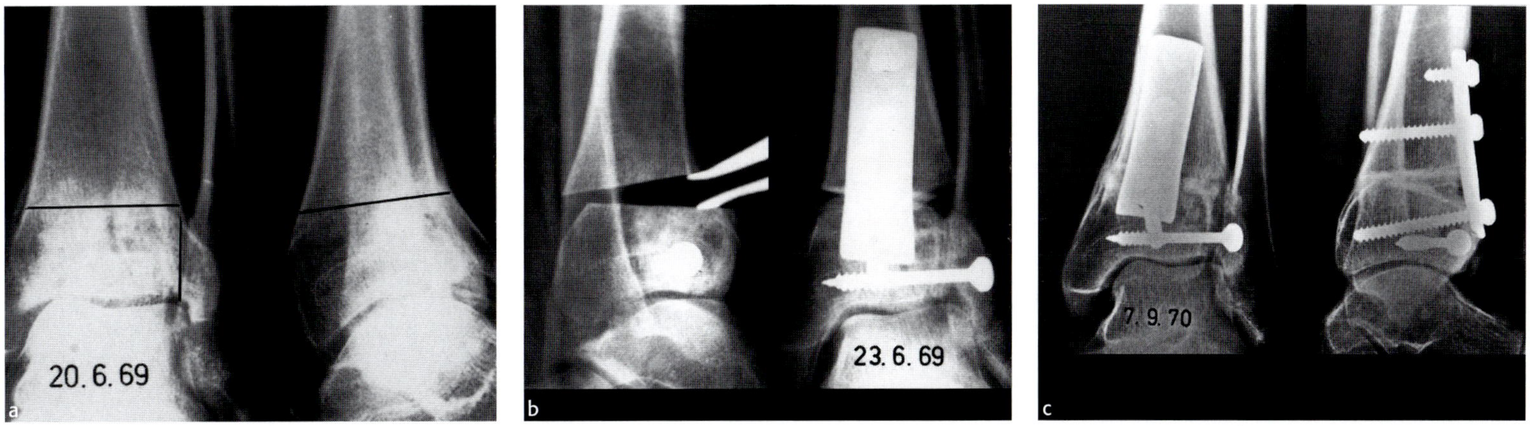

Fig. 5-16a–c

a The overlong fibula is connected by the syndesmotic ligaments to the fractured tibial tubercules. The tubercules stayed at the right level, while the pilon was pushed proximally. Additional angulation-recurvatum is present. Preoperative planning: lines of osteotomies, ie, sagittal osteotomy of the two tibial tubercules, horizontal osteotomy of the tibia.

b Perioperative control with spreader in situ. The osteomized tibial tubercules are already screwed to the right place. Lengthening and correction of angulation is performed, the defect is filled with an autogenous pelvic-wedged bone graft, an anterior contoured semitubular plate provides rigid fixation.

c 15 months later. Anatomy is restored.

Supramalleolar valgus osteotomy [6, 12]

When a supramalleolar tibial fracture has healed with slight varus deformity, a supramalleolar closed wedge osteotomy realigns the ankle joint (Fig. 5-17a–e).

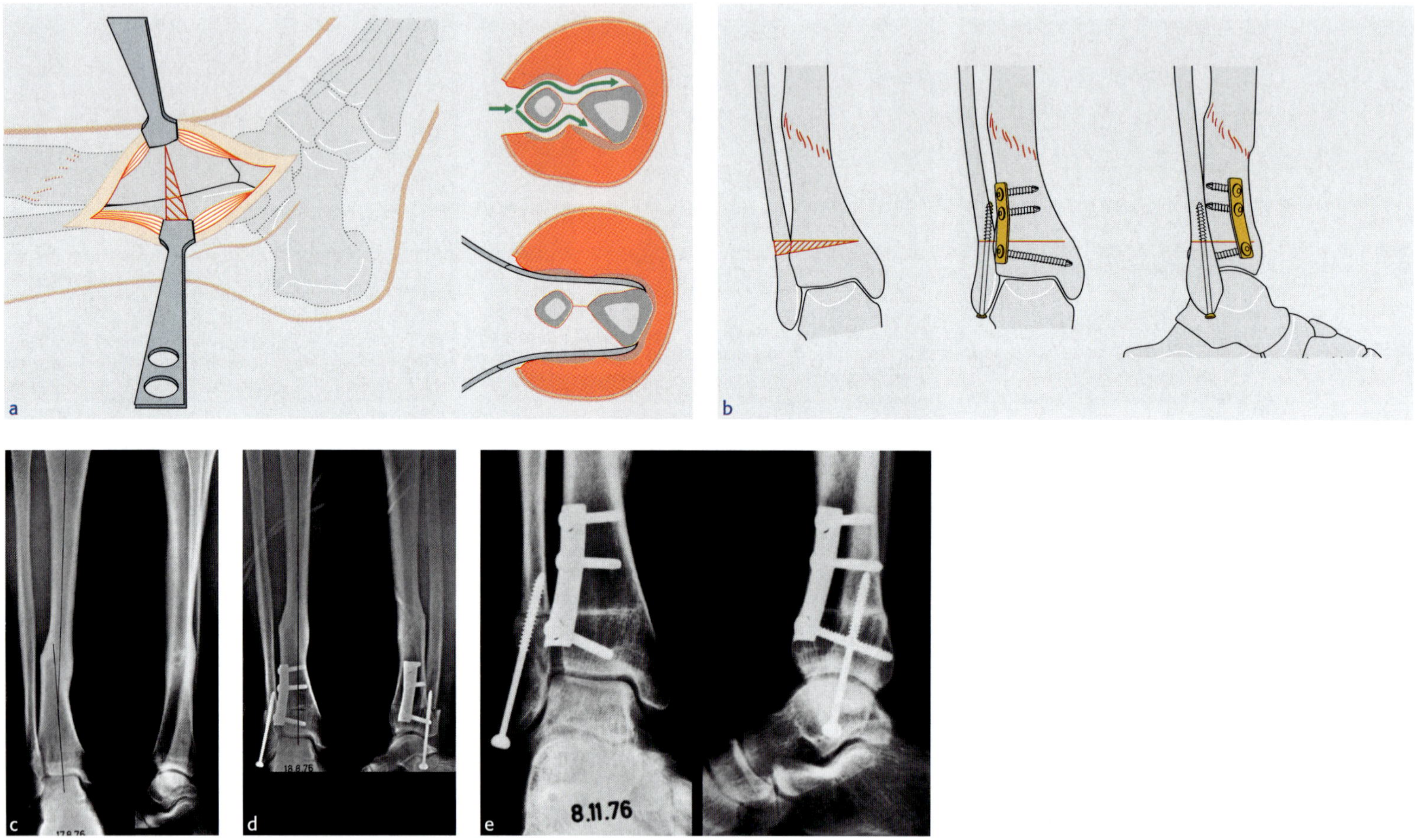

Fig. 5-17a–e

a Subperiosteal exposure of fibula and tibia from a lateral approach.

b The pseudo one-bone wedge resection with oscillating saw and internal fixation.

c Varus deformity following isolated tibia fracture.

d Realignment after surgery.

e 3 months after surgery: bone healing.

3.3 The fibulotibial synostosis

An acquired synostosis of the fibula to the tibia is painful: stiffness of the ankle fork, limited dorsiflection of the foot, damage to the joint cartilage resulting in osteoarthritis. The ankle fork needs rotational freedom of the fibula to accommodate the astragalus, which moderates the width of the mortise [6] (Fig. 5-18–20a–c).

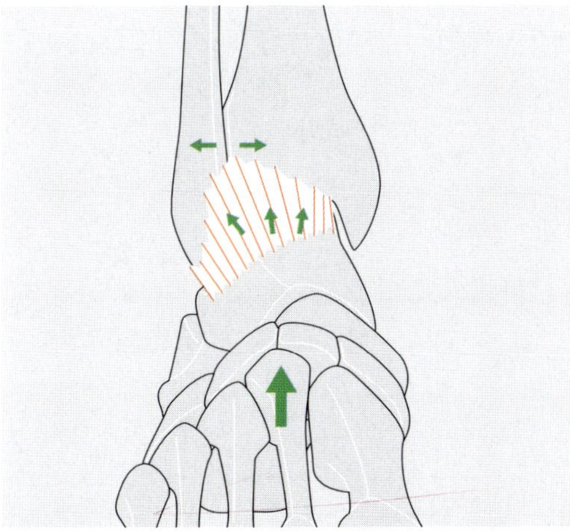

Fig. 5-18 Biomechanics of the ankle joint during stance phase [6]: the load is distributed to the fibula and shock-absorbed by the distal syndesmotic ligaments, the interosseous membrane and by the contraction of the peroneal muscles. The ankle fork is tightly elastic and not stiff.

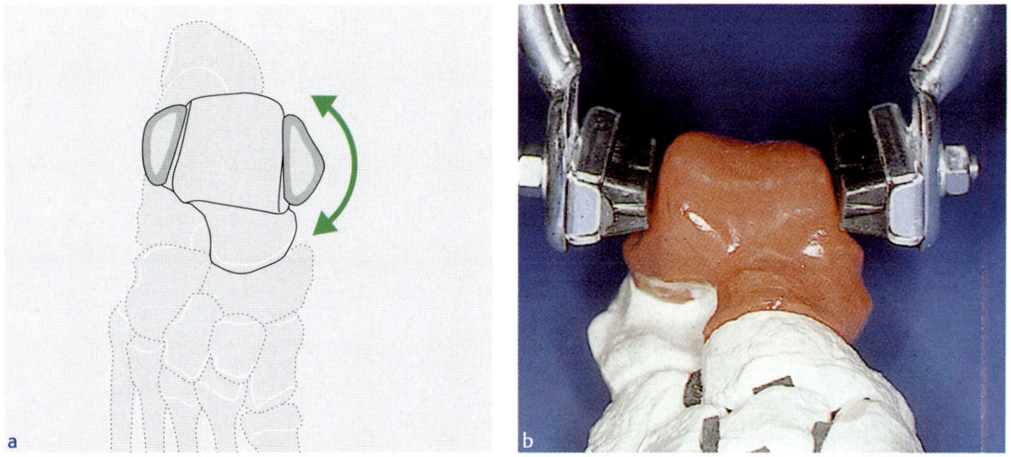

Fig. 5-19a–b The ankle mortise (right foot).

a Seen from the top: the astragalus is broader on the front than on the back. Dorsiflection widens, plantar flexion narrows the fork by adaptive mobility of the fibula (arrows).

b Seen from the front: dorsiflexion is comparable to a bicycle brake—the astragalus is squeezed in dorsiflexion when the fork (ie, the brake) is stiff.

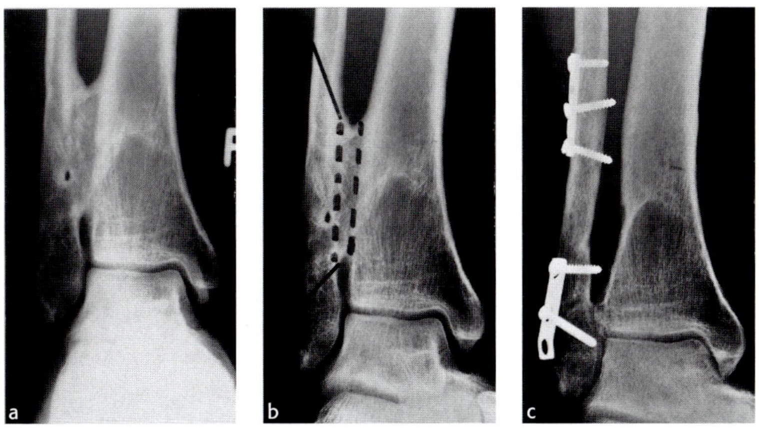

Fig. 5-20a–c Technique of resection of synostosis.

a Synostosis at 3 years following distal lower leg fracture. Persistant pain requires resection.

b Preoperative planning: two oblique osteotomies, block resection with ossified interosseous membrane, trimming off the synostosis on the instrument table (dotted lines). The fibula is replaced and fixed with two antigliding plates.

c 1 year after resection. No longer any pain, unrestricted function.

3.4 Ankle fusion

The ankle fusion technique of Charnley [13] with two Steinmann pins and an external fixator frame occasionally fails due to pivoting of the denuded talus against the denuded distal tibia. To prevent such instability, the following operative technique has proven successful for 35 years (Fig. 5-21–5-23).

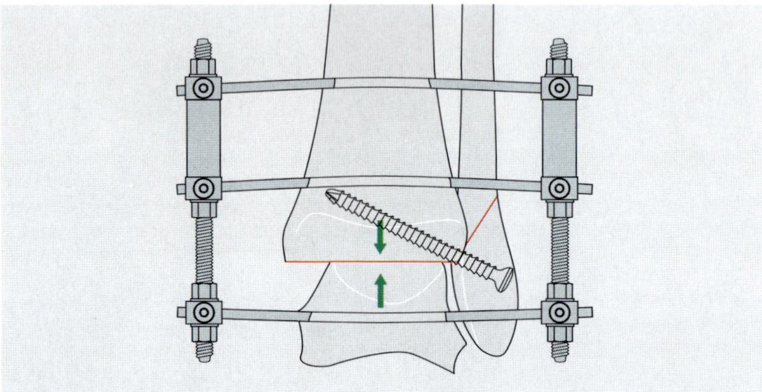

Fig. 5-21 Three-pin frame external fixator for fusion of the ankle joint [14].
The operation is performed from a lateral and a medial approach.
The lateral malleolus is temporarily osteotomized/removed and refixed after the fusion. The medial malleolus is excised.
Two 4.5 mm Steinmann pins in the proximal fragment are rigidly fixed with two double clamps. One Steinmann pin of 5 mm diameter crosses the talus and a compression frame is mounted. Such an external fixator is left in place for 5 weeks, the patient, progressively bears weight, using cruches. No additional or other type of fixation.
5 weeks after surgery the external fixator is removed, best in intravenous anesthesia. A scotch-cast for full weightbearing is applied for another 5 weeks (CAF).
10 weeks after surgery, when the cast is discarded, the patient walks free without orthopedic shoe correction. Ankle fusion is successful when it is at right angle or 5° below in calcaneus. Normal walking is regained 3–4 months after the operation. The lag screw for the fixation of lateral malleolus may be removed at any time from a stabwound under local or intravenous anesthesia.
The three-pin ankle fusion has the advantage that the patient has no major implant inserted that might need removal, such as fusions internally fixed with screws or plates.

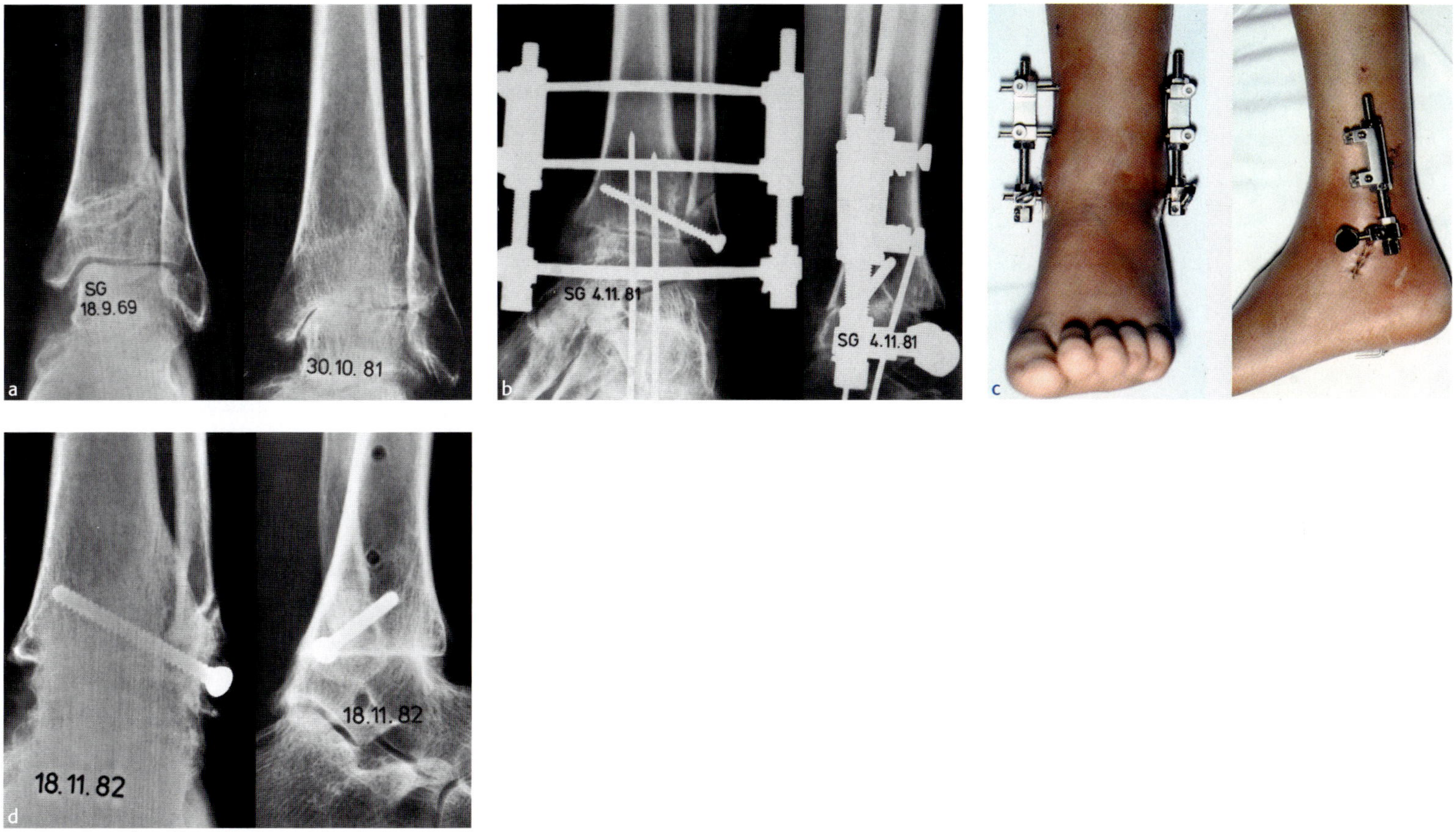

Fig. 5-22a–d Secondary late ankle fusion following tibia fracture [14].

a Preoperative x-rays. An isolated tibial fracture heals with an overlong fibula. Osteoarthritis 12 years later.

b Postoperative x-rays of fusion. Transfixation of the hindfoot at right angle with two K-wires for 2 weeks. They stabilise the talocalcaneal joint in neutral position and are removed 2 weeks after surgery together with the stitches with or without anesthesia.

c At 2 weeks, when the stitches and the two K-wires are removed.

d 1 year after fusion. Sound union, normal walking with normal shoes.

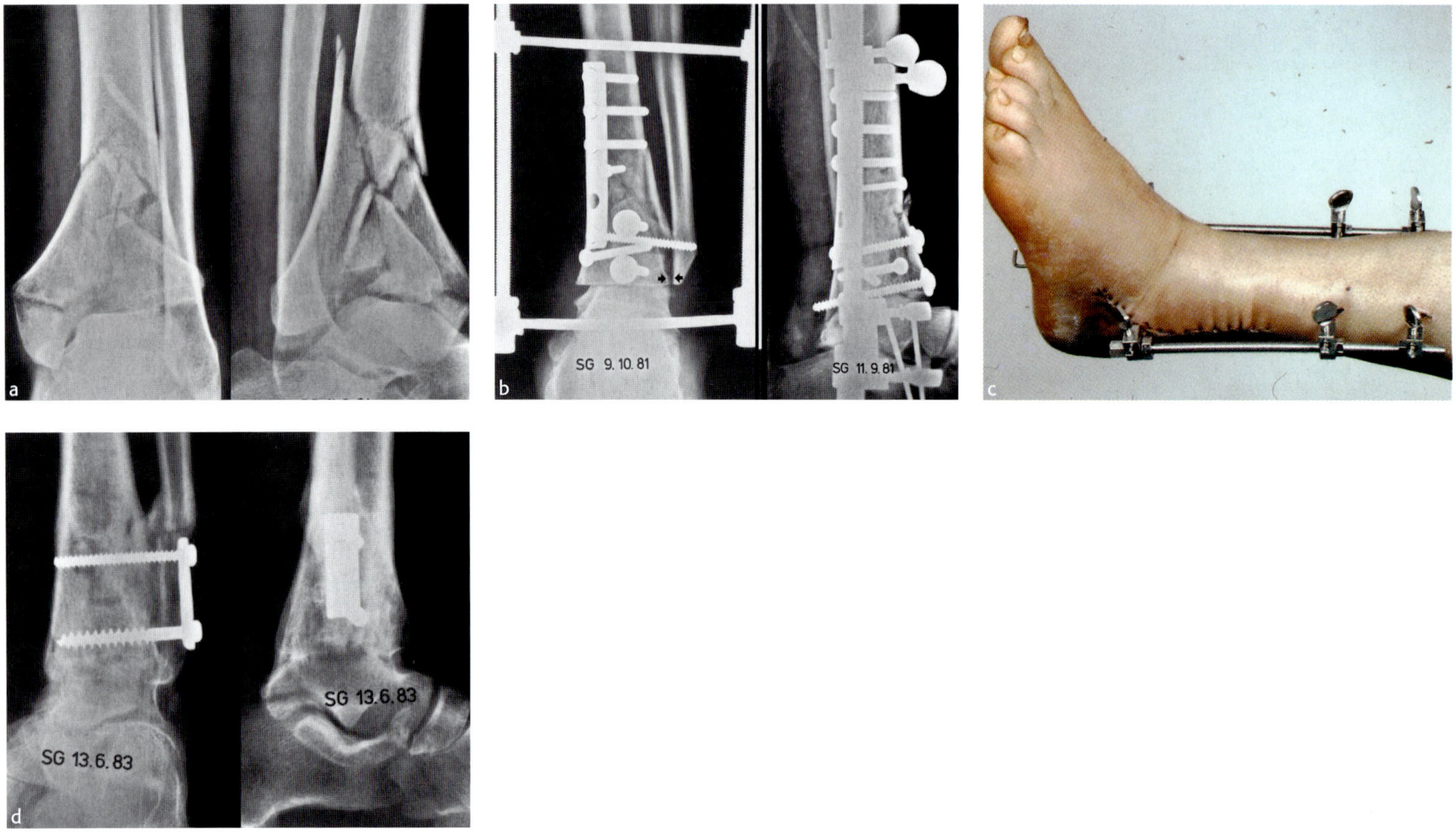

Fig. 5-23a–d Primary ankle fusion following pilon fracture of the tibia [14–16]. Pilon fractures are occasionally too bad for reconstruction. Primary fusion shortens the overall treatment time.

a The shattered pilon is too complex to allow 'waterproof' anatomical reconstruction of the tibial joint surface.

b Open reduction and internal fixation with primary fusion. The resected malleoli are used as bone grafts. Future painful fretting of fibula on tibia (arrows). Synostosis done 6 months later.

c The clinical aspect 3 weeks after injury. The stitches and the two transfixing K-wires are removed. A scotch-cast for 9 weeks is applied, allowing progressive weightbearing (CAF).

d At 1 year 8 months: sound healing of fractures, fusion, and fibulotibial synostosis.

Primary fusion following fracture of the talus

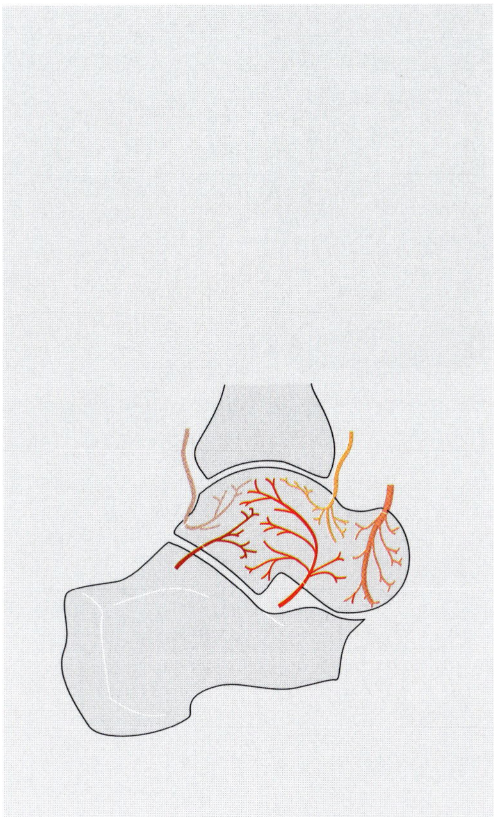

Fig. 5-24 The blood supply of the astragalus [16]. The blood supply of the body of the astragalus depends on one main artery that comes from the sinus tarsi. Small arteries along the capsule and ligaments are unable to compensate for a ruptured main artery.

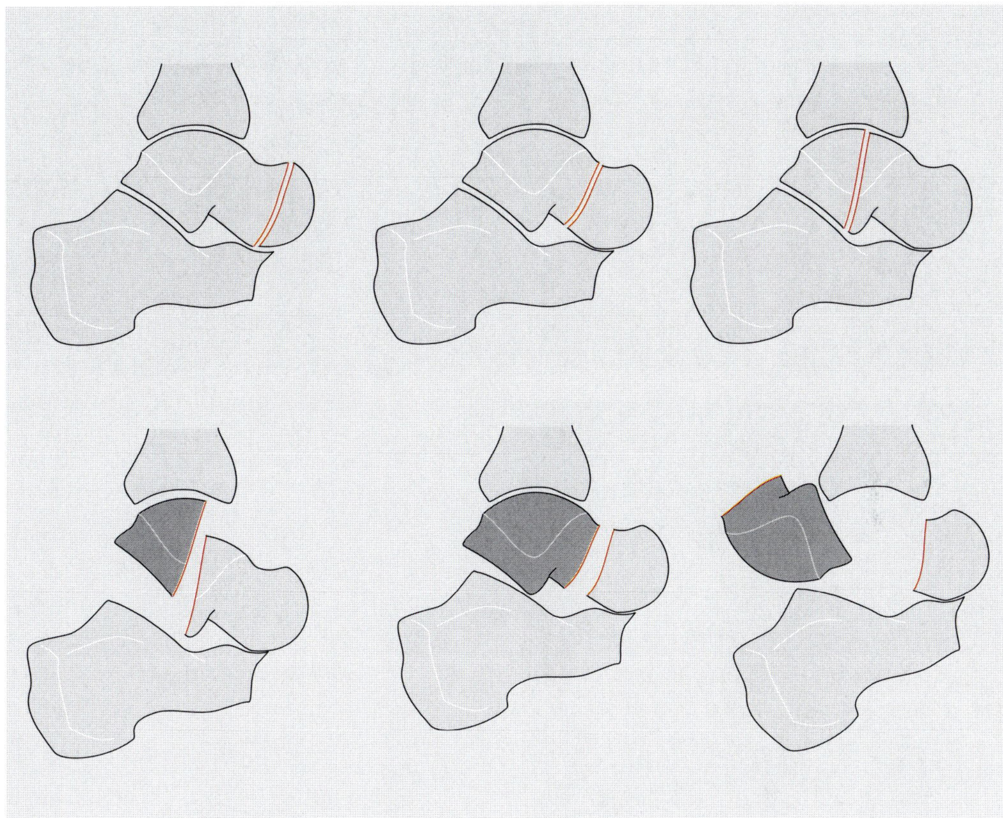

Fig. 5-25 Fracture types and risk of aseptic necrosis [8, 16, 17]. The more proximal a fracture in the astragalus and the more important the displacement of the fragments (mainly of the body of the talus), the more certain the talus is to undergo avascular necrosis, irrespective of an optimal reduction and fixation. Revascularization is only possible either from an ankle or from a subtalar fusion. Our experience is that the impairment of function and of life quality is smaller with a fusion of the ankle joint, than with a subtalar fusion. An ankle fusion in the worst talus fractures offers to the patient the best possible end result. Should the subastragalar joint undergo osteoarthritis at a later time, it can always be fused secondarily.

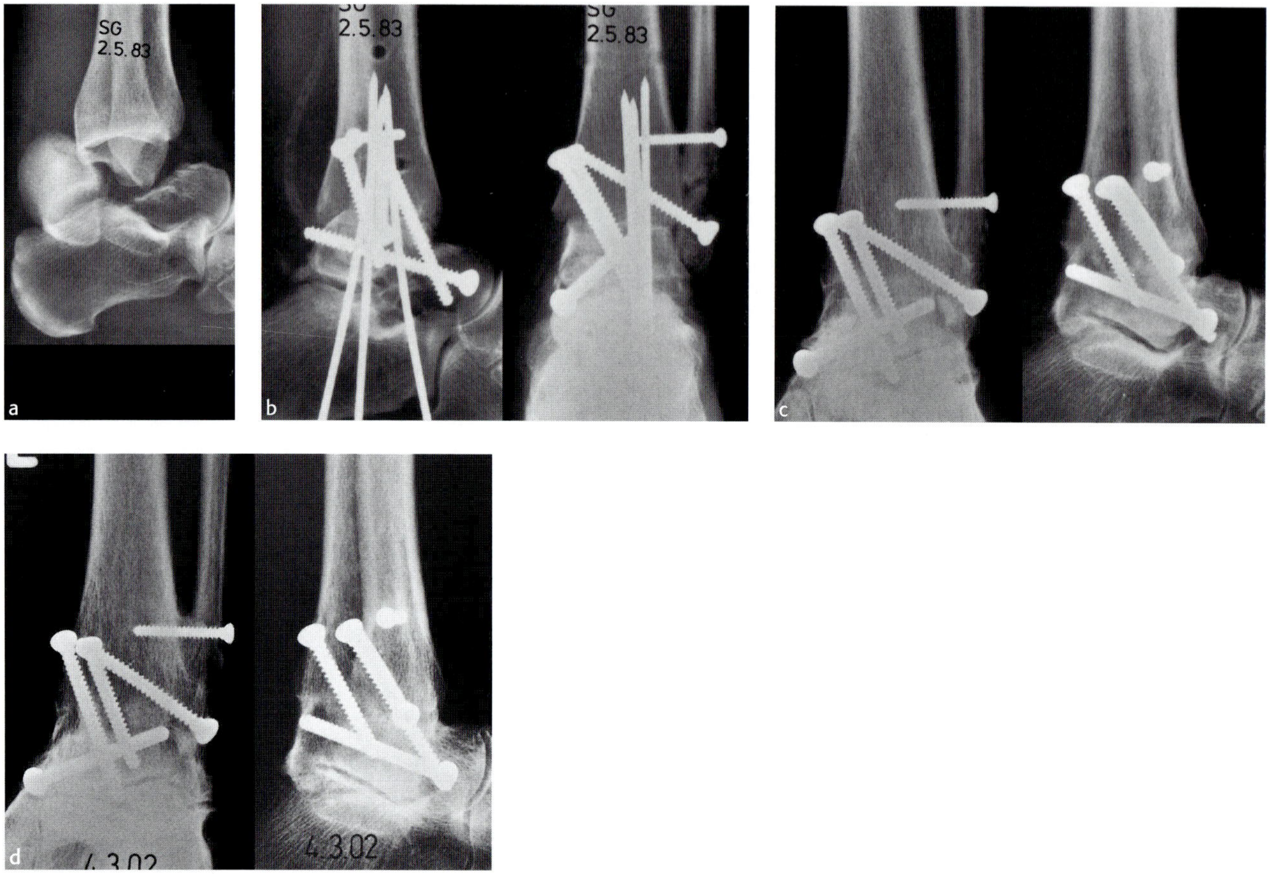

Fig. 5-26a–d Primary ankle fusion for fracture of the talus [8, 16].

a The injury: open dislocation fracture.

b Open reduction and internal fixation with primary resection of the ankle joint. Temporary transfixation of the hindfoot.

c Result 2 years after injury.

d At 19 years: no complaints, almost normal function and activity. The subtalar joint is asymptomatic, but has stiffened due to residual partial necrosis of the talus. The patient (lady) plays recreational sports, including mountaineering (Mt. Kilimanjaro one year ago).

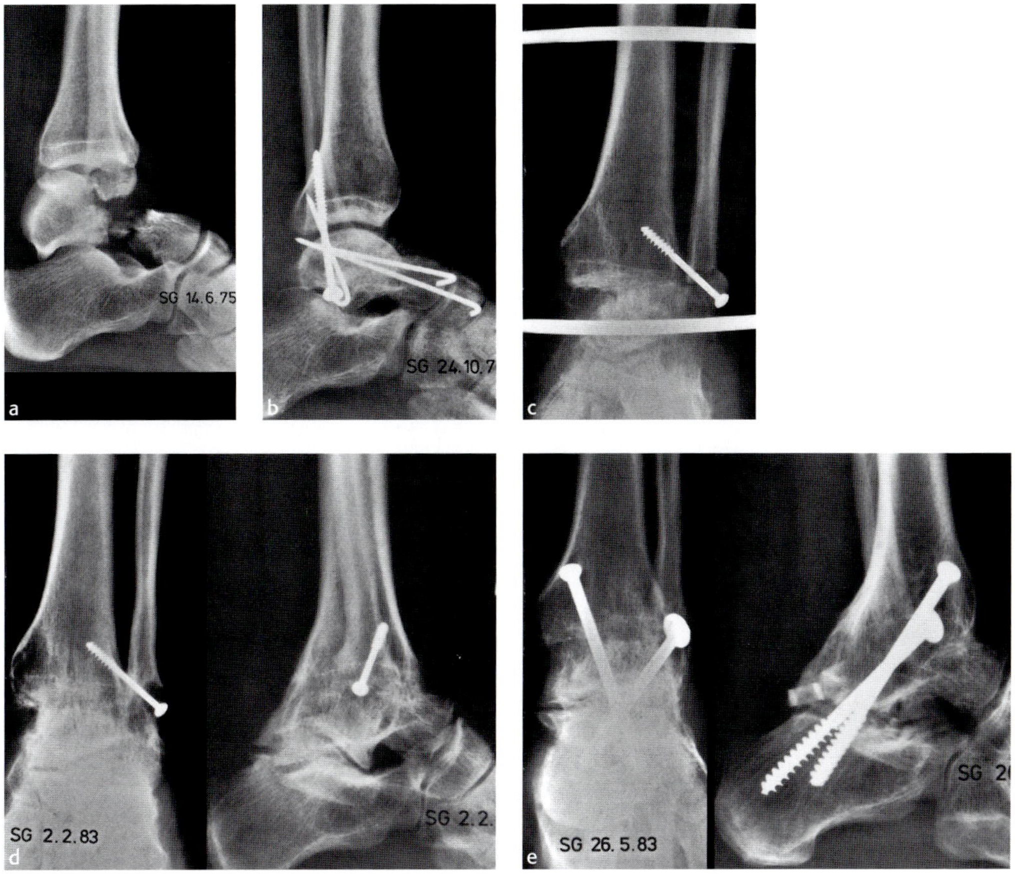

Fig. 5-27a–e Senseless open reduction and internal fixation of the severest talus fracture. Talus necrosis. Secondary ankle fusion and late subtalar fusion.

a Talus necrosis is programmed.

b Unsuccessful trial to avoid necrosis.

c Secondary ankle fusion 2 years later.

d 6 years after the fusion, 8 years after the original injury: painful subtalar osteoarthritis.

e Subtalar fusion with screw fixation and with autogenous grafts from the ilium 8 years after the injury. During all that time, pain and loss of life quality were present. Primary ankle fusion would have been better.

3.5 Secondary clubfoot following Salter III/IV fracture of the medial malleolus (excision of epiphyseal fusion)

The result of fractures that cross the growth plate depends on the precision of the reduction [18–22].

In both situations described below (Fig. 5-28–5-29), the fracture gap is closed completely, no metal crosses the growth plate, and further growth will be undisturbed.

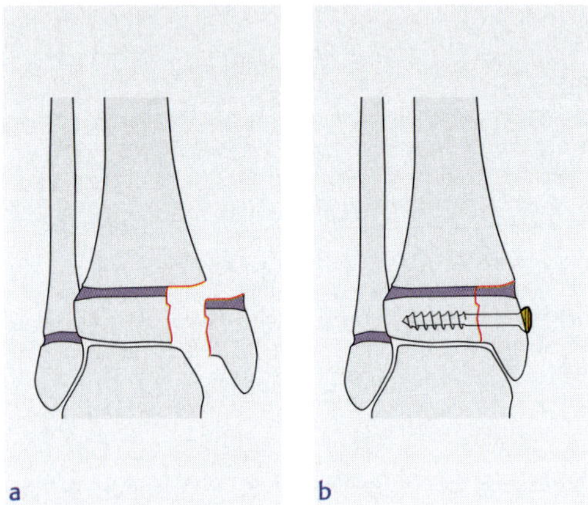

Fig. 5-28a–b
a Salter III fracture.
b Waterproof open reduction and internal fixation. The prognosis is good.

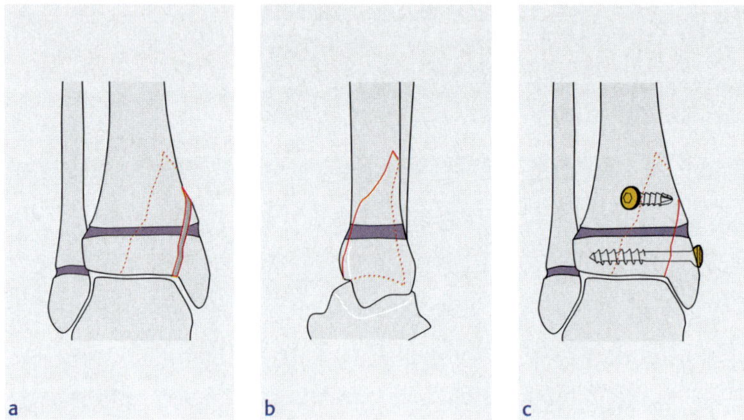

Fig. 5-29a–c
a Salter IV fracture.
bc Waterproof open reduction and internal fixation. The prognosis is good.

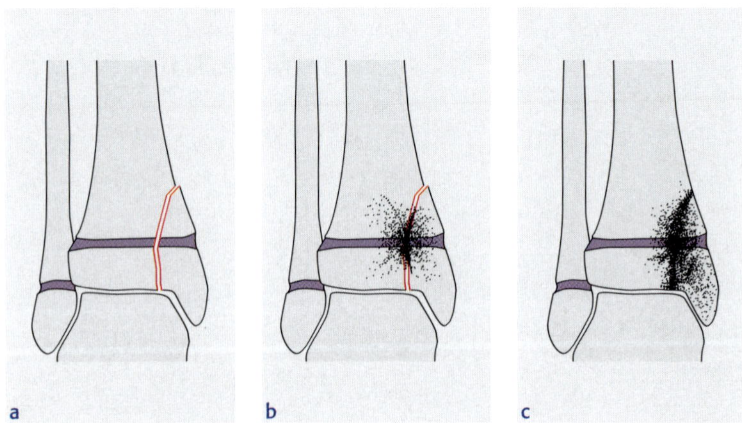

Fig. 5-30a–c
a Salter III or IV fractures may be reduced incompletely.
b Along the fracture gap, a bony bar develops.
c The physeal bar, peripherally located, causes excentric growth arrest, posttraumatic clubfoot, and leg shortening.

The amount of secondary deformity depends on the age of the child: The closer the end of growth is, the lesser the shortening and varus deviation—ankle joint incongruency, however, remains since the fracture reaches the pilon of the tibia. Open reduction and internal fixation is indicated to prevent the consequences of incongruency.

The younger the child, the longer the growth arrest ahead, so the more seriously the deformity develops, shortening and varus. Ankle joint incongruency may be hindered by tibiatalar adaptation. Joint deformity, however, will increase with time.

Langenskjöld [23, 24] has recommended resecting the physeal bar and filling the defect with fat from the buttock. Improvement in the deformity and return of growth were observed with time.

The following examples demonstrate our procedure:

- A supramalleolar open wedge osteotom with 3–5° of overcorrection is performed and finally a pelvic graft is inserted.

- From the osteotomy, close and parallel to the growth plate, the bar is resected and the resulting defect filled with a fingerpacked bone-cement plug.

- When shortening is more than 1–2 cm, typical in young children, leg lengthening is performed as a separate procedure before the excision of epiphyseal fusion.

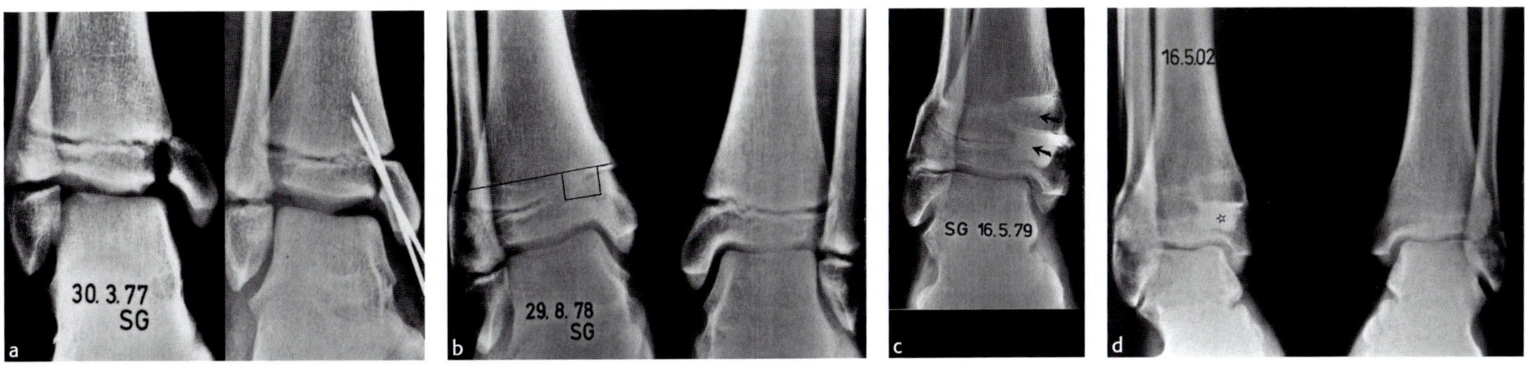

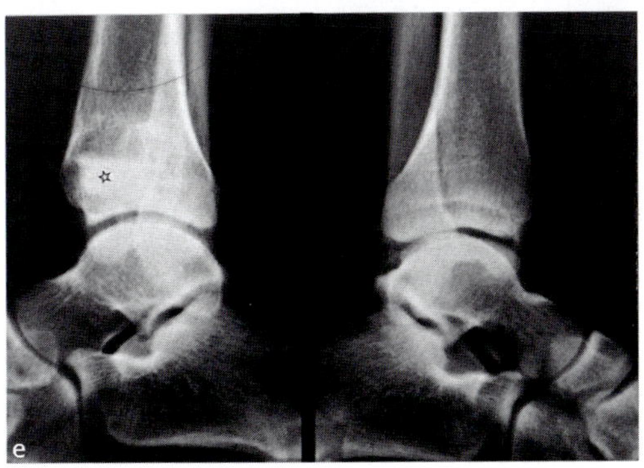

Fig. 5-31a–e 12-year-old boy.
a Salter III fracture medially, Salter I fracture of fibula. Incomplete, not waterproof reduction, minimal invasive fixation.
b 18 months later: typical deformity compared with opposite side. Preoperative planning: osteotomy plus excision of epiphyseal fusion.
c 6 months after surgery. The leg no longer shows any deformity. The graft has been incorporated (arrow). The remaining growth plate is producing leg length, like the distal fibular physis. The cement block prevents the development of a physeal bar (arrow).
de 23 years after surgery: Normal anatomy and function, no complaints. 'Silent' cement plug (starlets).

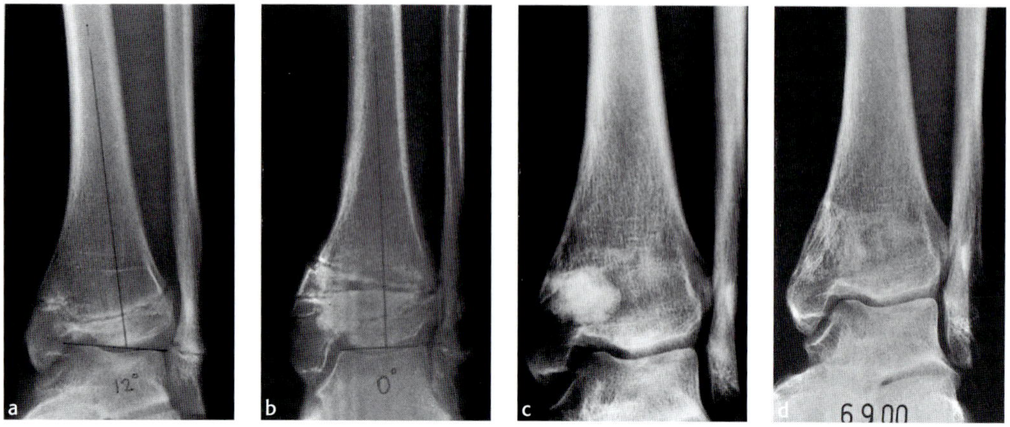

Fig. 5-32a–d 12-year-old girl.

a 6 years ago Salter III fracture. Deformity and 2 cm leg shortening.

b 2 months after surgery.

c 5 years later: no recurrence of deformity, shortening now 1 cm, ie, growth took place until growth arrest on both sides. At that stage the bone-cement plug was removed and replaced with bone from the iliac crest.

d 10 years after surgery, at age 22: aspect and function are normal, leg is 1 cm shorter.

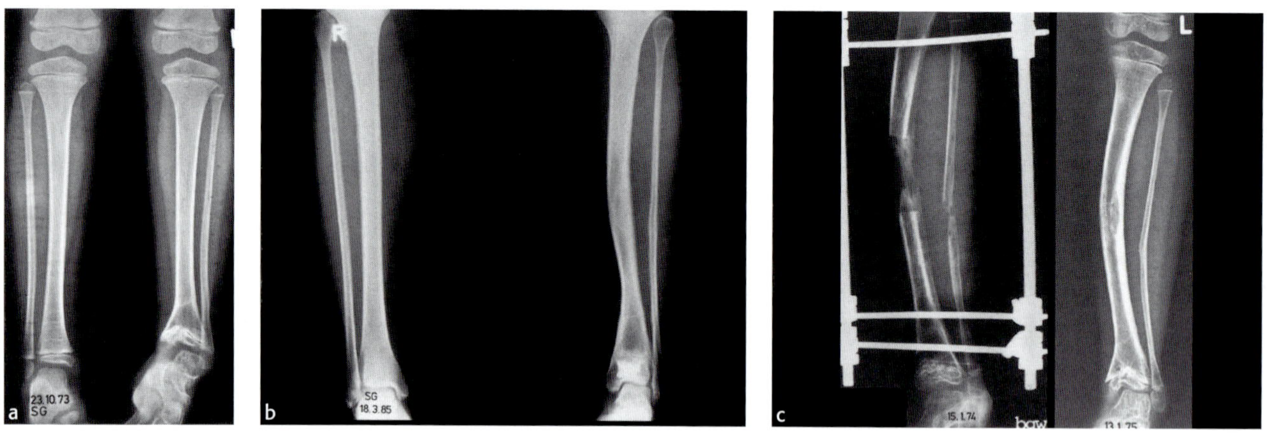

Fig. 5-33a–i 5-year-old girl.

a 18 months ago Salter III or IV fracture: serious clubfoot and 4.5 cm shortening.

b Late result after 12 years at the end of growth. 1 cm shortening, residual ankle joint tilt of 4° varus. No complaints.

c Lengthening with intended tibia varus and with overlengthening 4 cm. Leg 1 year after lengthening.

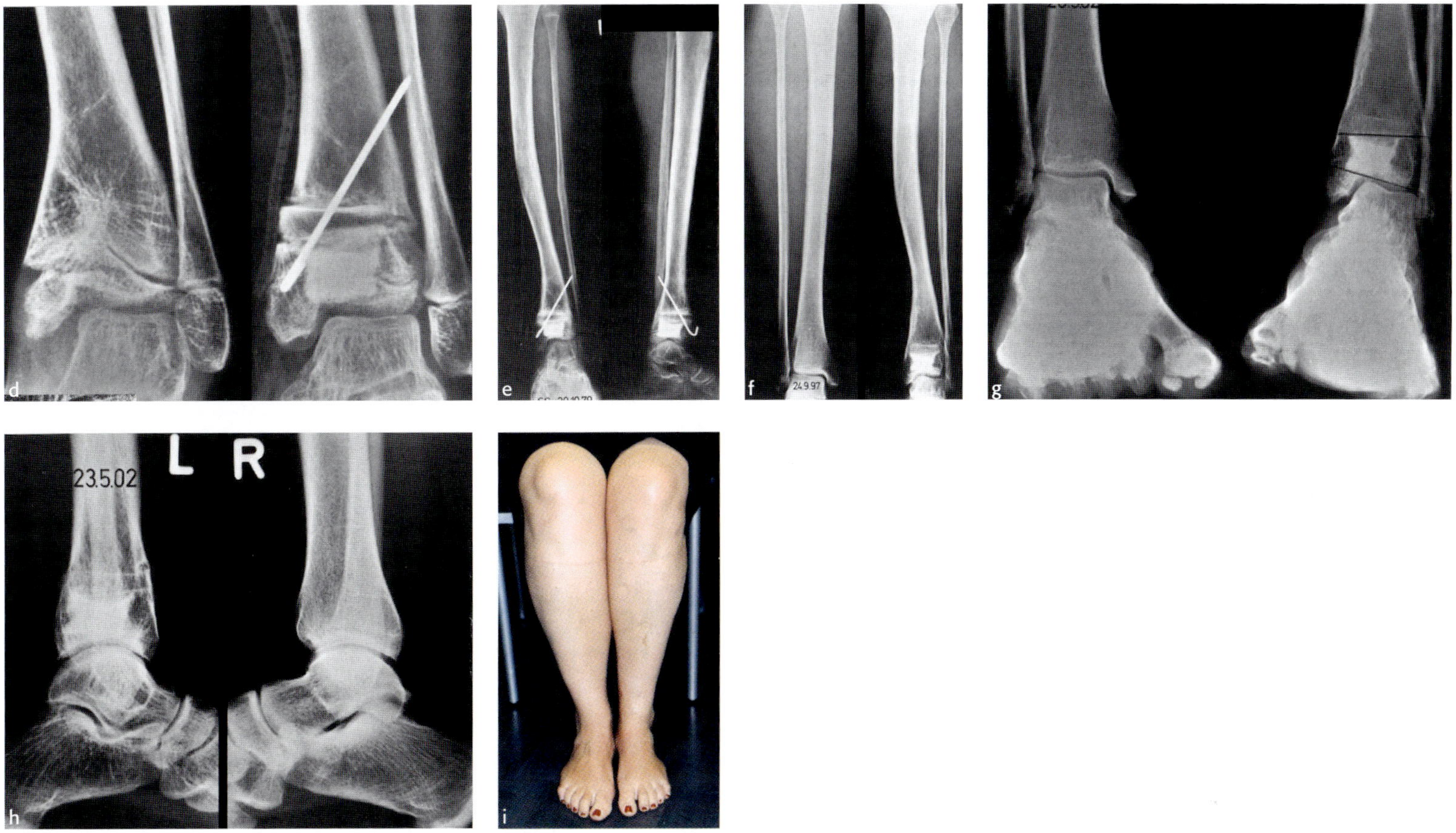

Fig. 5-33a–i cont.

d The excision of epiphyseal fusion, pre- and postoperatively.

e 3 months after surgery. Leg-ankle axis corrected.
The K-wire is now removed.

f 18 years after surgery.

gh After surgery. Varus of ankle joint 4°, no complaints. Open wedge supramalleolar osteotomy is planned (tracing of deformity).

1 Identical lower legs.

4 Achilles tendon

Surgery on the Achilles tendon is loaded with infection risk. Infection repercussions are difficult to cure. The healing potential is limited by the fact that the blood supply of the Achilles tendon is very different from other tissues like muscle, skin, and bone. The tendon depends on the rete calcaneare, arriving from the posterior tibial artery and from small other arteries some centimeters proximally. Damaged tendon tissue hardly bleeds. When contaminated, local infection defense and antibiotic afflux are poor, which explains the defensive policy of treatment, the preference for minimal invasive suture for acute rupture and for conservative casting with the foot in equinus.

For those of us who have been performing most orthopedic surgery under sterile enclosure conditions since 1970 [25], Achilles tendon surgery is not minimal, but done according to the MINIMAX principle [26] so it is more than minimal: open surgery, respecting the critical blood supply and still striving for full anatomical and functional restoration [27, 28].

The following points should be understood under the noted premise of contamination prevention [25], which avoids the otherwise risk of dramatic infections and permits refusal of equinus of the foot at any time of treatment.

4.1 Acute Achilles tendon rupture and repair

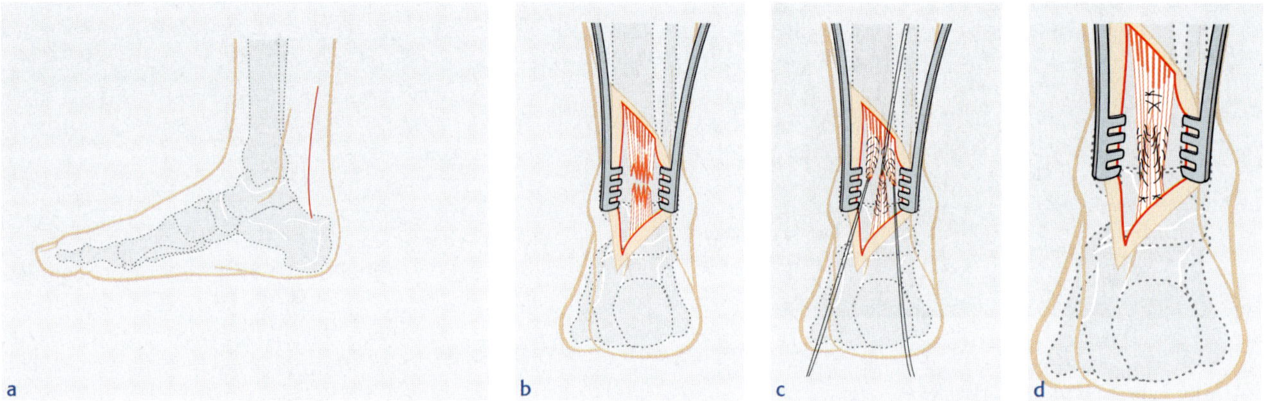

a b c d

Fig. 5-34a–f Three-strand suture for Achilles tendon rupture [28].

a The patient is operated on in a prone position, with a tourniquet. The tendon is exposed from a medial incision parallel to the Achilles tendon.

bcd The disrupted tendon fibers are organised into three strands, one distal, two proximal. The three strands are each seized with resorbeable No. 2 thread. The suture technique is copied from sail makers. The six free ends of the three threads are countersutured upwards and downwards. Two running conjoining No. 000 resorbeable sutures are added. Measurement of the pull-strength on a cadaver resulted in 30–40 kg resistence. This is by far enough to resist continuous active function (CAF) in a walking scotch-cast.

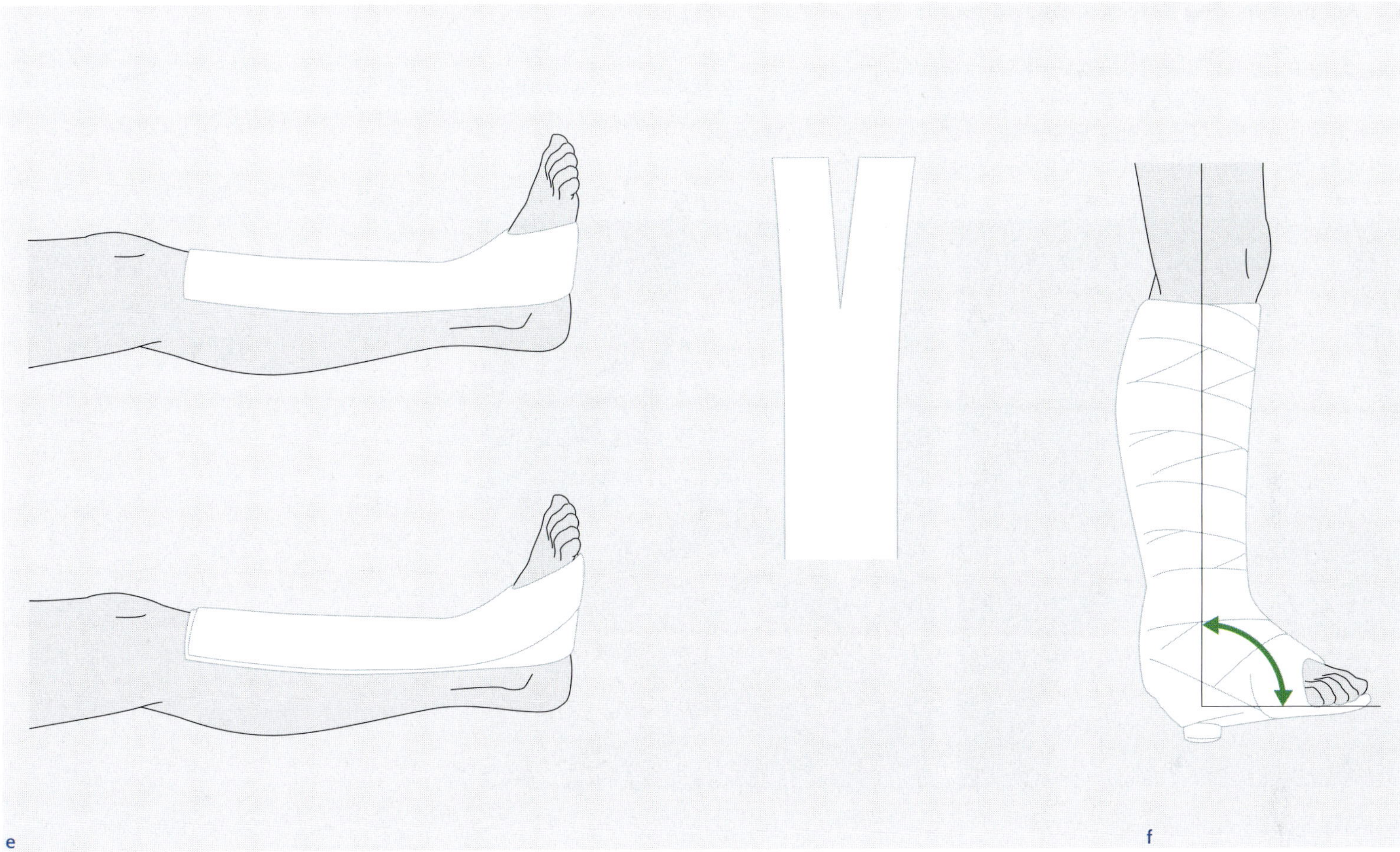

Fig. 5-34a–f cont.

e The padded postoperative stirrup plaster splint for 2 weeks—the patient walking with it, with partial weightbearing, with ground touch of the whole foot sole.

f Right-angled brace for full weightbearing for 8 weeks from 2 weeks post surgery. 10 weeks after surgery, the brace is removed, the patient walks free, physiotherapy is unnecessary, full function is back 3–4 months after injury and surgery.

4.2 Achilles tendon defect reconstruction

Typical defects of the Achilles tendon remain from neglected ruptures, from failed surgery, and most often from infection after surgery. Before reconstruction, infected necrotic tissue must be removed. End of drainage and sound wound healing must be awaited first (Fig. 5-35).

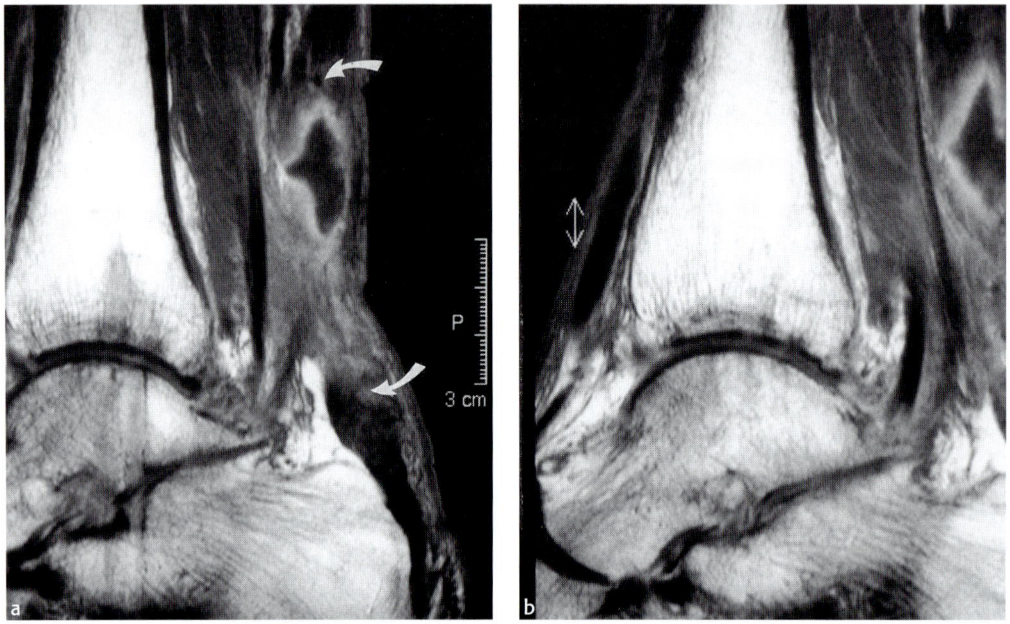

Fig. 5-35a–b Defect with drainage.
A professional mountain guide and ski instructor had acute Achilles tendon rupture and suture in a conventional operating room one year ago, followed by infection, in spite of massive antibiotic medication. The problem is threefold: infection, defect compensation, and revascularization at the reconstruction site.

a Debridement to be done to 7 cm of necrotic tissue (arrows).
b Central abscess and drainage (arrow). The surgical eradication of infected necrotic tissue, the cure from infection is supported with local Gentamycin foam and systemic antibiotic medication.

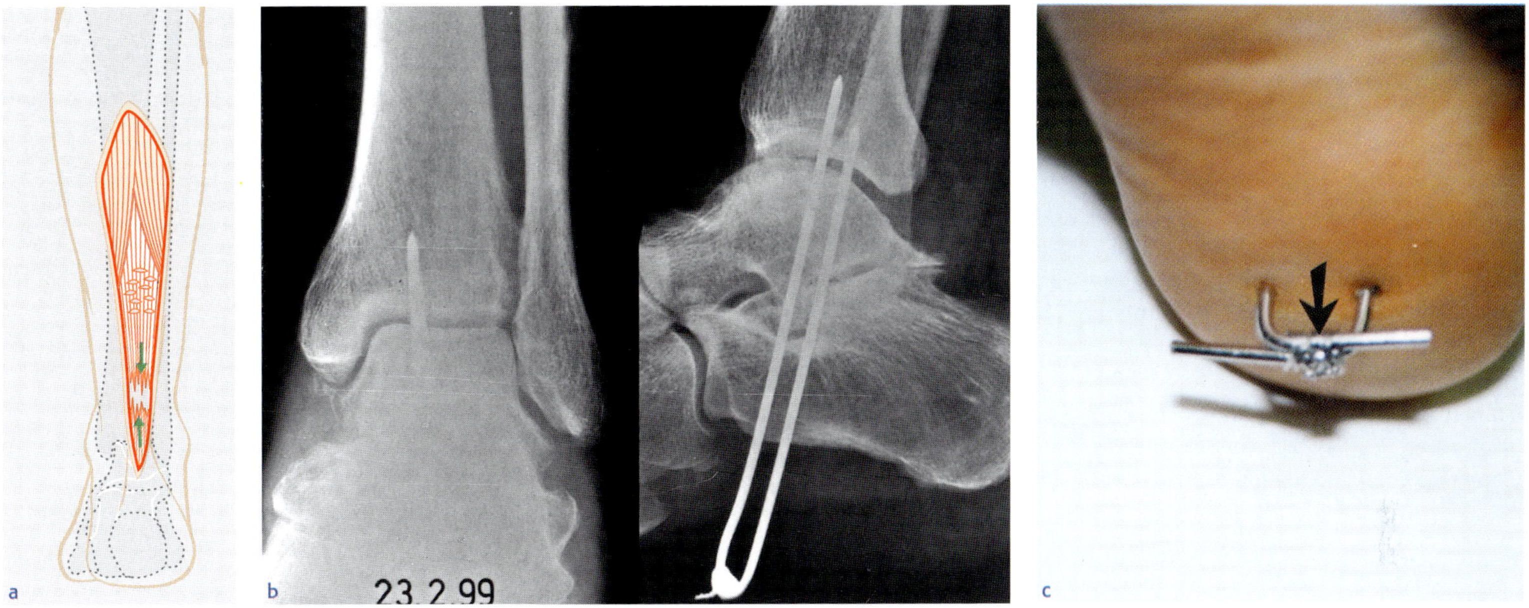

Fig. 5-36a–c Compensation of Achilles tendon defect.

a The gastrocnemius fascia is incised in V-shape, singular or double parallel. 3–5 cm can be gained with gastrocnemius slide length by harmonica-like gaping. The end-to-end suture is performed in analogy to the acute repair with resorbeable No. 2 thread (arrows).

bc The hindfoot is transfixed with two parallel 2.5 mm K-wires for 6 weeks to stabilize the suture area. To prevent pull-out, the two K-wires are bent 90° and fastened together with a continuous thin wire-cerclage (arrow). A brace with a heel hole for daily desinfection with isopropylic alcohol spray is applied. At 6 weeks, the two K-wires are removed and a second scotch-cast for another 6 weeks is applied.

4.3 ST Hansen muscle transfer (slightly modified)

Hansen [29] transfers the flexor hallucis longus muscle belli to an Achilles tendon for achillodynia and for rupture to stimulate the healing process. Revascularization is promoted by vascular ingrowth from the muscle to the Achilles tendon. Hansen [29] uses the severed flexor tendon to fasten to the calcaneus or to the rupture area, as a tendon augmentation.

The tendon is not severed in our technique—active big toe flexion comes back in about 1 year. The same technique is also used for achillodynia and for rupture following achillodynia.

For all three indications a postoperative brace-protection is recommended for 8–12 weeks. CAF, ie, partial followed by full weightbearing, favors blood perfusion and tendon healing—in analogy to fracture healing.

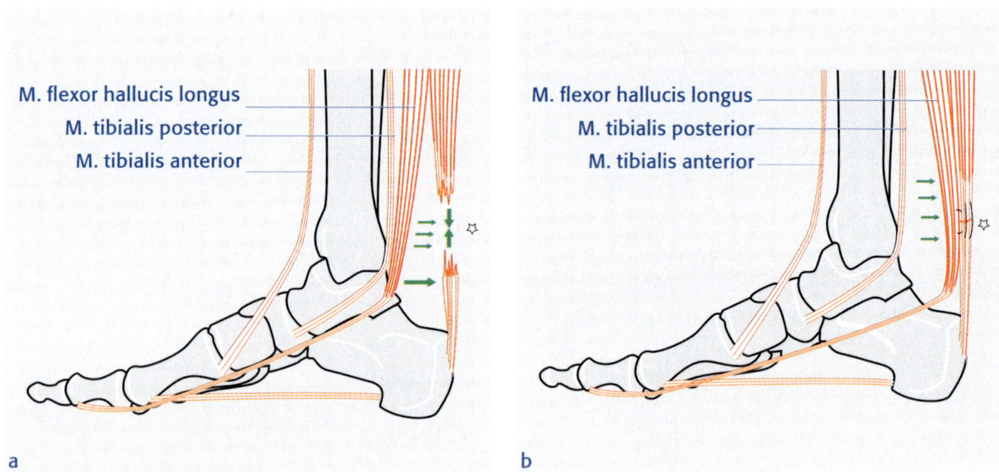

Fig. 5-37a–b Transfer of flexor hallucis longus muscle without cutting its tendon.

a The defect (starlet) is to be closed according to Fig. 36 (2 fat arrows). The flexor hallucis longus muscle and tendon are freed and provided for transfer (other arrows).

b The defect is closed (starlet). The flexor hallucis longus muscle and its tendon are transferred to the lesion. The muscle belli is sutured onto the lesion (fine arrows). The flexor hallucis longus tendon is sutured onto the distal Achilles tendon (curved fat arrow).

4.4 Foot flexors stretching with external fixator [14]

Shortened muscles and other soft tissues at different locations (foot, knee, elbow) need lengthening when physiotherapy fails. Progressive stretching or lengthening with an external fixator is an option, either alone or following surgical release or lengthening.

Full correction in one move without continuous stretching may be hazardous for blood circulation and innervation, the typical risk of all lengthening or shortening procedures. In contrast, the stretching in small increments with an external fixator allows permanent observation and risk elimination [14] (Fig. 5-38).

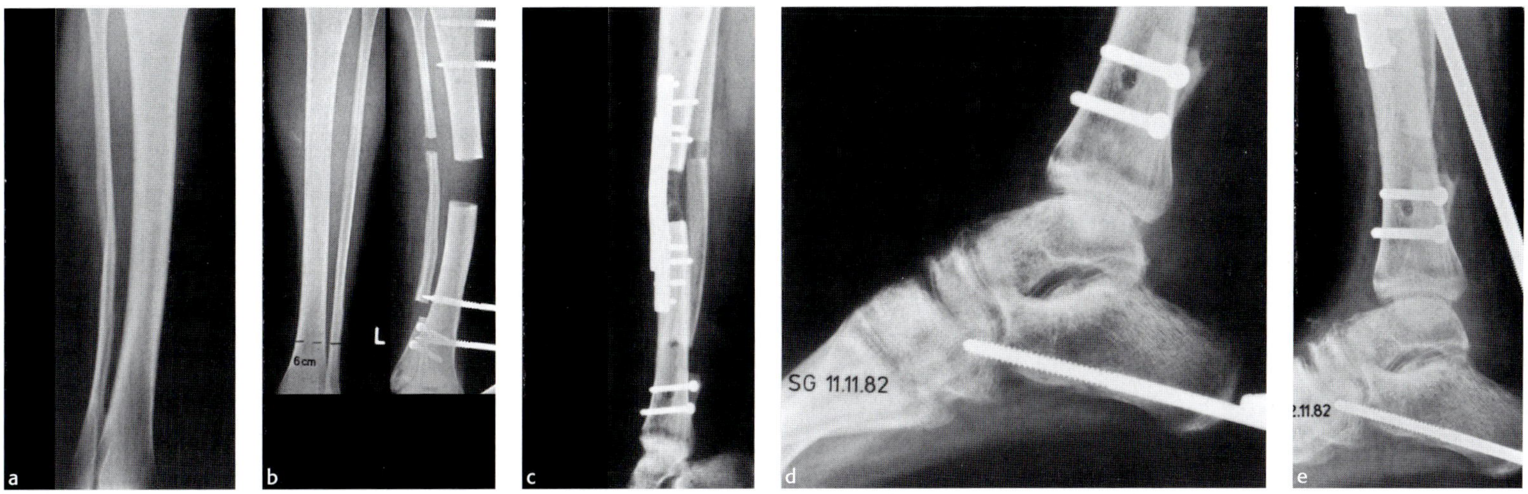

Fig. 5-38a–i Foot flexor lengthening with an external fixator (17-year-old woman).

a Congenital shortening of lower leg at age 17, difference 6 cm.

b Lengthening with Wagner lengthening device, with plating and autogenous bone graft. Note: double osteotomy of fibula to hinder valgus tethering.

c 3 months later: foot equinus of 35°.
Note: Callus distraction on tibia and fibula.

d Stretching with external fixator has started one week ago following sliding tenotomies of all foot flexors. Gain of dorsiflexion 35° in 3 weeks.
Note: Schanz screw through the calcaneus.

e 11th day of stretching.

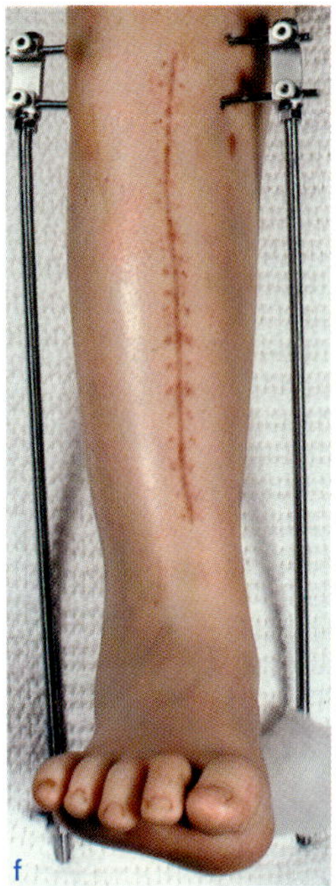

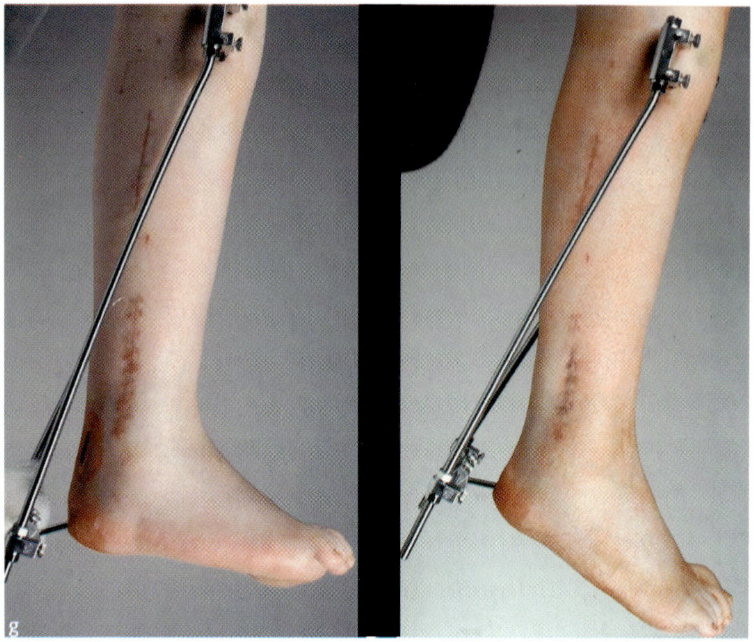

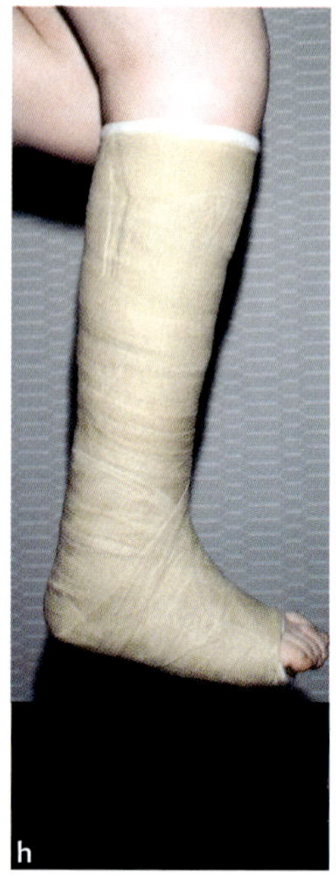

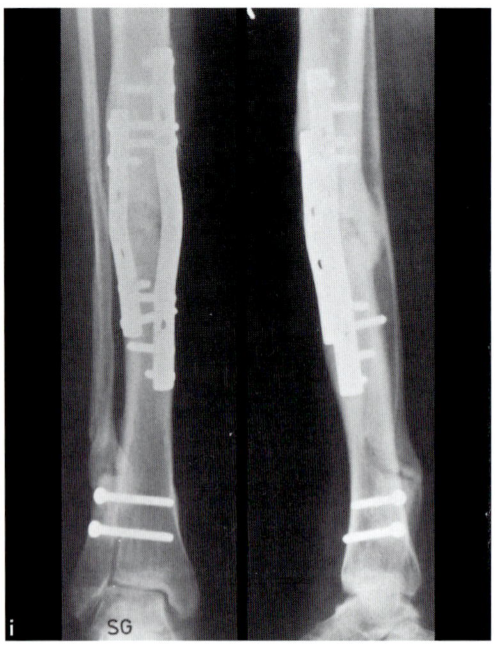

Fig. 5-38a–i cont.

f Frame external fixator: the proximal anchorage is a prestrained frame with two Steinmann pins.

g 35° correction in 3 weeks.

h The brace for full weightbearing till 10 weeks after the start of muscle-tendon lengthening and stretching.

i 1 year after starting reconstruction: bone healed, foot function flexion-extension 10/0/30. The two distal transfixation screws are now removed, the two tibial plates year later.
Note: The distraction callus is bridged with two wave plates.

5 Acute and recurrent ankle sprain

5.1 Diagnosis of acute and chronic ankle sprain [6]

The history of trauma and local findings may require more precise assessment of ligament damage. Stressed x-rays are done for comparison without, or better with, local or general anesthesia (Fig. 5-39–5-42).

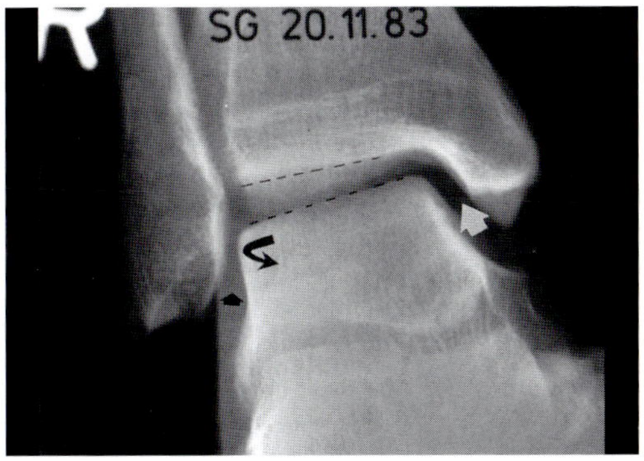

Fig. 5-39 Isolated fresh rupture of the anterior fibulotalar ligament. The joint space between fibula and talus is mildly widened due to anterior rotation of the lateral talus in the ankle fork. The talus is tilted less than 5°, the joint space medially is normal (arrows).

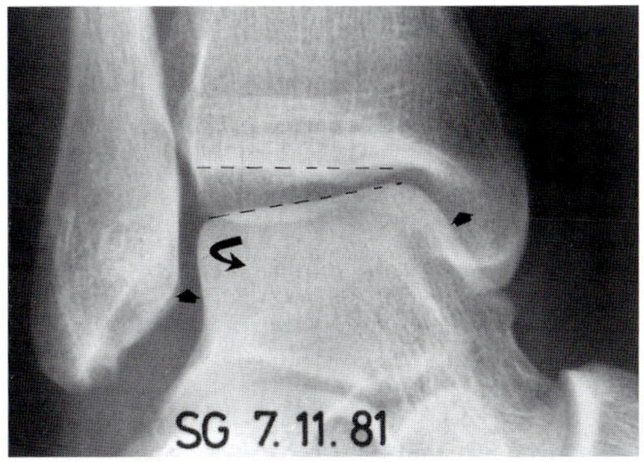

Fig. 5-40 Fresh rupture of the anterior fibulotalar, fibulocalcaneal, and posterior fibulotalar ligaments. The astragalus is rotated and markedly tilted in supination 5° and more, the joint space medially is not normal (arrows).

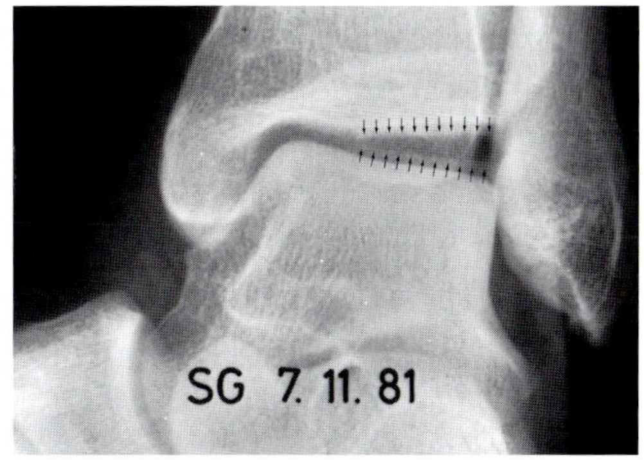

Fig. 5-41 Chronic insufficient anterior fibulotalar ligament, ie, rotatory instability of the talus. 'Gas' phenomenon. Bilateral stressed x-rays are done to clarify the diagnosis without anesthesia between recurrent sprain episodes. The joint space between talus and fibula is mildly widened, the talus is only slightly tilted. A narrow wedge of a vacuum phenomenon 'gas' is present (arrows).

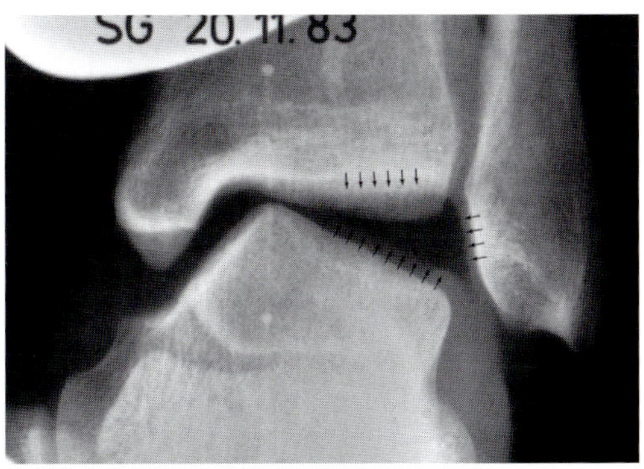

Fig. 5-42 Subtotal or total insufficiency of the fibular collateral ligaments 'Gas' phenomenon. The lateral joint space is markedly widened, the astragalus is strongly tilted. An impressive vacuum 'gas' phenomenon is present (arrows).

Widening of ankle joint space and talar tilt without vacuum phenomenon is proof of an acute lesion. Blood in the ankle joint prevents vacuum and therefore 'gas' formation is impossible. When a vacuum phenomenon is present, effusion is missing. Together with widening of the joint space and eventually with talar tilt, a chronic ankle sprain can be diagnosed, especially when the 'gas' phenomenon is unilateral. Is it bilateral? Then joint laxity is present on both sides.

5.2 Treatment of acute ankle sprain

Conservative treatment of acute ankle sprain is the treatment of choice for many doctors [30].

At our institution, acute ruptures of the fibular collateral ligaments have been sutured systematically since 1960. With the availability of clean-air operating rooms and the body-exhaust system in 1970, postoperative infection has disappeared.

Secondary reconstructions for recurrent ankle sprain are the result of conservative treatment in patients who are referred to us. Recurrent ankle sprain is absent with accurate suture [31–33].

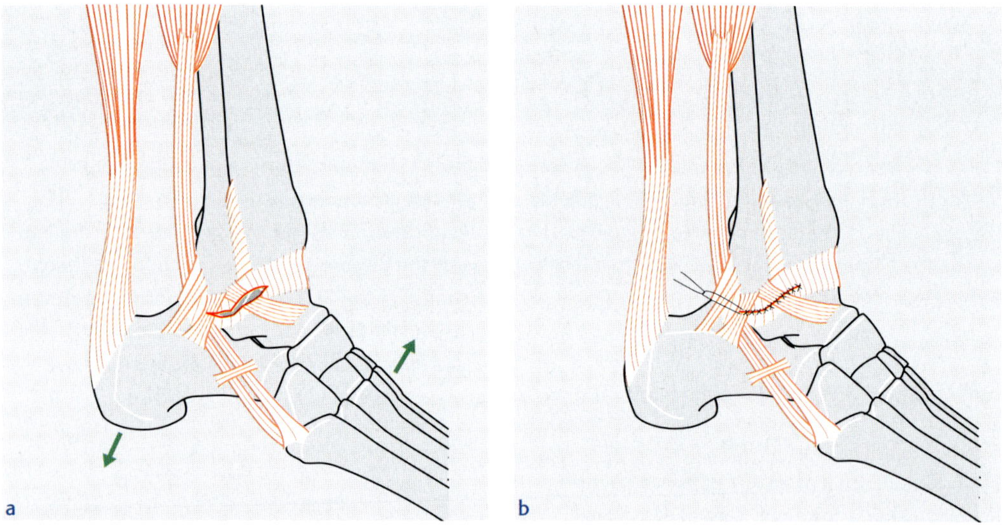

Fig. 5-43a–b Suture of fresh fibular ligament rupture [6, 31].

a Less or more extended rupture of the joint capsule and ligaments. Watch for lateral dome damage of the talus!

b From a standard incision, a running shoelace suture with resorbeable thread is made. Stirrup splint for 2 weeks, followed by a brace at right angle for full weightbearing for 5–6 weeks after surgery.

5.3 Treatment of recurrent ankle sprain [6, 31–33]

Our two procedures minimize surgical tissue insult to avoid prolonged swelling of the ankle region.The first procedure is provided for the deficiency of the isolated anterior fibulotalar ligament and for the rotatory instability of the talus in the ankle fork. The second procedure is for more serious instabilities after rupture of two or of all three collateral fibular ligaments, for instability of the ankle, subtralar, and occasionally also of the calcaneocuboidal joint.

The postoperative treatment is the same for both procedures: Postoperative padded stirrup splint for 12 days. The stitches are removed and a below-knee-walking brace for full weightbearing is applied. 8 weeks after surgery, the brace is removed. Normal walking and motion of the foot are back at three months after surgery. Physiotherapy is not necessary because of the full weightbearing with the brace. Regain of normal function is prepared (CPM and CAF), and muscle wasting is minimal and compensated for automatically with unprotected physical performance.

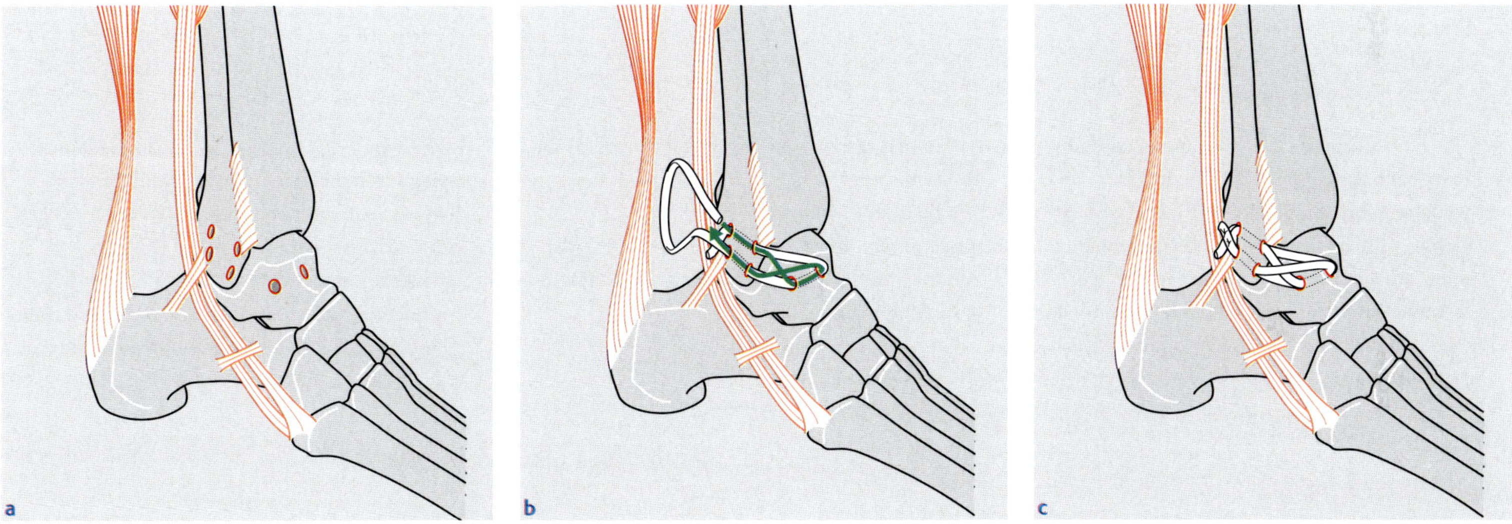

Fig. 5-44a–c Reconstruction for anterior fibulotalar ligament deficiency [33].

a The plantaris muscle tendon is harvested from a small para-achillar medial incision proximal to the calcaneal tuberosity with a tendon stripper. My personal preference is a second 3 cm incision, where the posterior crest of the tibial ends at the base of the tibial head. The index finger splits the soleus and gastrocnemius muscles and easily finds the tendon next to its small muscle belly. At that stage, the distal end of the tendon is severed. The 20–25 cm long tendon is now pulled upwards with the index finger into the proximal incision and is harvested. Drillholes in the distal fibula and in the neck of the talus with 4.5 mm drill bit are made.

bc The plantaris muscle tendon is inserted through the holes (arrows) twice. The strands are tightened and finally stabilized with resorbeable thread No. 0.

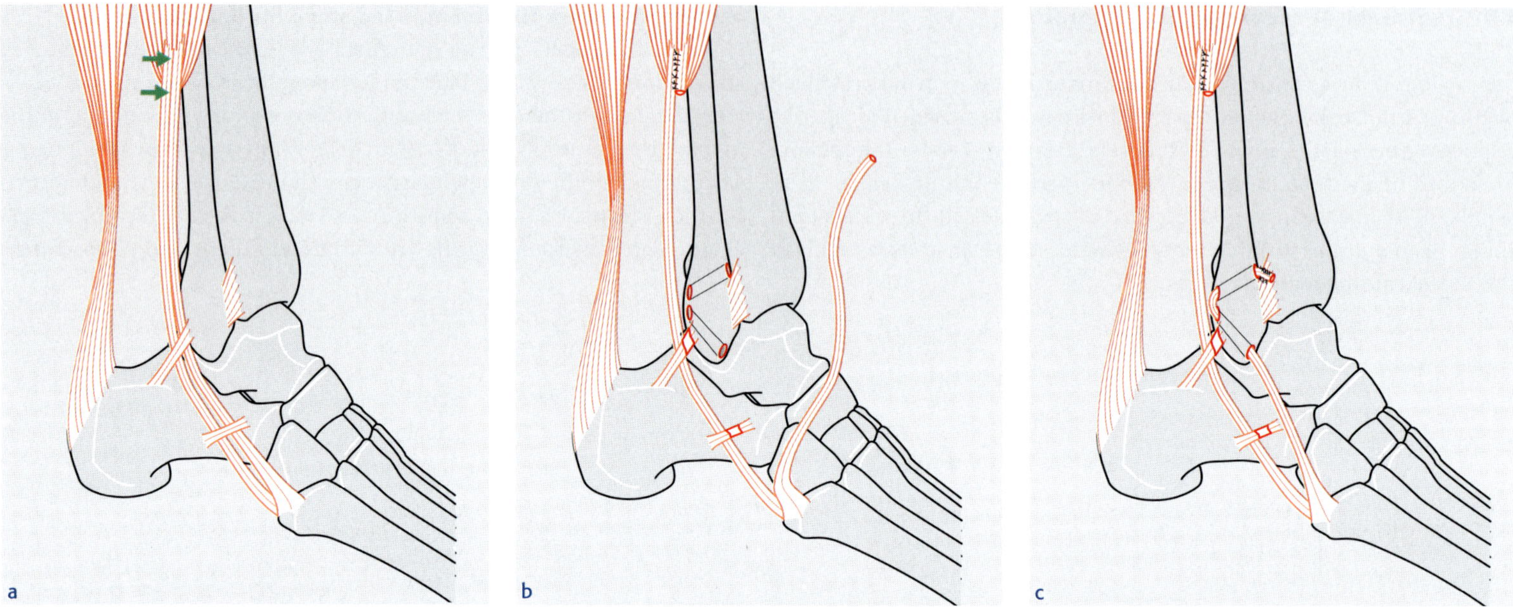

Fig. 5-45a–c Reconstruction for more extended deficiency of fibular collateral ligaments [33].

a 8–9 cm long incision parallel to the lateral malleolus from its tip upwards. The peroneal tendons are sutured together with No. 2 resorbable thread (arrows). The deeper tendon in the wound, the tendon of the peroneus brevis muscle is severed.

b A second 3 cm incision proximal of the tip of the 5th metacarpal bone is made parallel to the tendon of the peroneus brevis muscle. The tendon is identified, isolated, and pulled down into the wound. It remains pedicled to the base of the 5th metatarsal bone.

c Two 4.5 mm drill holes are made in the lateral malleolus and widened up to about 6 mm diameter with a Kocher clamp. The tendon's end, fastened to a resorbable thread No. 2, is subcutaneously directed to the lateral malleolus. It is guided through the two drill holes and under mild tension applied to the periosteum and the fascia cruris.

6 Bibliography

Blue references indicate links to abstracts of articles online available through Medline (www.nlm.nih.gov).

1. **Müller ME, Allgöwer M, Willenegger H** (1963) *Technik der operativen Frakturbehandlung.* Berlin Göttingen Heidelberg: Springer-Verlag.
2. **Müller ME, Allgöwer M, Schneider R, et al.** (1991) *Manual of Internal Fixation.* Berlin Heidelberg New York: Springer-Verlag.
3. **Rüedi TP, Murphy WM, Colton CL, et al.** (2000) *AO Principles of Fracture Management.* Stuttgart New York: Thieme.
4. **Danis R** (1949) *Théorie et pratique de l'ostéosynthèse.* Paris: Masson.
5. **Weber BG** (1964) Behandlung der Luxationsfrakturen des oberen Sprunggelenkes. *Aerztliche Praxis;* XVI (38):1554.
6. **Weber BG** (1972) *Die Verletzungen des oberen Sprunggelenkes.* Bern Stuttgart Wien: Hans Huber.
7. **Brunner ChF, Weber BG** (1982) *Special Techniques in Internal Fixation.* Berlin Heidelberg New York: Springer-Verlag.
8. **Weber BG** (1981) 58. Brüche von Knöcheln und Talus. Bewährtes und Neues in Diagnostik und Therapie Langebecks. *Arch Chir (Kongressbericht);* 355:421–425.
9. **Winkler B, Weber BG, Simpson LA** (1990) The dorsal antiglide plate in the treatment of Danis-Weber type-B fractures of the distal fibula. *Clin Orthop;* (259):204–209.
10. **Weber BG** (1981) Lengthening osteotomy of the fibula to correct a wiened mortice of the ankle after fracture. *Intern. Orthopaedics (SICOT);* 4:289–293.
11. **Weber BG, Simpson LA** (1985) Corrective lengthening osteotomy of the fibula. *Clin Orthop;* (199):61–67.
12. **Weber BG** (1977) Zur Operationstechnik der supramalleolären valgisierenden Osteotomie beim Erwachsenen. *Unfallheilkunde;* 80:191–193.
13. **Charnley J** (1953) *Compression arthrodesis.* Edinburgh and London: E & S Livingstone Ltd.
14. **Weber BG, Magerl F** (1985) *The external fixator.* Berlin Heidelberg New York Toky: Springer-Verlag.
15. **Weber BG** (1964) Die Behandlung der Sprunggelenks-Stauchungsbrüche nach biomechanischen Gesichtspunkten. *Hefte zur Unfallheilkunde;* 81:176–179.
16. **Weber BG** (1974) Knöchel, Fusswurzel und Mittelfuss: Frakturen und Bandverletzungen im oberen Sprunggelenk. Chirurgie der Gegenwart. München Berlin Wien: Urban & Schwarzenberg. Band 4, Unfallchirurgie: 1–46.
17. **Grob D, Simpson LA, Weber BG, et al.** (1985) Operative treatment of displaced talus fractures. *Clin Orthop;* (199): 88–96.
18. **Weber BG** (1964) Epiphysenfugen-Verletzungen. *Helv Chir Acta;* 31 (2):103–118.
19. **Weber BG** (1972) *Epiphyseal injuries: internal fixation of fractures of Aitken type 2 and 3.* Intern. Congress, Series No. 291. Excerpta Medica, Amsterdam: 867–868.
20. **Weber BG** (1974) Die Osteosynthesen epiphysennaher Frakturen einschliesslich der Korrektureingriffe: Die Osteosynthesen im Sprunggelenksbereich. *Aktuelle Traumatologie.* Stuttgart: Georg Thieme Verlag; 2:109–112.
21. **Weber BG** (1975) Das Besondere bei der Behandlung der Frakturen im Kindesalter. *Mschr. Unfallheilk;* 78:193–198.
22. **Weber BG, Brunner Ch, Freuler F** (1980) *Treatment of Fractures in Children and Adolescents.* Berlin Heidelberg New York: Springer-Verlag.
23. **Langenskiöld A** (1975) An operation for partial closure of an epiphyseal plate in children, and its experimental basis. *J Bone Joint Surg [Br];* 57 (3):325–330.
24. **Langenskiöld A, Videman T, Nevalainen T** (1986) The fate of fat transplants in operations for partial closure of the growth plate. Clinical examples and an experimental study. *J Bone Joint Surg [Br];* 68 (2):234–238.
25. **Weber BG** (1984) Reinraumtechnik in der orthopädischen Chirurgie. In: Draenert K, Rütt A, editors. *Erfahrungen mit dem operativen Gelenkersatz.* München: Art and Science: 117–123.
26. **Weber BG** (2000) MINIMAX-Prinzip für Osteosynthesen beim Erwachsenen. In: Dubs L, editor. *Orthopädie an der Schwelle.* Bern Göttingen Toronto Seattle: Huber: 19–133.
27. Kerkhoffs GM, Struijs PA, Raaymakers EL, et al. (2002) Functional treatment after surgical repair of acute Achilles tendon rupture: wrap vs walking cast. *Arch Orthop Trauma Surg;* 122 (2): 102–105.
28. **Weber BG, Marti R** (1972) *Rupture of the Achilles tendon. Suture and fuctional aftertreatment.* Intern. Congress, Series No. 291. Excerpta Medica, Amsterdam: 857–859.
29. **Hansen ST Jr** (2000) *Functional reconstruction of the foot and ankle.* Philadelphia: Lippincott Williams & Wilkins.
30. **Kerkhoffs GM, Rowe BH, Assendelft WJ, et al.** (2001) Immobilisation for acute ankle sprain. A systematic review. *Arch Orthop Trauma Surg;* 121 (8):462–471.
31. **Grob D, Weber BG** (1981) [Primary suturing of fresh fibular ligament ruptures—technique and results of 500 cases.] *Z Unfallmed Berufskr;* 74 (1/2):63–64.
32. **Weber BG** (1968) Fussdistorsion. *Z Unfallmed Berufskr;* 130–136.
33. **Weber BG** (1977) Ligament injuries of the foot and their repair. In: Injuries of the ligaments and their repairs. Stuttgart: Thieme: 186–190.

6 Biodynamics, classification, and treatment of nonunions

1 Introduction

The healing process of a fresh fracture depends on three factors [1]:

1. The vascularity of the fragments, since without vascularity, osteogenesis does not begin.
2. The reduction or anatomical approximation of the fragments.
3. The stability of the fracture.

These three requirements or preconditions are equally important for both conservative and surgical fracture treatment.

If fracture ossification does not occur, the result is nonunion. The cause of such nonunion is usually related to the three above-mentioned factors; or rather, to the absence of one or more of these factors [2].

Current treatment of fractures leads to fewer nonunions and pseudarthroses than previous treatment regimens. After conservative management (or non surgical treatment), nonunions that typically develop are hypertrophic nonunions; after surgical treatment, hypertrophy is not seen very often. In fact, the opposite occurs with a certain atrophy of the fragments recognized on x-rays.

The scintigraphic and scintometric studies at our former institution illustrate the following points [3–6] (Fig. 6-1a–b).

- Non-infected nonunions are, as a rule, better vascularized than an fresh fracture, independent of whether the nonunion shows a hypertrophic or an atrophic change of the bone on the x-ray (Fig. 6-1a).
- Infected nonunions, as a rule, are more poorly vascularized than a fresh fracture (Fig. 6-1b).

In other words, one nonunion is biologically hyperactive or active, and the other is biologically inactive. The physician must plan the treatment of the nonunion based on the bioactivity. Therefore, a reliable classification of nonunions is of utmost importance.

Vascularized—ie, active nonunion	
• Hypertrophy • Porosis • Atrophy	• Vascularity BETTER than normal

Poorly vascularized—ie, inactive nonunion	
• Necrosis • Resorption • Defect	• Vascularity POORER than normal

Fig. 6-1a–b The two groups of nonunions based on x-ray appearance and scintography-scintometry.
a Biologically active nonunions.
b Biologically inactive nonunions.

2 The biodynamic classification of nonunions [7, 8]

The radiological history of a nonunion and, if needed, scintographic studies have led to the following classification of nonunions:

- **Biologically active nonunions** are, as a rule, aseptic (Fig. 6-2a).
- **Biologically inactive nonunions** are, as a rule, septic or have been septic sometime in their history.

Particularly typical of this condition are nonunions with a defect (Fig. 6-2b).

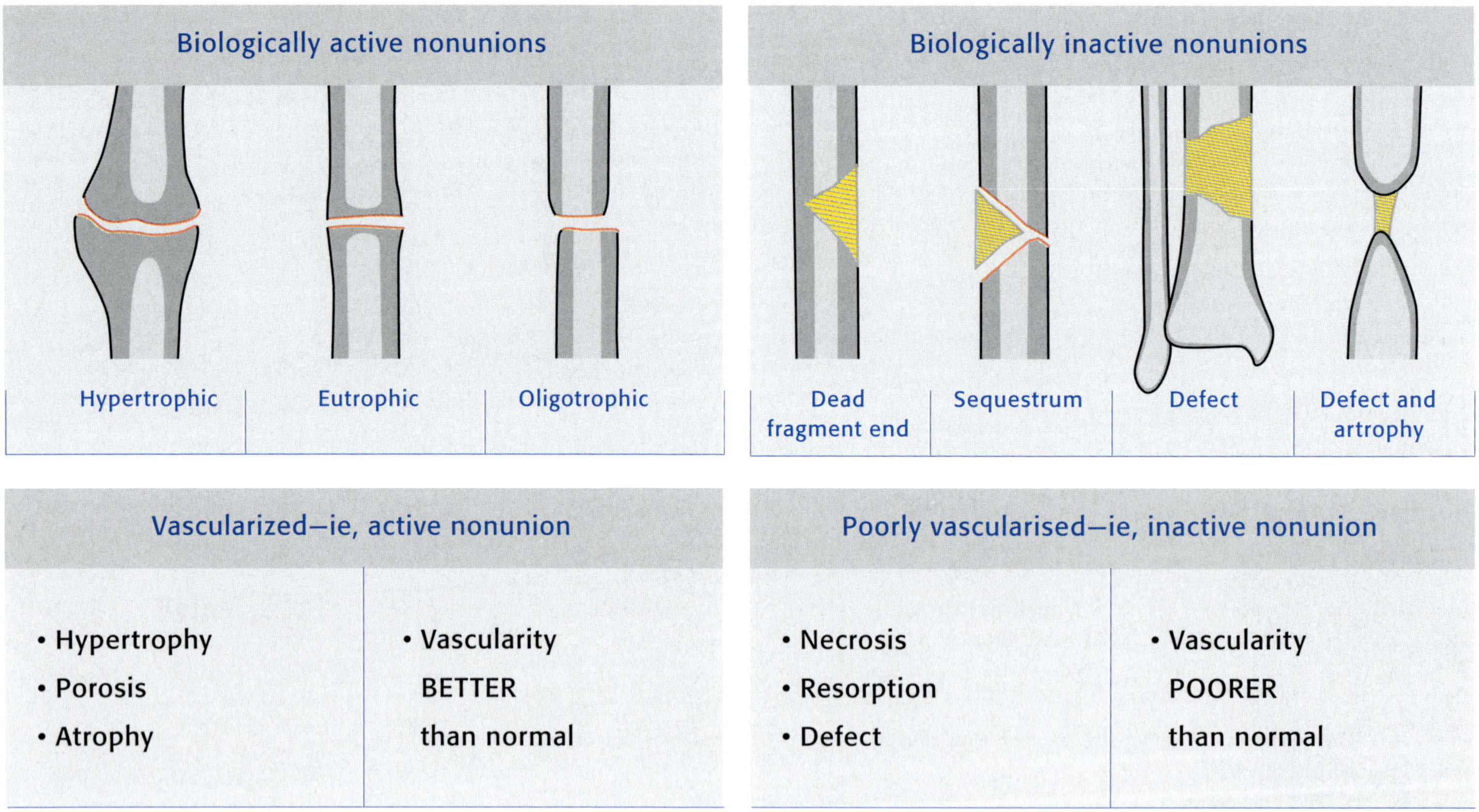

Fig. 6-2a–b X-ray appearance of nonunions.
a Biologically active nonunions.
b Biologically inactive nonunions.

3 The treatment of nonunions based on their bioactivity [2, 7, 8]

The treatment of a nonunion must be directed along the bioactivity of the fragment ends. In addition to the bioactivity of the fragment ends, the treating physician must take into consideration the septic vs aseptic property of the nonunion [9].

3.1 The treatment of aseptic nonunions

Fig. 6-3a–b show how the treatment must be directed for the aseptic nonunion. Fig. 6-4–6-5 are typical case examples.

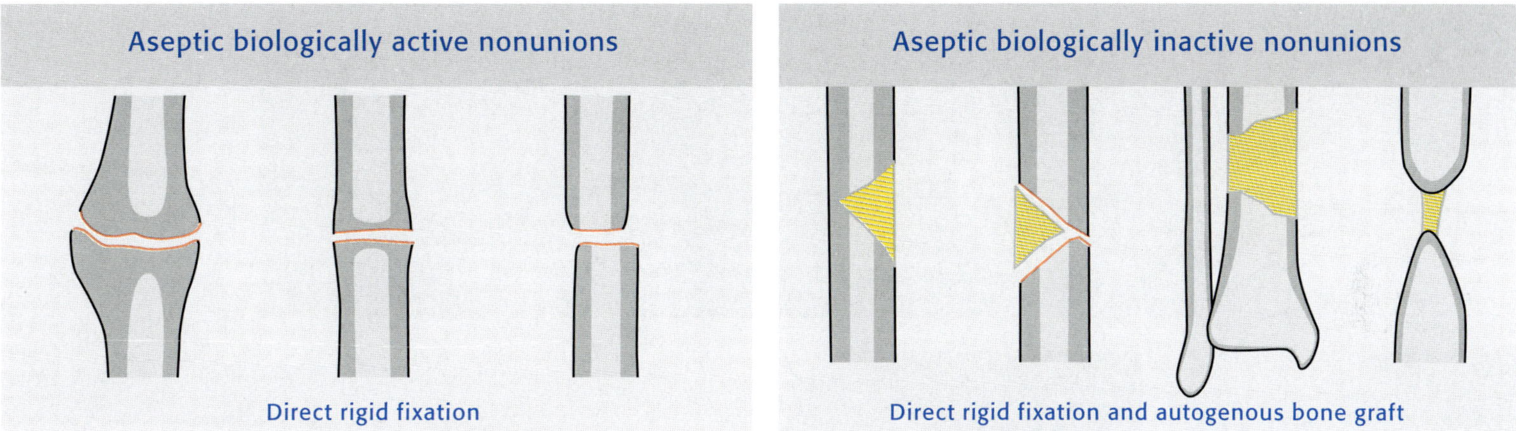

Fig. 6-3a–b The basic treatment of aseptic nonunions.
a Biologically active nonunions.
b Biologically inactive nonunions.

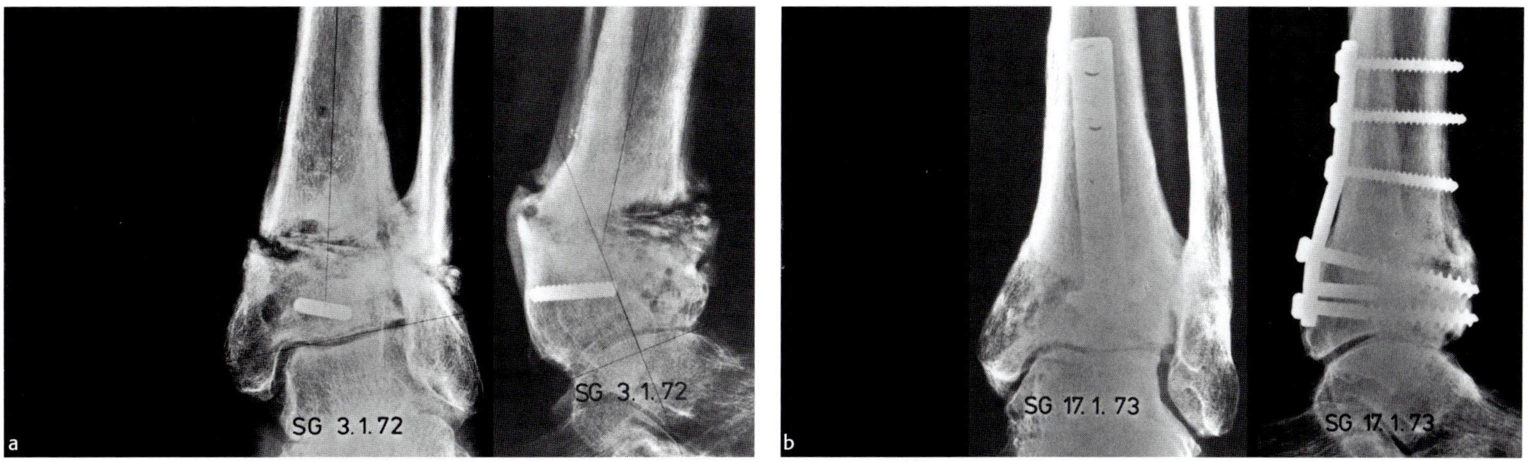

Fig. 6-4a–b Hypertrophic aseptic nonunion.
a 3 years after fracture, internal fixation, and metal removal.
b 1 year after compression plating.

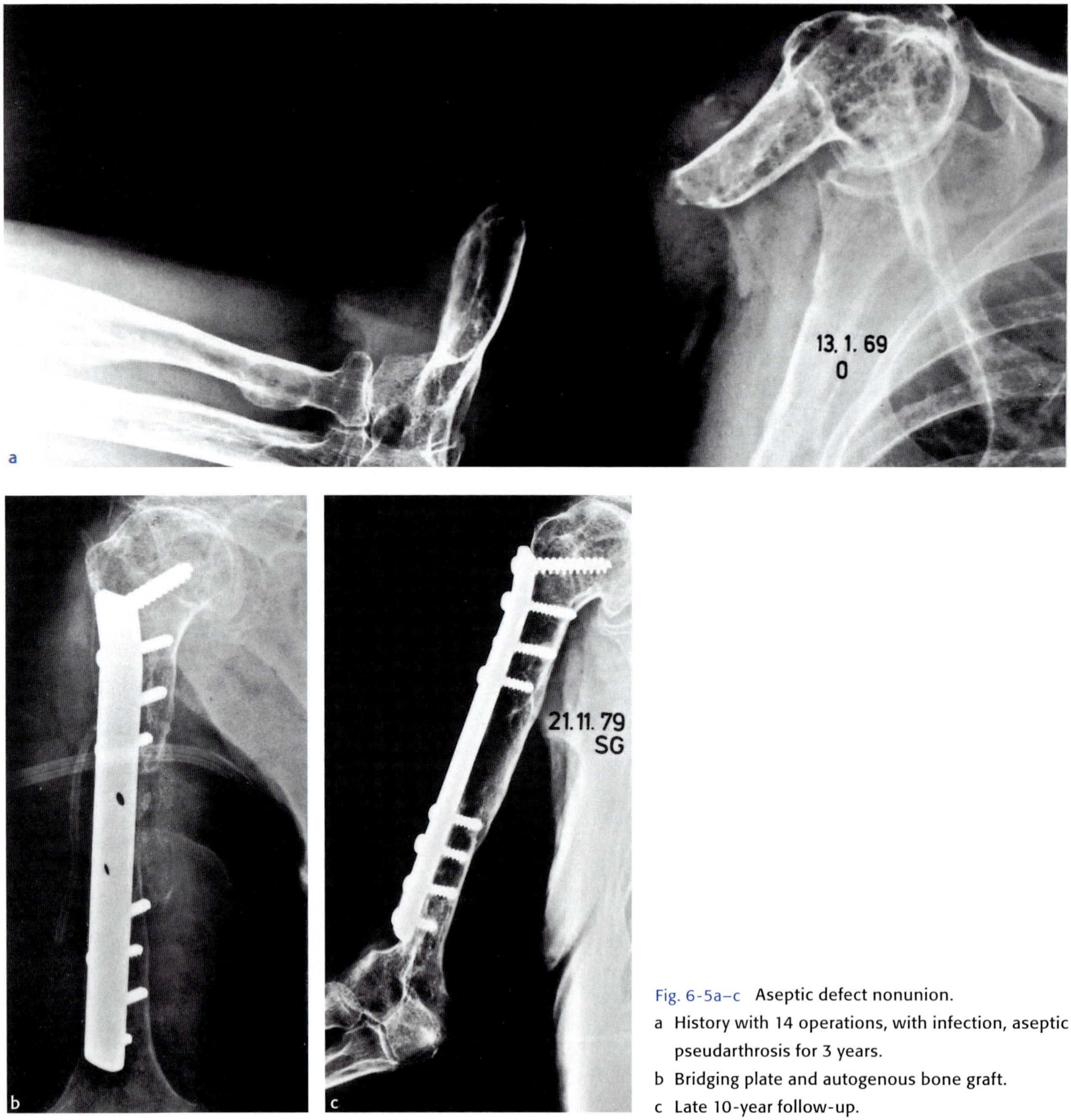

Fig. 6-5a–c Aseptic defect nonunion.

a History with 14 operations, with infection, aseptic pseudarthrosis for 3 years.

b Bridging plate and autogenous bone graft.

c Late 10-year follow-up.

3.2 The treatment of septic nonunions

Fig. 6-6a–b summarize the treatment needs for septic nonunions. The three case examples in Fig. 6-7–6-9 are typical for that treatment.

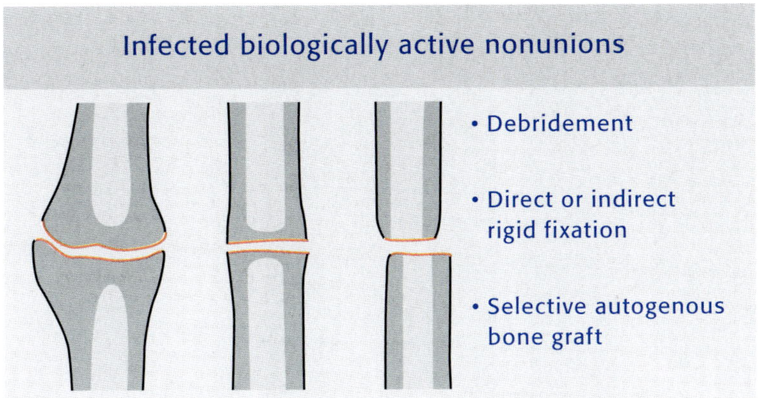

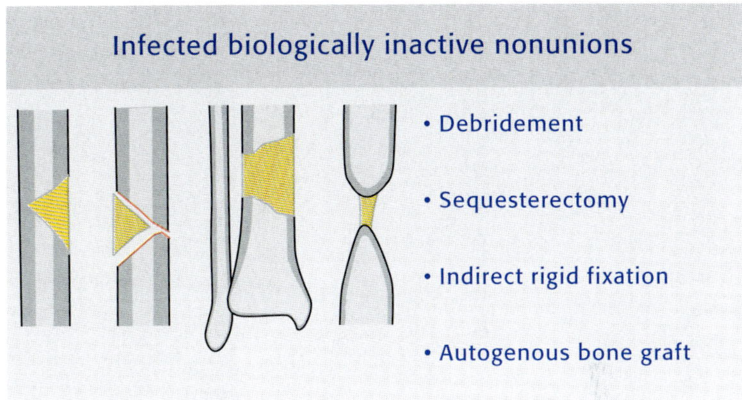

Fig. 6-6a–b The basic treatment of infected nonunions.
a Biologically active nonunions.
b Biologically inactive nonunions.

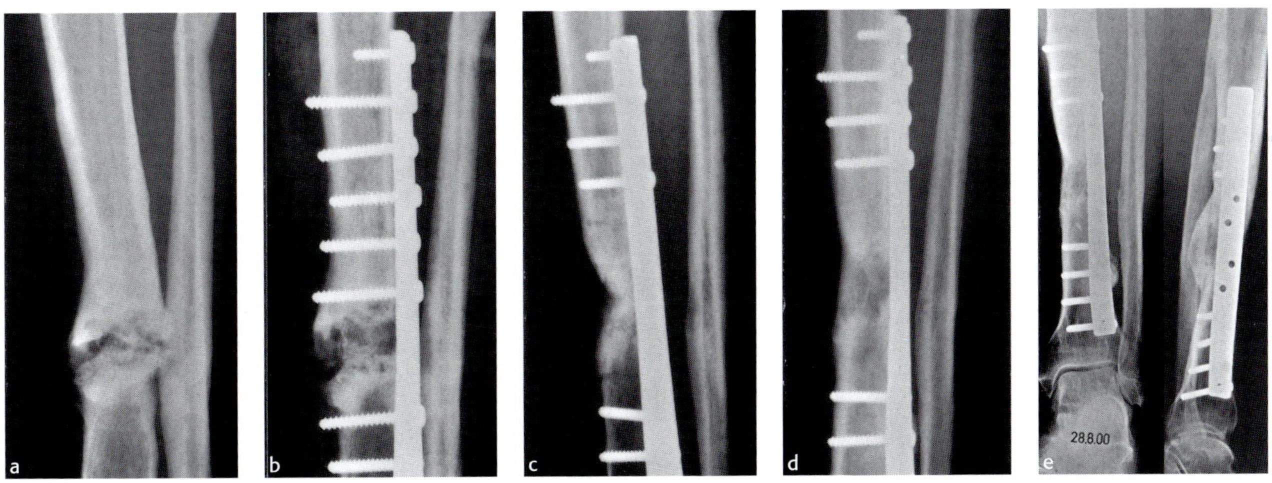

Fig. 6-7a–e Hypertrophic infected nonunion.
a 4 years after open fracture, septic drainage.
b Bridging plate from a sound lateral approach. 3 weeks later, debridement.
c 1 year later, three screws near the nonunion are removed. Posteromedial bone grafting.
d 4-year result.
e Late 20-year follow-up. No symptoms left.

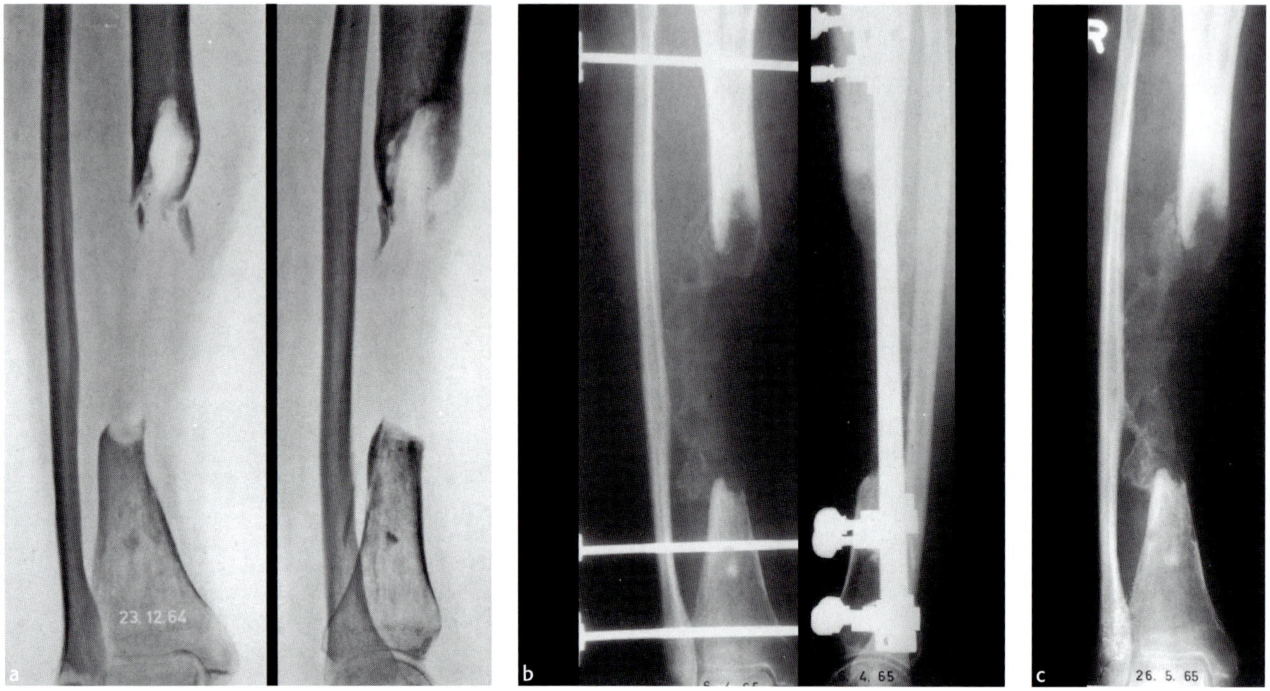

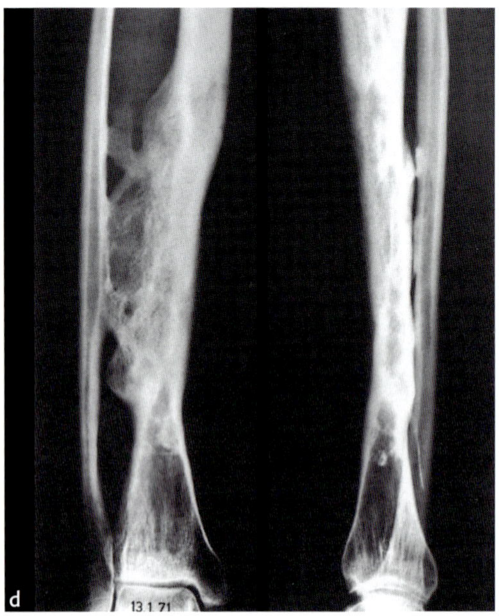

Fig. 6-8a–d Infected defect nonunion.

a Defect, sequestra, drainage. 3 years after fracture, plating, and sequestration of midshaft.

b External fixator (frame), sequestrectomy and autogenous bone graft from a sound lateral approach (Harmon approach). External fixator for 5 months.

c 18 months after inicial treatment.

d Late 6-year follow-up. Restored tibia.

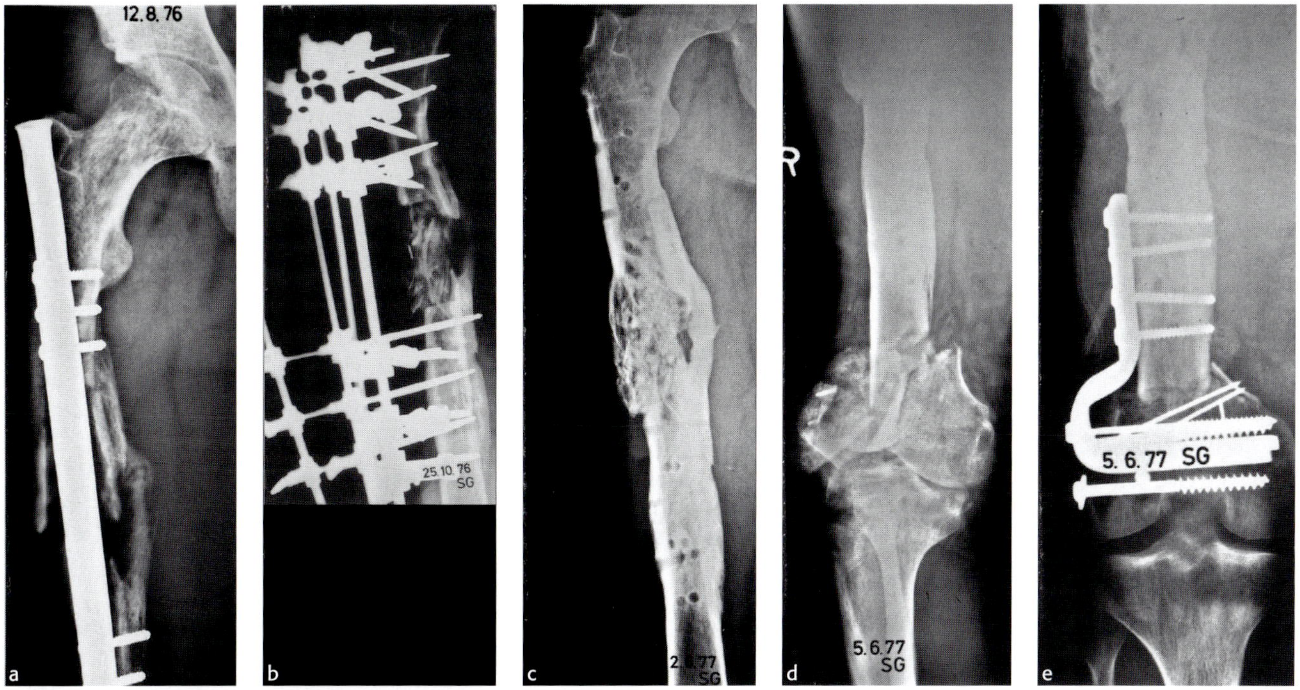

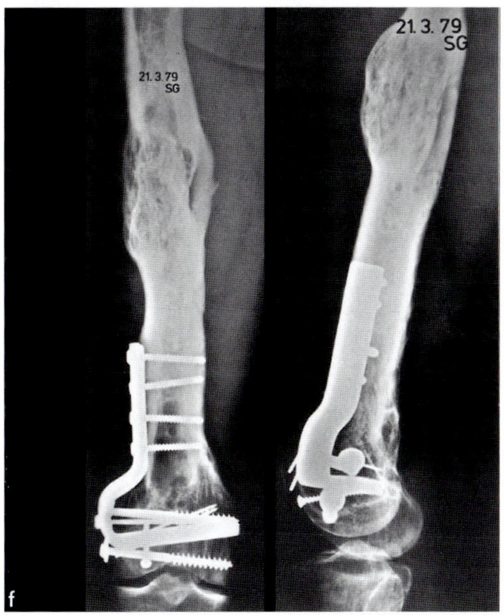

Fig. 6-9a–f Infected nonunion with extensive sequestration.

a The nonunion 2 years after fracture and internal fixation. Sequestra, drainage.

b Biplane unilateral external fixator. Sequestrectomy. Autogenous bone graft.

c The incorporation of the graft within 8 months.

de 8 months after the treatment of the nonunion: new motorcycle fracture and internal fixation.

f 2 1/2-year follow-up: nonunion and wfracture are healed.

4 Treatment knowledge and treatment results

In the setting of this article, we cannot enter into the complex treatment, operative technique, antibiotic regimens, and aftercare for handling nonunions. These areas are well discussed in other publications and the literature [2, 7, 8, 10].
As an example, the tibial nonunion selected from our monograph [7, 8] "Pseudarthroses" shows the following:

4.1 The treatment methods of tibial pseudarthrosis (Fig. 6-10–6-11)

Rigid fixation with a 'pressure' plate is predominantly used for treating aseptic pseudarthroses (Fig. 6-10). Only seldom is the intramedullary nail used, and when it is used, the rule is to use a thicker, more rigid nail rather than a thin intramedullary nail with insufficient stability. Only very seldom is a bone graft needed because the aseptic nonunion shows high bioactivity. It is almost always healed with one operation.

The majority of the infected nonunions (Fig. 6-11a) are stabilized with an external fixator [10]. Frequently one, sometimes two, and seldom a third operation with autogenous bone graft substitute are needed for lost bone substance. I prefer, for the most part, to use the autogenous bone graft over a fragment transport in the manner of Ilizarov.

The fragment transfer, which is of most interest biologically, can under certain circumstances (worst case) lead to an adventure for the patients, who are generally already sufficiently challenged. The healing of an infected nonunion almost always requires more operations than the initial procedure.

4.2 The results (Fig. 6-10–6-11)

The results are, as one would expect, better for the aseptic than the septic nonunions.

Surgery in 127 non-infected nonunions of the tibia		
• Plate	61	48.0%
• Nail	50	39.4%
• External fixator	8	6.3%
• Bone graft	8	6.3%
Consolidated with		
• 1 operation	112	88.0%
• >1 operation	15	12.0%

Results of 127 non-infected nonunions of the tibia	
• Sound union	126
• 'Rigid' nonunion	1

Fig. 6-10 The treatment means and results of 127 aseptic nonunions in the tibia.

Surgery in 122 infected nonunions of the tibia		
• External fixator	118	96%
• Plate	4	3%
• Bone graft	122	100%

Results of 122 infected nonunions of the tibia	
• Sound union without drainage	117
• 'Rigid' nonunion and drainage	2
• Amputation	3

Fig. 6-11 The treatment means and results of 122 infected nonunions of the tibia.

5 Conclusion

The treatment of nonunions based on the bioactivity of the fragments promises a very high success rate if the treatment used is surgically perfect. Under these circumstances, the healing process of a nonunion is in every case a biomechanically reproducible experiment with almost certain healing success. In the case of a Biologically active nonunion, which is the majority, results actually show faster ossification than a comparable fresh fracture. This is because the fragment ends have a better blood supply than they did at the time of the fresh injury. In the infected nonunion, it needs 3–4 times longer to heal because either the ends of the fragments are poorly vascularized or additionally the bone transplant first needs to vascularize and then be converted through functional stress rising (Wolff's law). Often, more operations are needed, but here the healing rate is also high.

6 Bibliography

Blue references indicate links to abstracts of articles online available through Medline (www.nlm.nih.gov).

1. **Cech O, Segmüller G** (1973) [Physiopathology of pseudoarthrosis.] *Helv Chir Acta;* 40 (1):259–262.
2. **Weber BG, Brunner C** (1981) The treatment of nonunions without electrical stimulation. *Clin Orthop;* (161):24–32.
3. **Segmüller G, Cech O, Bekier A** (1970) Diagnostic use of 85 strontium in the preoperative evaluation of nonunion. *Acta Orthop Scand;* 41 (2): 150–160.
4. **Segmüller G, Cech O, Bekier A** (1970) 85-Sr uptake study in nonunion in man. *Eur Surg Res;* 2 (3):226–232.
5. **Segmüller G** (1971) [Functional diagnosis of pseudarthrosis with the use of 85-Sr-scintimetry.] *Ther Umsch;* 28 (5):329–332.
6. **Segmüller G** (1973) Spätphasen der Frakturheilung ermittelt mit Hilfe der Szintimetrie. *Hefte zur Unfallheilkunde;* 117:263–270.
7. **Weber BG, Cech O** (1973) *Pseudarthrosen.* Bern Stuttgart Wien: Hans Huber.
8. **Weber BG, Cech O** (1976) *Pseudarthrosis.* Bern Stuttgart Wien: Hans Huber.
9. **Segmüller G, Cech O, Bekier A** (1969) [Osteogenetic activity in the area of pseudarthroses of the long tubular bones.] *Z Orthop Ihre Grenzgeb;* 106 (3):599–609.
10. **Weber BG, Magerl F** (1985) *The External Fixator.* Berlin Heidelberg New York Tokyo: Springer-Verlag.

7 Autogenous bone transplantation

1 Introduction

Autogenous bone is the best available material to compensate for local bone defect. When harvested and instantly transplanted to a new vascularized site, autogenous bone continues to live. It does not cause immunological rejection phenomena and does not transmit foreign diseases.

Autogenous bone remodels under the new local strain into an optimal architectural structure according to Wolff's law.

In all respects, autogenous bone is superior to all other currently available substances.

Autogenous bone has three inconveniences, however:

1. Limited quantities available.
2. Potential morbidity at the harvest site.
3. Bone harvest is an additional operation, not only for the patient but also for the surgeon.

These three inconveniences of autogenous bone explain our use of substitutes, which are ready made and available from the shelf in unlimited quantity.

2 Purpose of the chapter on autogenous bone

The purpose of this chapter is to demonstrate the potential of autogenous bone grafting, which has been stupendous for me over some 45 years of professional activity.

Three aspects are discussed in this chapter:
1. Harvesting of autogenous bone.
2. The preparation of the host site.
3. Clinical examples to demonstrate the biological potential of transplanted autogenous bone.

Ilizarov callus distraction is beyond my personal experience. For lengthening, the Synthes threaded-rod external fixator or the Wagner device were preferred.

3 Harvesting sites of autogenous bone

According to the individual requirements, different harvest sites are used:

1. Bone is harvested next to the host site when only a small amount of bone is required: proximal ulna, distal radius, greater trochanter, tibial head, distal tibia (Fig. 7-1a–b).
2. The medial tibial surface may offer a long corticocancellous graft defect (Fig. 7-2).
3. Vascular pedicled graft: iliac crest, fibular shaft.
4. The most frequently used donor site is the ilium for larger amounts of autogenous bone, either from an anterior or a posterior approach. As a rule one donor site offers enough bone, however, sometimes two iliac crests are exploited in the same session or in stages (Fig. 7-3a–d).

To reduce local morbidity, the harvesting operation needs meticulous technical performance: exposure of the iliac crest, anatomical reconstruction of soft tissues, prevention of hematoma by bleeding control, and suction drainage.

The most serious morbidity is damage to the lateral femoral cutaneous nerve, the iliohypogastric nerve, and the ilioinguinal nerve, all of which are on their course to the periphery in close relationship to the spina iliaca ventralis and the iliac crest (Lanz and Wachsmuth).

The anterior iliac crest is safely exposed from a skin incision 2 cm distal and parallel to the crest. The spina iliaca ventralis is localized by palpation only, but strictly spared from further preparation.

The abdominal muscles along the crest are dissected. The medial wall of the ilium is cleared subperiosteally.

In contrast, the approach to the posterior donor site should strictly concentrate on the spina ilica dorsalis cranialis by blunt preparation after skin incision, aiming not to damage the nervi clunium craniales. The origin of the musculus gluteus maximus is detached and the outer surface of the ilium next to the spina ilica dorsalis cranialis is superiostally exposed.

At both sites, bone is harvested with various chisels or with an oscillating saw. Whenever possible, the iliac crest is respected and detached muscles are sutured back anatomically, if needed, transosseally.

Prior to muscle reconstruction, the donor site is packed with gel-foam (gelatine) and a suction drain prevents postoperative hematoma.

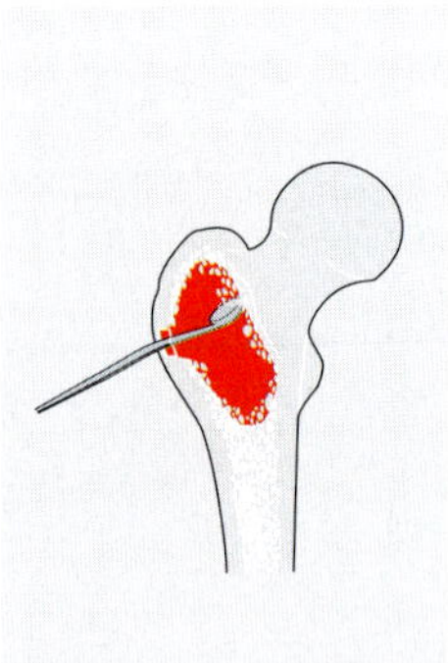

a

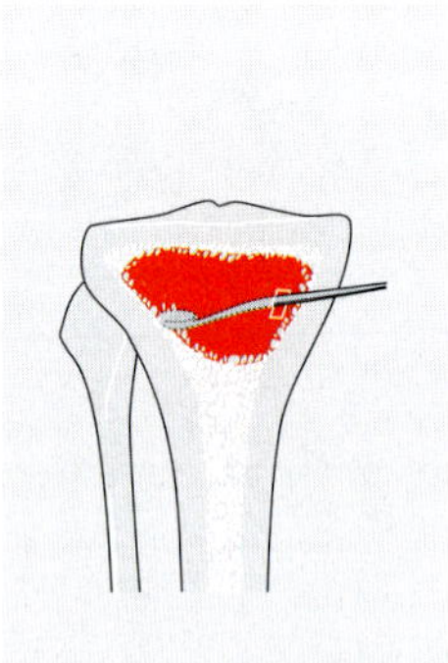

b

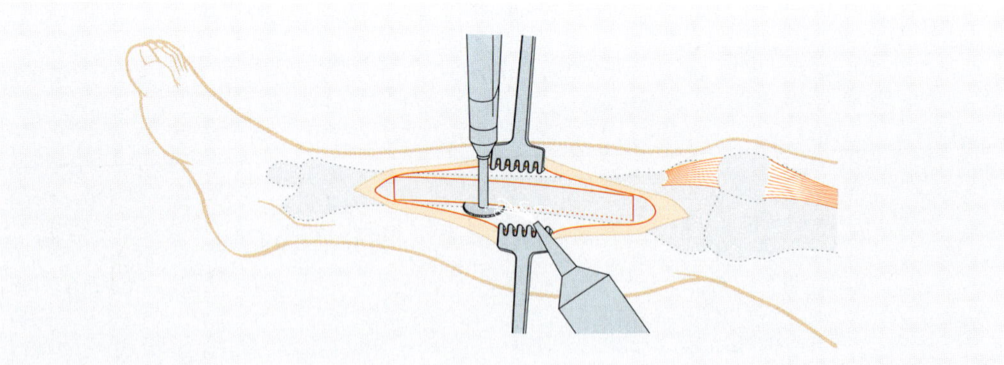

Fig. 7-1a–b Bone is harvested next to the host site, when only a small amount of bone is required.

Fig. 7-2 Medial tibial surface may offer a long corticocancellous graft defect

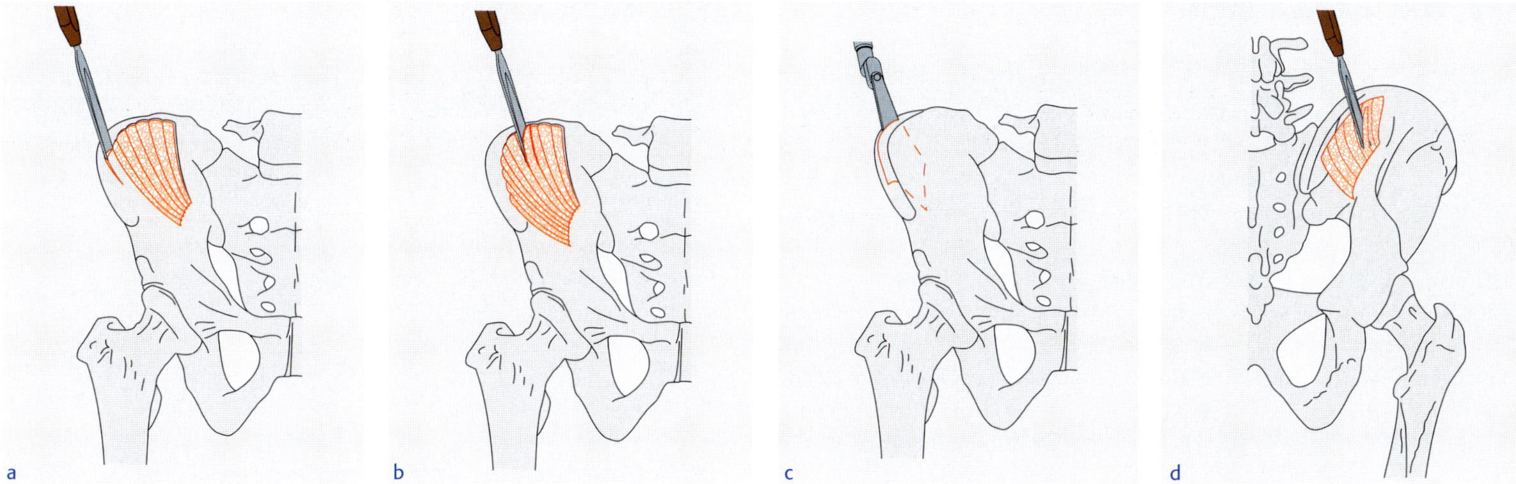

Fig. 7-3a–d Bone grafts taken from the ilium.

ab Patient in supine position. Grafts taken from the inner wall of the ilium with graft chisels, in layers.

c Corticocancellous graft cut with the saw. The outer rim of the crest is left intact for reattachment of muscles.

d The patient in a prone position. The grafts are taken from the outer iliac wall. One third of the iliac crest should be spared for anatomical reconstruction.

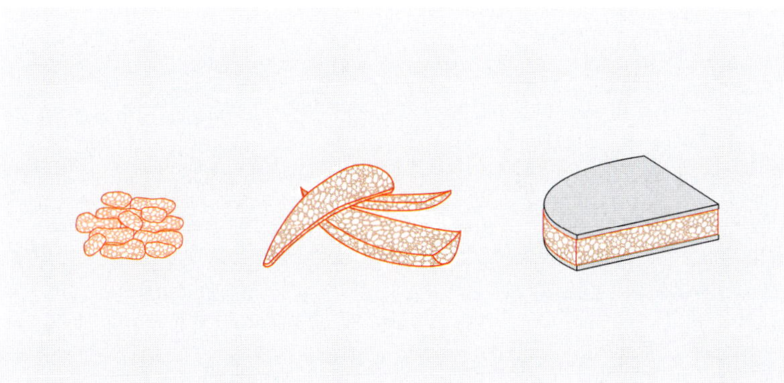

Fig. 7-4 Graft configuration.
Small cancellous pieces, strips or flakes. Corticocancellous blocks.

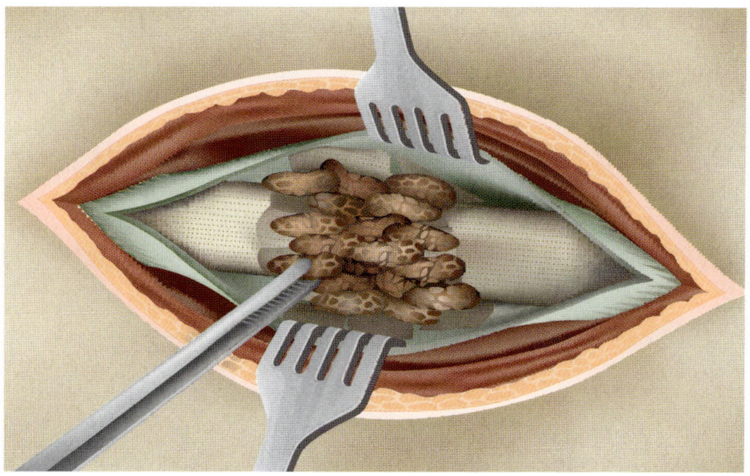

Fig. 7-5 Decortication.
The shaft bone is shingled to create a pouch of small vascularized fragments. The pouch is filled with autogenous cancellous grafts.

4 Host site preparation

The host site should be aseptic, well vascularized, and mechanically stable, which will allow the transplanted autogenous bone to be incorporated and revascularized rapidly. It undergoes remodeling according to Wolff's law under the condition that the transplant area is submitted to increasing normal strain and stress, ie, to continuous active function (CAF).

The only indications for grafting under septic conditions are selected septic nonunions and selected cases of osteomyelitis (Judet, Weber and Cech, Papineau). Nowadays, instead of bone grafting in the septic area, flap coverage is first performed. Bone compensation is delayed until the infection has disappeared. Nevertheless, we report our experience with one example out of many successes without additional flap surgery.

The sooner the blood perfuses from the surrounding tissues to the bone grafts, the better the mechanical stability at the host site, and the faster the grafts are integrated. The better the CAF, the quicker the graft remodels and self-augments the transplanted bone mass.

In contrast: Bone grafts that are not submitted to strain, suffering from blood supply and mechanical protection, undergo resorption.

5 Clinical examples

The main purpose of the examples is to demonstrate the behavior of transplanted autogenous bone, its integration and its transformation, independent of location and indication. The examples also demonstrate the indications for autogenous bone grafting to solve orthopedic and trauma problems.

The examples may confirm or develop confidence in autogenous bone grafting. It is self evident that every example opens the question of an alternative treatment.

5.1 Spine fusions

According to the underlying pathology, fusions of spine segments, singular or multiple, are either performed in situ, with distraction of intervertebral space, after reduction of deformity, or to compensate for a defect.

Tumor-related problems are not discussed here. The specific stabilizations are mainly mechanical or instrumental without the use of autogenous bone.

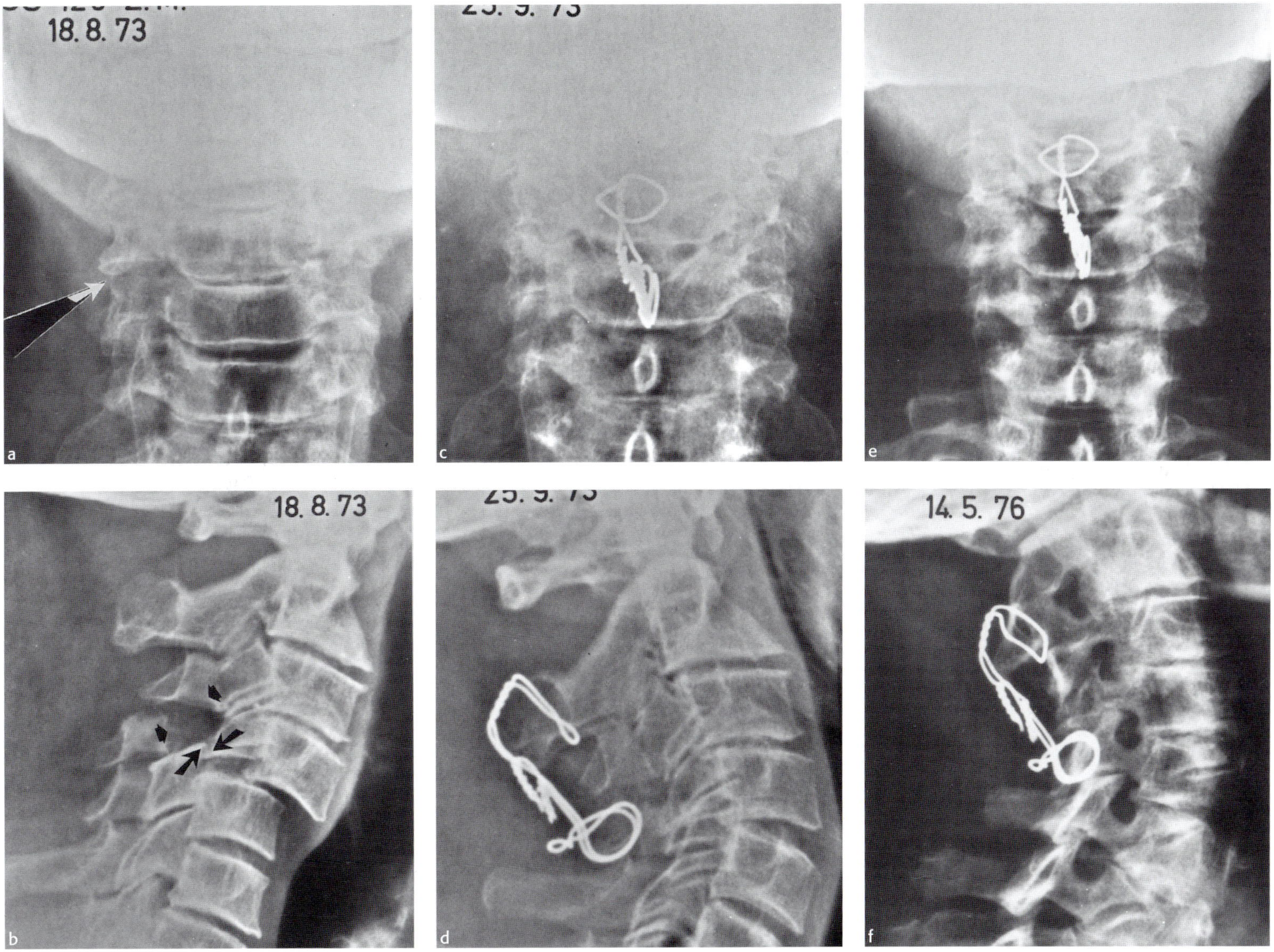

Fig. 7-6a–f Dislocation fracture C4/C5 with tetraparesis.

ab Forward displacement 50% of C4, dislocation of the facet joints (arrows), fracture of the arch that saved the medulla oblongata from crash (arrows).

cd 7 weeks postoperative: excision of the broken arch and the spinous process C5, open reduction of dislocation of the facet joints. The spinous process of C2 is banded to the arch of C5, the resected arch C4 and the spinous process C5 are used for local posterior grafting, together with cancellous grafts from the posterior iliac spine.

ef At 2 years 9 months: stability is present, the wire loop is unbroken, therefore the grafts have fused the segments C2/C3/C4/C5.

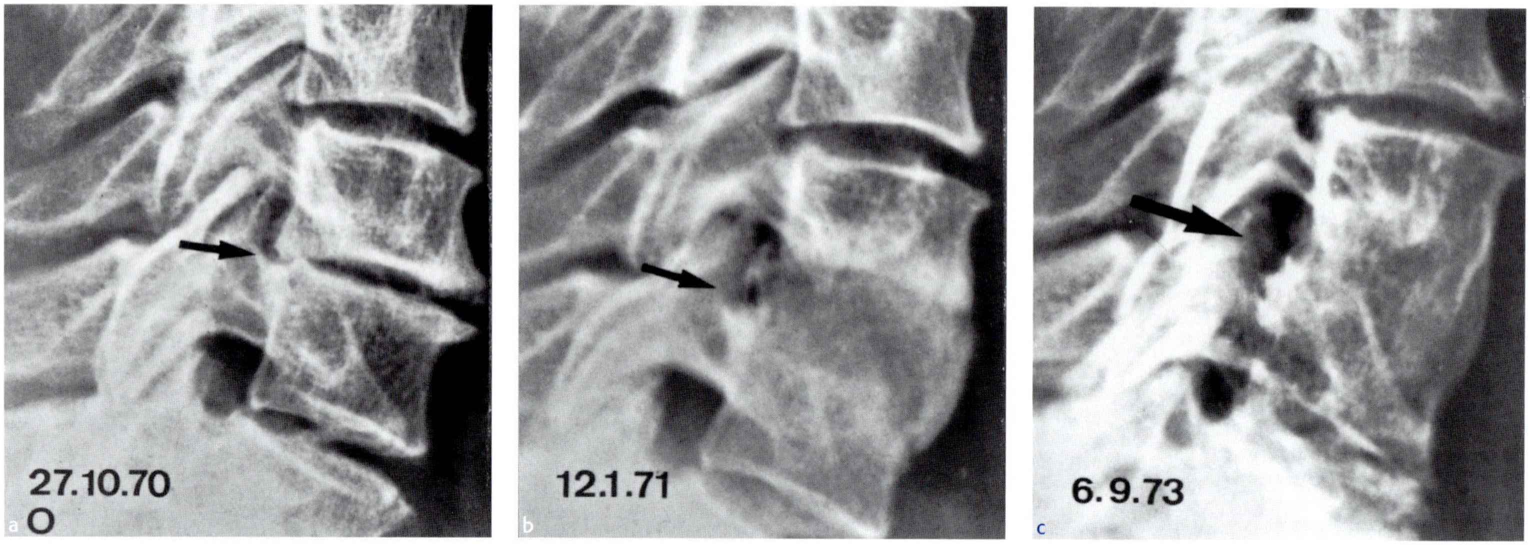

Fig. 7-7a–c Degenerated disc C5/C6 with neurological symptoms root C6.

a Degenerated disk with posterior spondylotic spur (arrow) and with narrowing of the intervertebral foramen.

b 2 months after transdiscal decompression (arrow) and fusion with distraction, ie, widening the intervertebral space.

c At 3 years: sound fusion, widened intervertebral foramen (arrow).

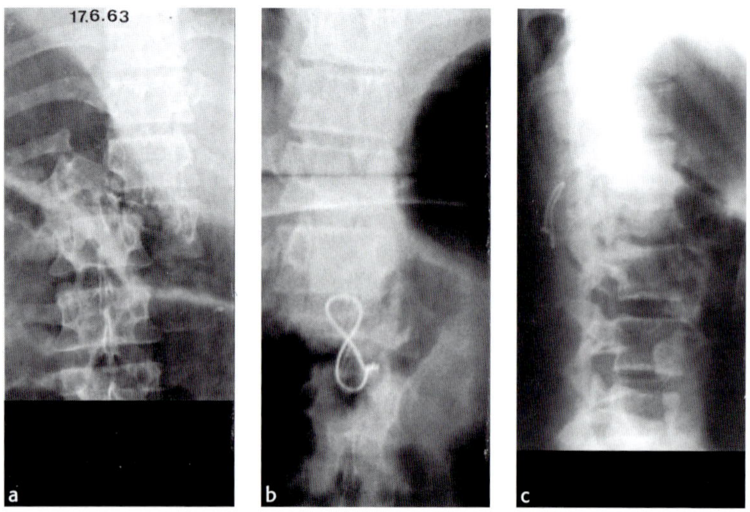

Fig. 7-8a–h Fracture dislocation L1 with complete paraplegia.

a The fracture. Lumbar puncture: yellow liquor, no blood. Queckenstedt negative, ie, neural structures are not disrupted, there is a chance of recovery with decompression.

bc Open reduction, decompression, hemivertebrectomy L1, preliminary fixation with interspinous wire loop and bone cement: dural sack was found intact, but contused or stretched.

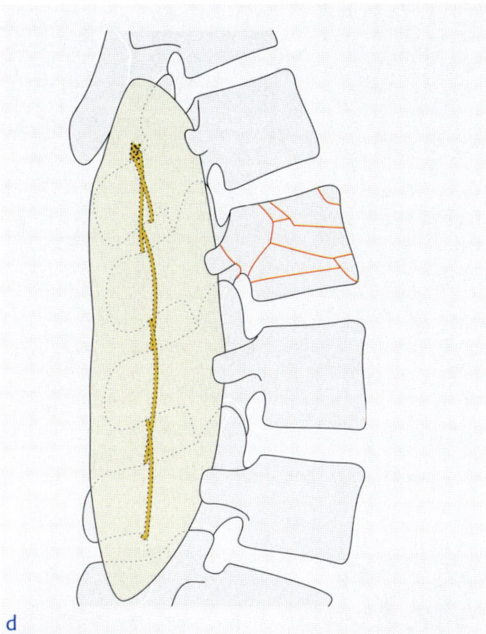

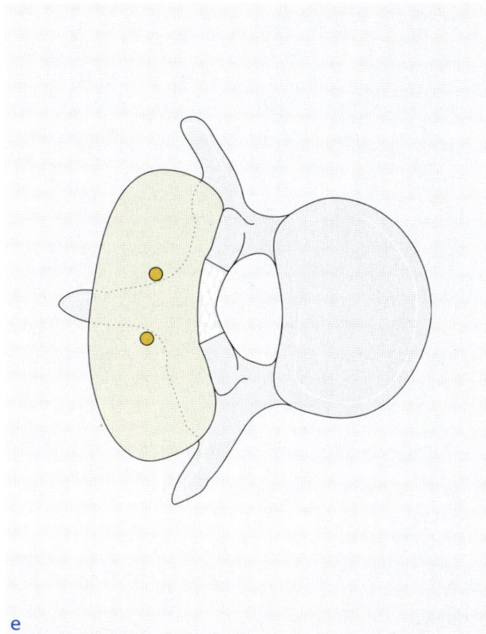

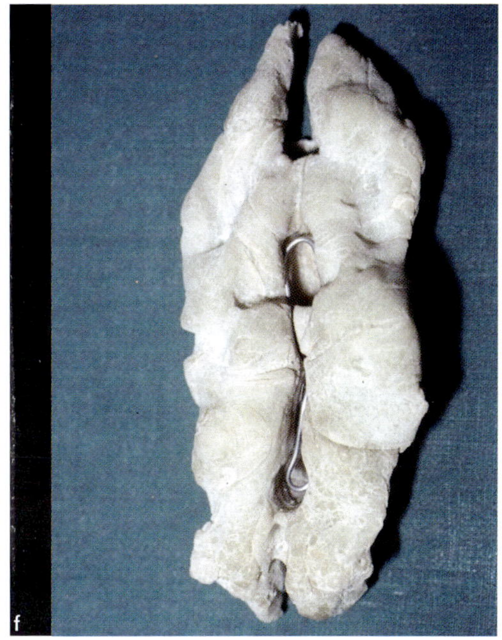

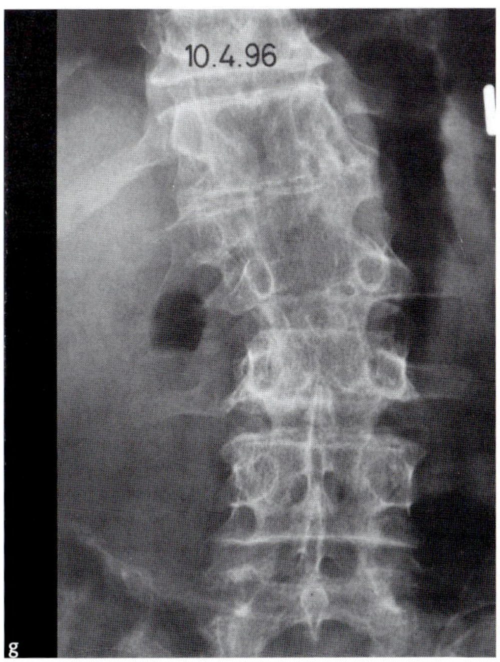

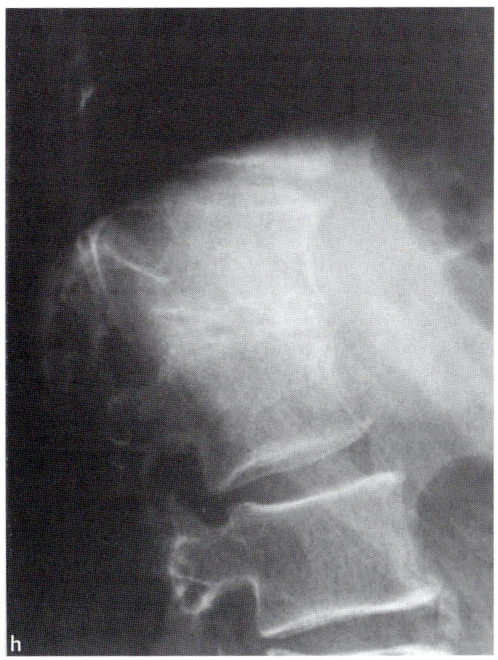

Fig. 7-8a–h cont.

de Preliminary fixation with wire loop and bone cement mass that incorporates the adjacent spinous processes.

f The removed preliminary fixation device 10 weeks after injury. It is replaced with autogenous posterior grafting. Neurological recovery has started at that stage.

gh At 33 years: The spine is fused between T12 and L2 after subtotal vertebrectomy L1 and posterior fusion. Remaining neurological consequence: mild peroneal palsy on one side.

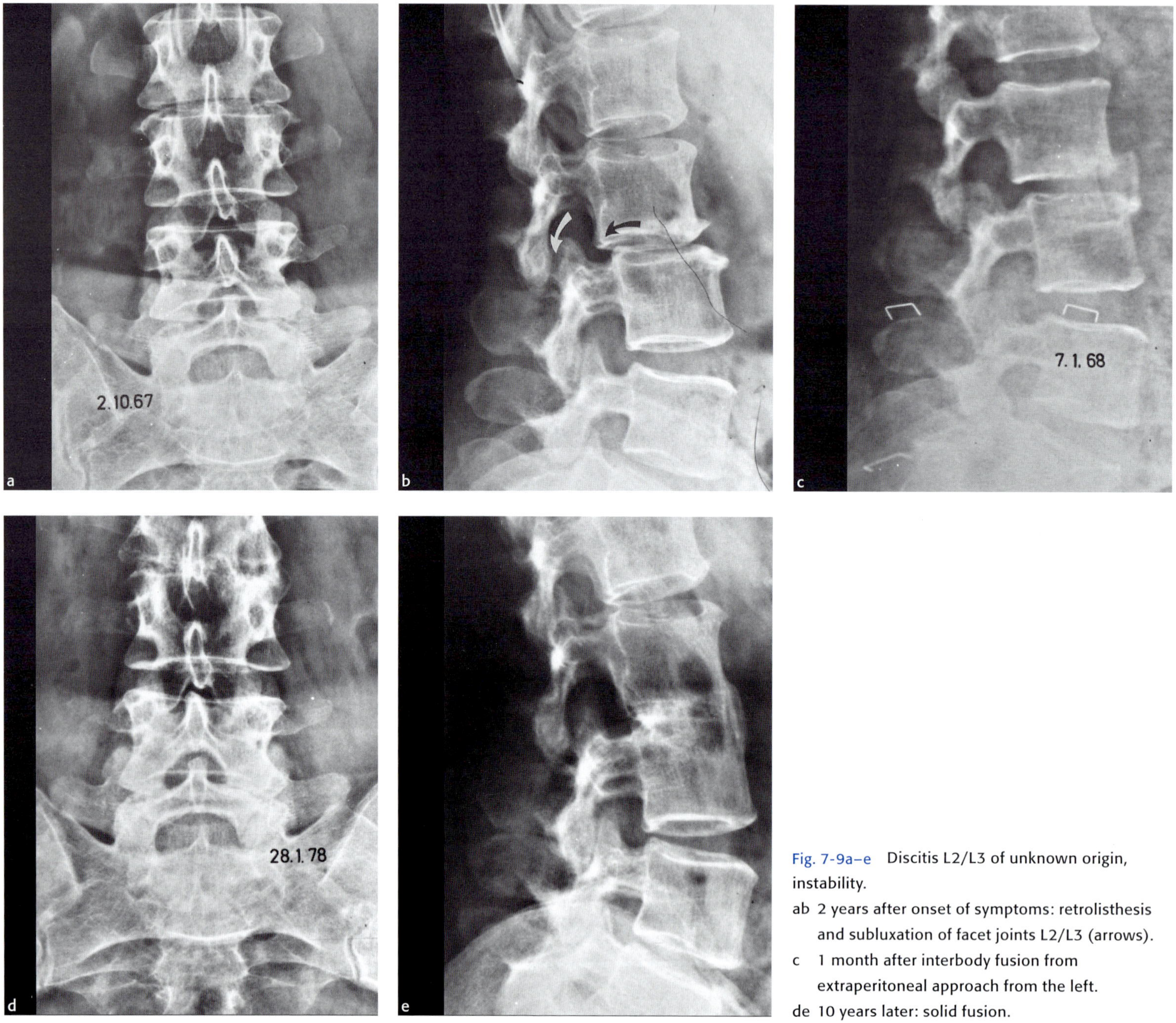

Fig. 7-9a–e Discitis L2/L3 of unknown origin, instability.

ab 2 years after onset of symptoms: retrolisthesis and subluxation of facet joints L2/L3 (arrows).

c 1 month after interbody fusion from extraperitoneal approach from the left.

de 10 years later: solid fusion.

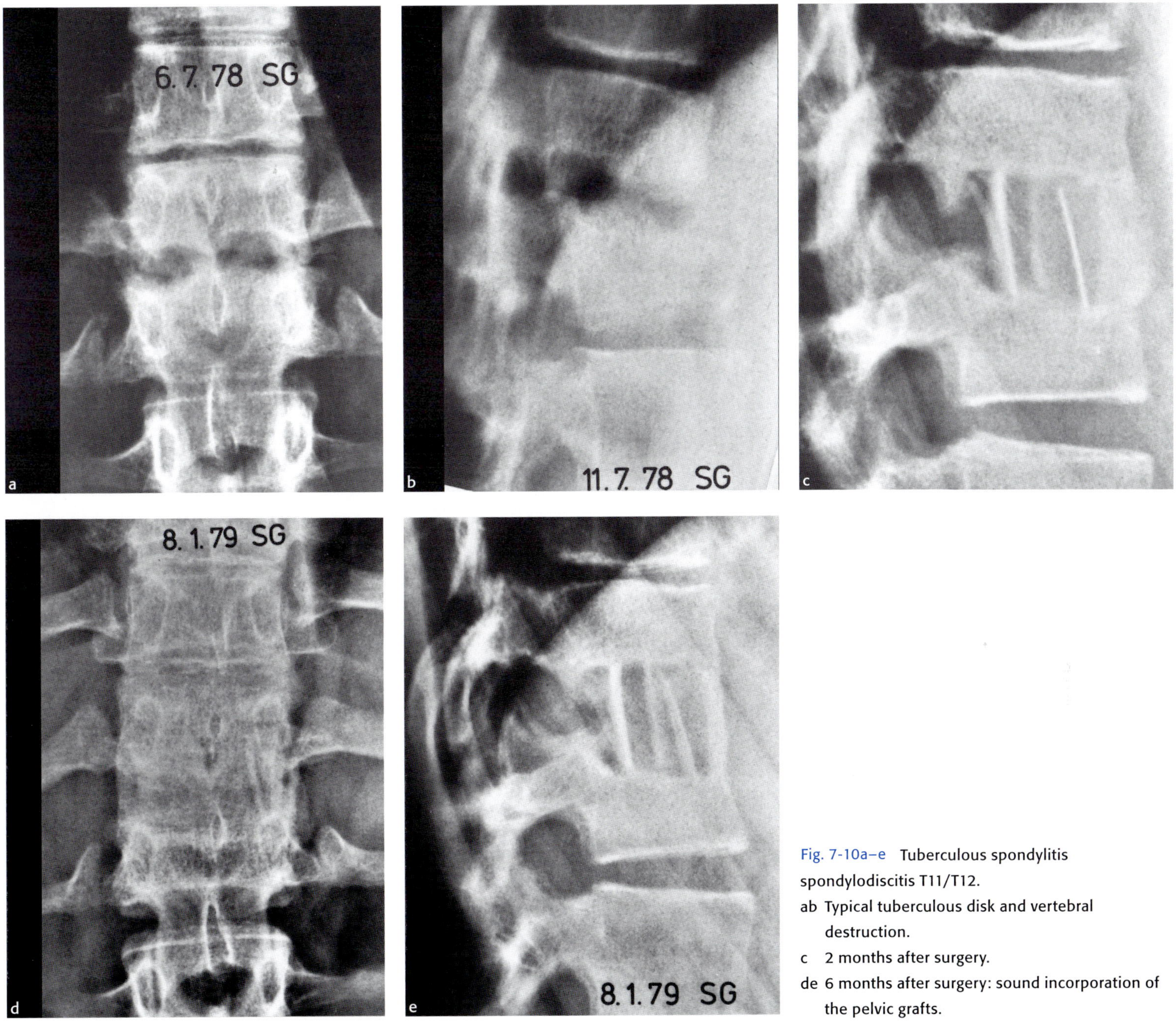

Fig. 7-10a–e Tuberculous spondylitis spondylodiscitis T11/T12.

ab Typical tuberculous disk and vertebral destruction.

c 2 months after surgery.

de 6 months after surgery: sound incorporation of the pelvic grafts.

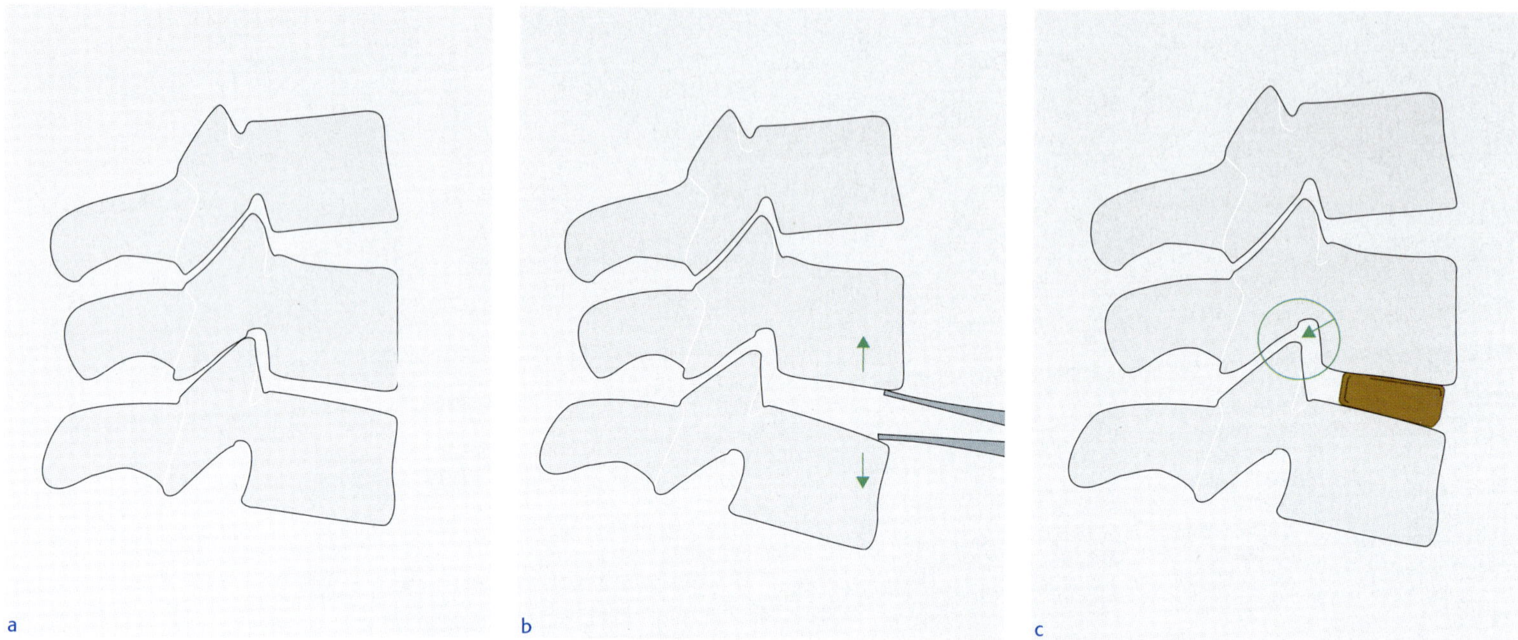

Fig. 7-11a–c Technique of interbody fusion with distraction to enlarge the intervertebral foramen.

a The narrowed disk space and intervertebral foramen.

b Spreading or distraction after disk resection.

c The distraction is maintained with pelvic grafts. The intervertebral foramen is widened (arrow).

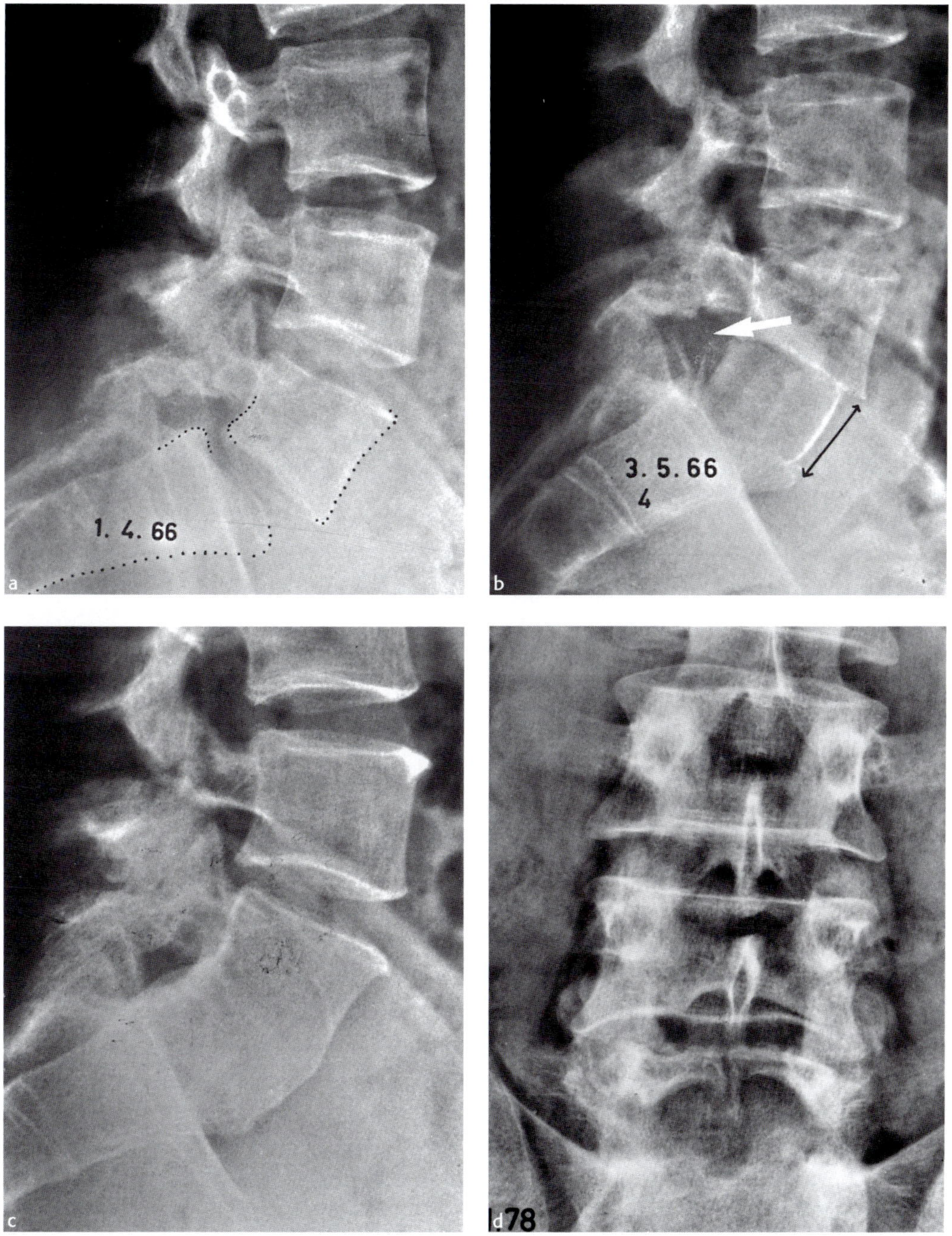

Fig. 7-12a–d Disk degeneration L5/S1, distraction-fusion.

a Narrowing of disk space and intervertebral foramen, pseudolisthesis.

b Distraction fusion with corticocancellous bone blocks. Widened intervertebral foramen (arrow).

cd 12 years later: solid distraction-fusion.

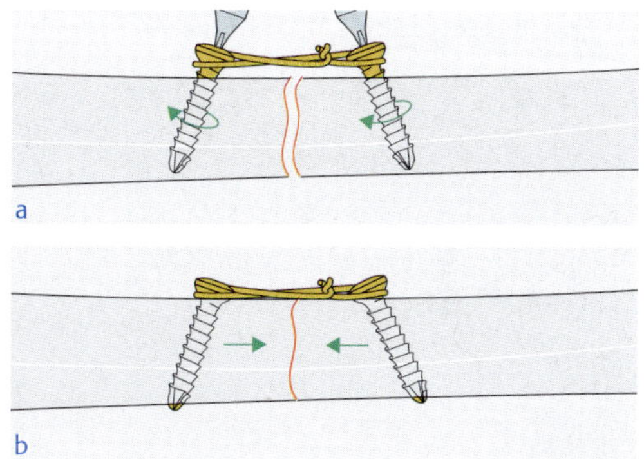

Fig. 7-13a–b Technique of tension-band fixation. When intrinsic stability of an intervertebral fusion is doubtful, a metallic internal fixation is added.

a Two divergent screws, not yet tightened, are joined with a tight wire-loop.

b When the screws are tightened, the two fragments are compressed and stabilized in accordance with the tension-band principle.

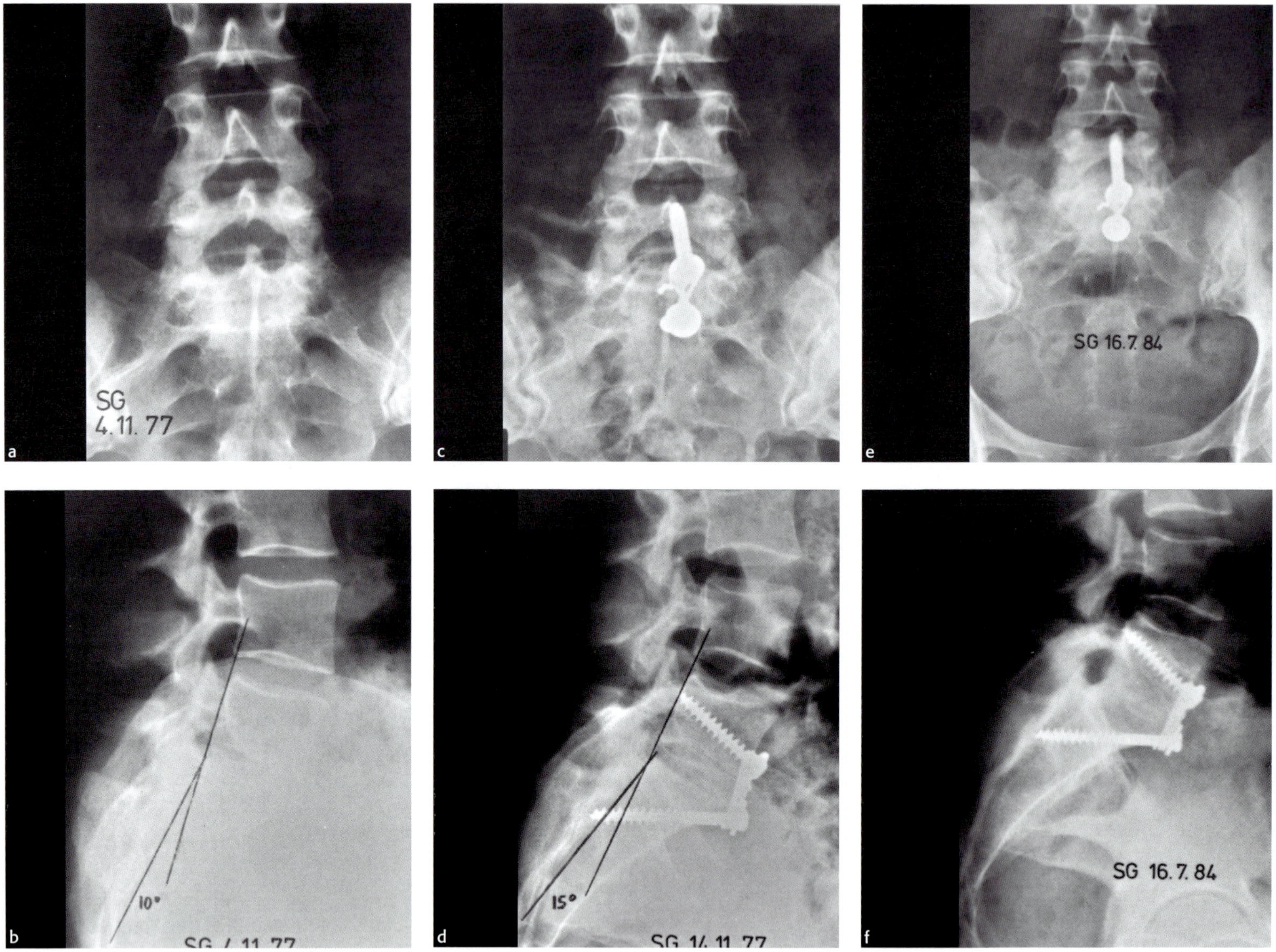

Fig. 7-14a–f Distraction-fusion and tension-band fixation for disk degeneration L5/S1.

ab Narrowed disk space and narrowed intervertebral foramen.

cd The distraction-fusion and the tension-band fixation.

ef 7 years later: Solid interbody fusion and wide open intervertebral foramen.

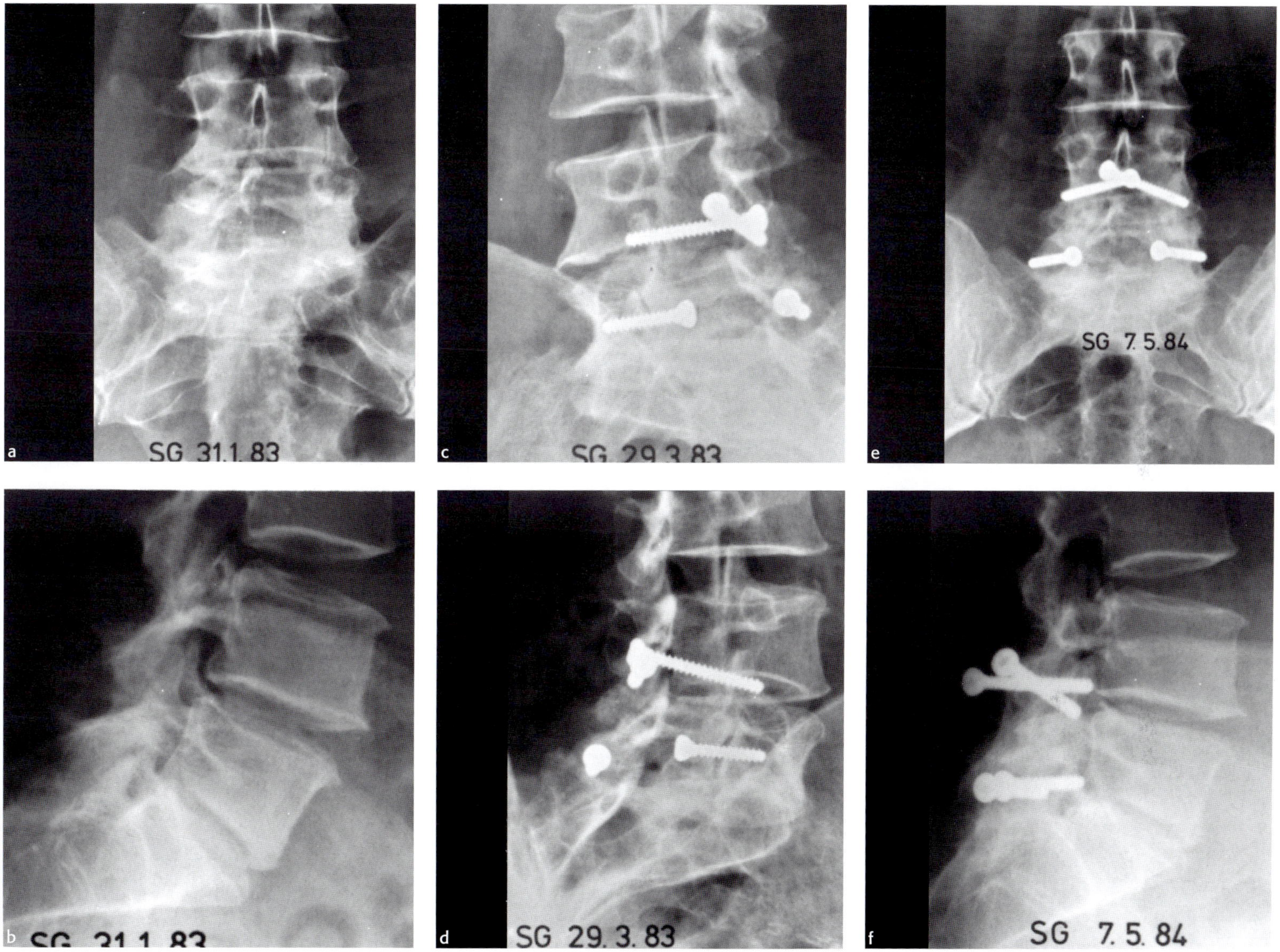

Fig. 7-15a–f Two-level posterior fusion in situ. For low back pain, when radicular symptoms are absent and normal lordosis is present, a posterior fusion in situ is adequate.

ab Narrowed disk spaces L4/L5/S1, normal lordosis. 3 years earlier: two-level disk surgery for disk herniation.

cd 2 months after surgery: the facet joints L5/S1 are stabilized directly, L4/L5 with translaminar screws. Posterolateral and interspinous cancellous bone grafting is performed.

ef 1-year result: solid fusion L4/L5/S1 by posterior transplanted bone mass.

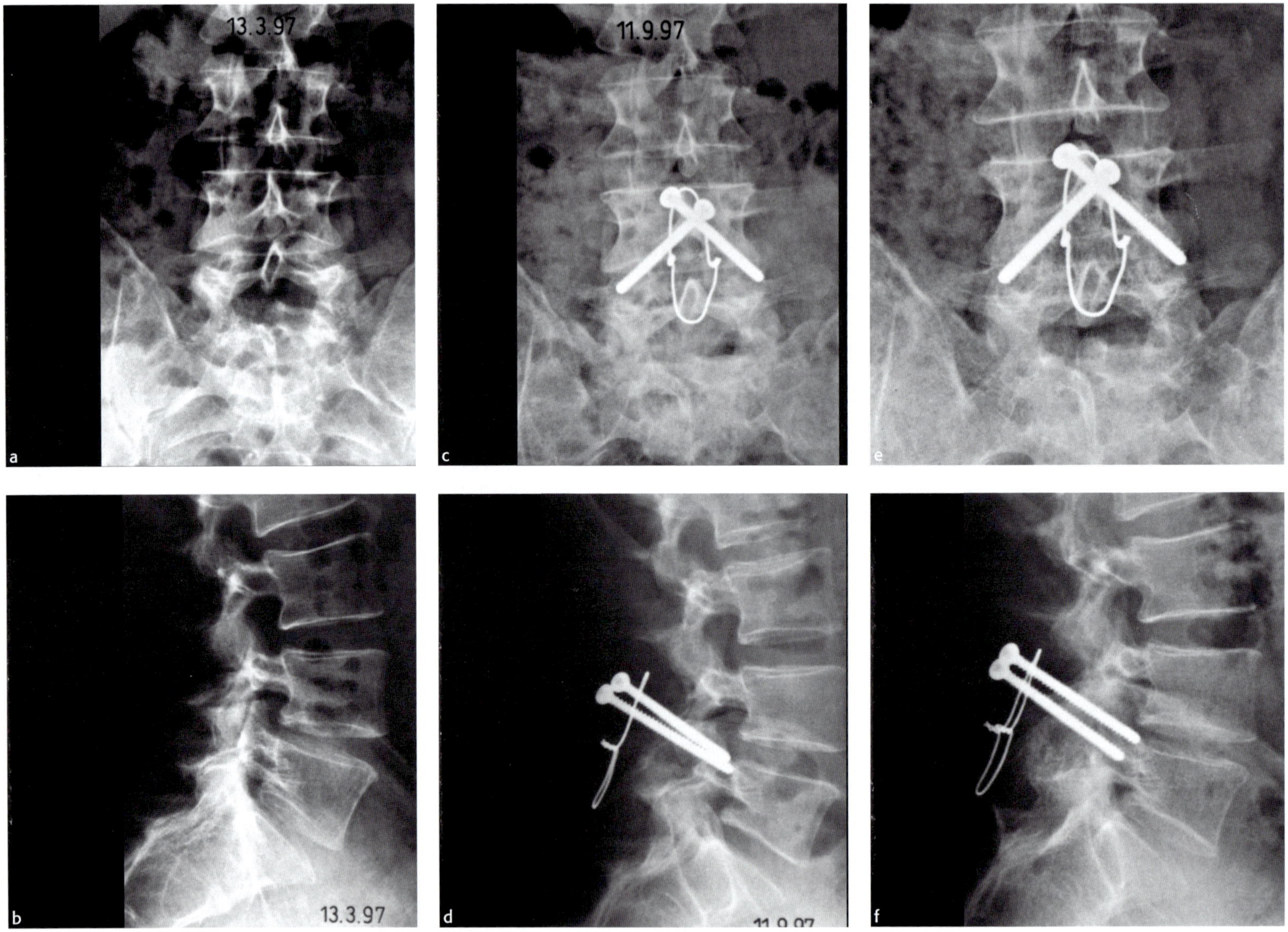

Fig. 7-16a–f L4/L5 disk degeneration. Posterior distraction-fusion and translaminar facet joint fixation (Magerl) and interspinous graft fixation with wire loop.

ab Disk space narrowing L4/L5 and narrowed intervertebral foramen.

cd The spinous processes L4 and L5 were spread to distract the disk space. Translaminar facet joint screw fixation. A corticocancellous bone graft is locked between the two spinous processes and held in place with a tight wire loop. Cancellous bone grafts are placed posterolaterally.

ef 4 1/2 years later: solid posterior bony fusion L4/L5. The fixation-fusion of the spinous processes protects the two screws from bending stress and fatigue fracture. It makes a three-point fixation out of a two-point fixation.

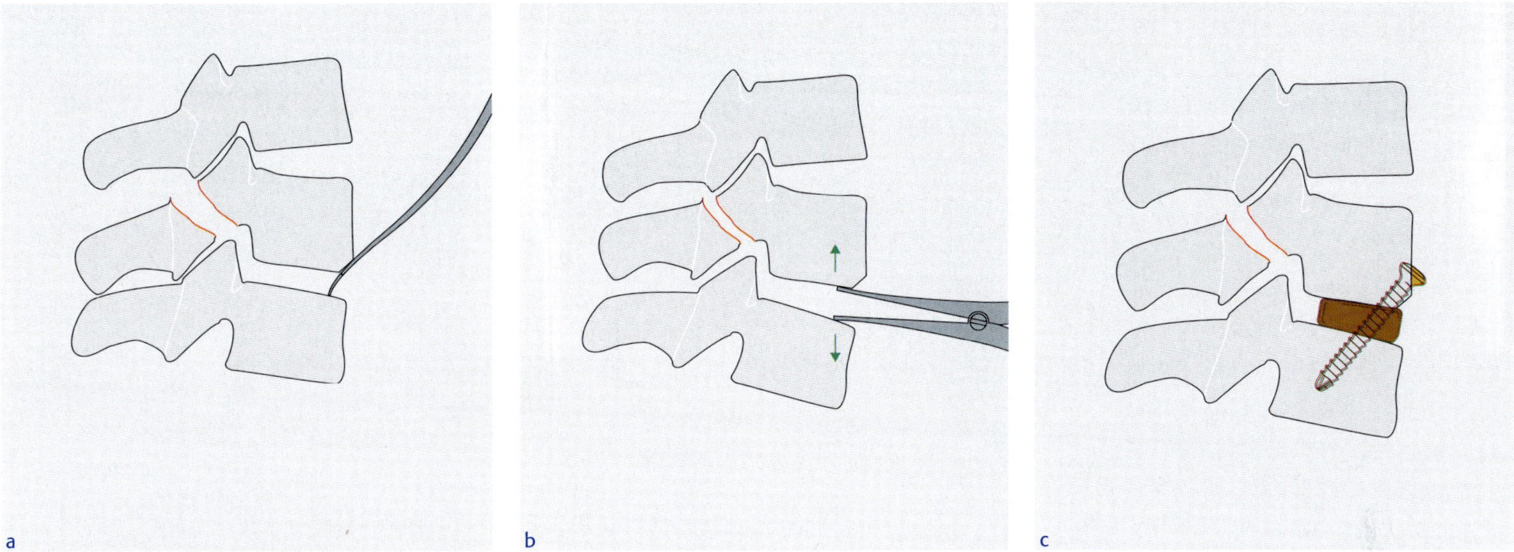

a b c

Fig. 7-17a–c Technique of interbody fusion for spondylolysis and spondylolisthesis.
In disk disease with intact posterior vertebral elements, an interbody fusion with massive pelvic grafts may be successful without internal metallic fixation. The interrupted interarticular portion of the posterior elements in spondylolysis/spondylolisthesis reduce interbody stability. Interbody fusion alone may fail due to insufficient intrinsic stability. Metallic fixation is therefore mandatory to compensate shear forces.

a Disk resection is followed by reduction of listhesis. In cases of radicular symptoms, posterior decompression by resection of the corresponding vertebral arch is performed first.

b Spreading of the intervertebral space after disk resection.

c When bone blocks are inserted, stability is ensured with screw fixation.

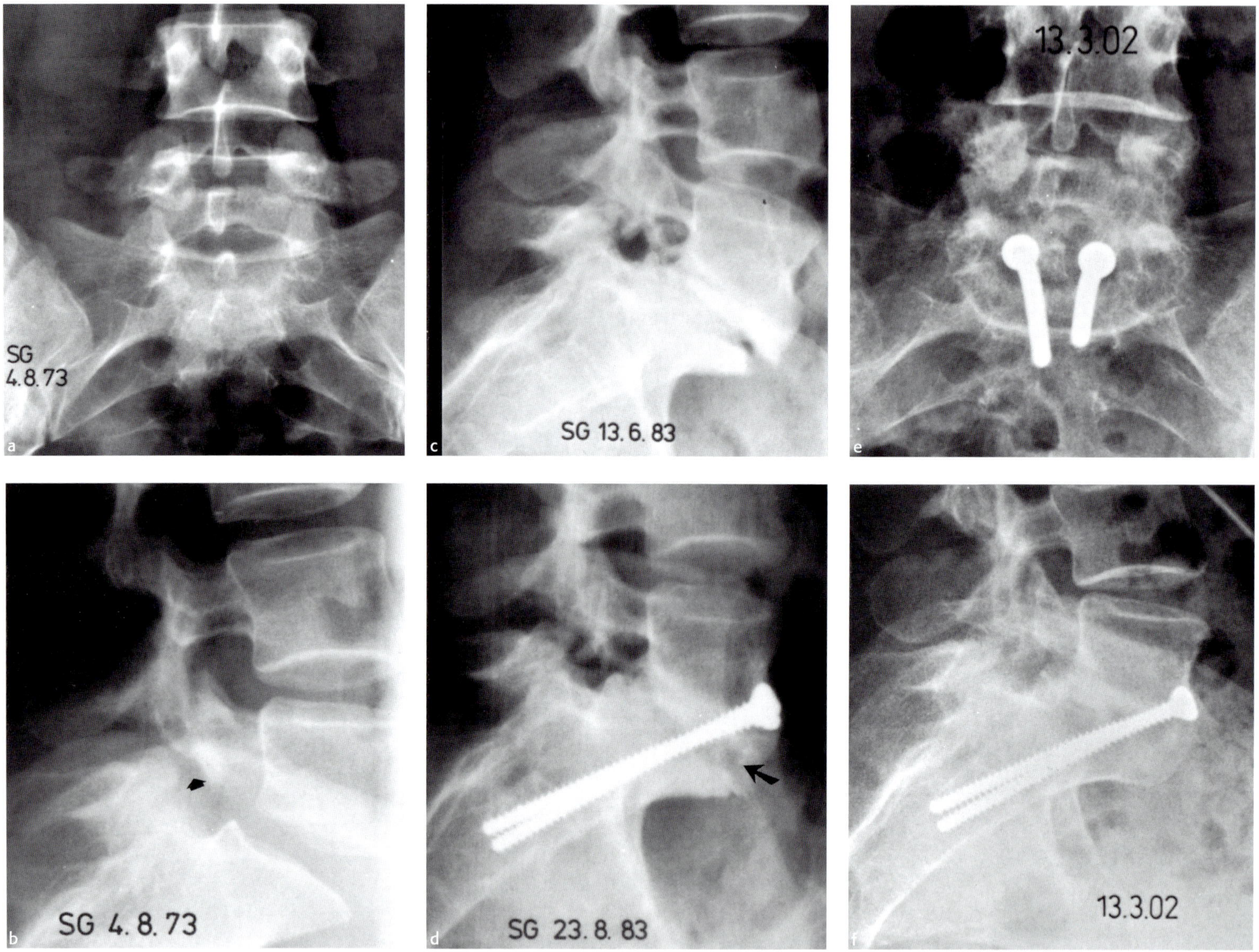

Fig. 7-18a–f Unsuccessful interbody fusion. Treatment of nonunions with secondary screw fixation at the time of revision.

ab Spondylolyses (arrow), mild listhesis L5 on S1.

c 10 years after interbody fusion: nonunion, chronic low back pain.

d Transperitoneal revision: a small new pelvic bone block is inserted (arrow), the nonunion is compressed with two lag screws.

ef 19 years after revision: sound union of the pseudarthrosis of interbody fusion L5/S1.

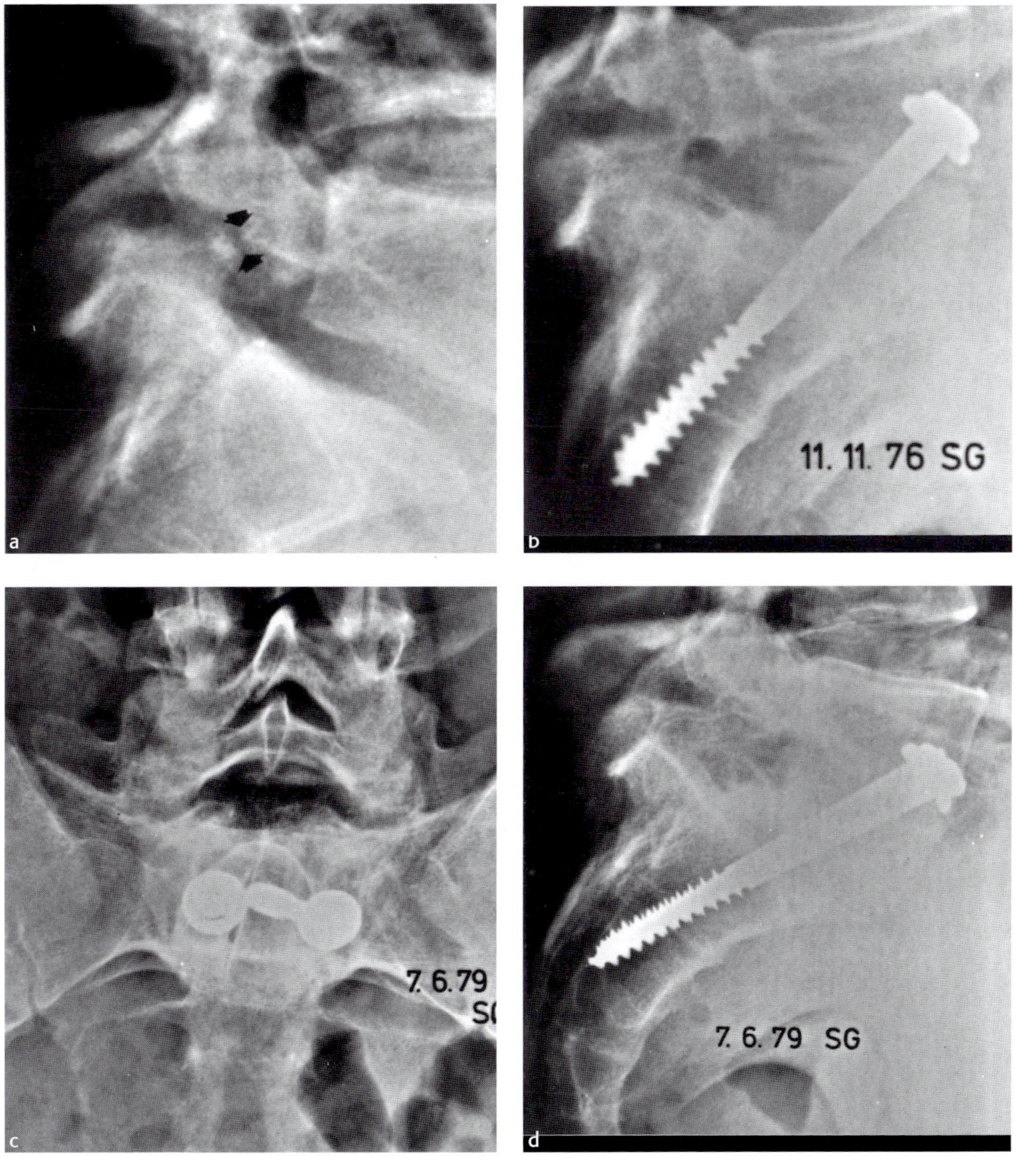

Fig. 7-19a–d Correct interbody fusion in spondylolisthesis: grafting and rigid fixation.

a Identical pathology as shown in Fig. 7-18b: mild listhesis and lysis of interarticular portion (arrows).

b Reduction distraction, fusion with pelvic bone blocks and primary internal fixation.

dc 3 years later: sound interbody fusion.

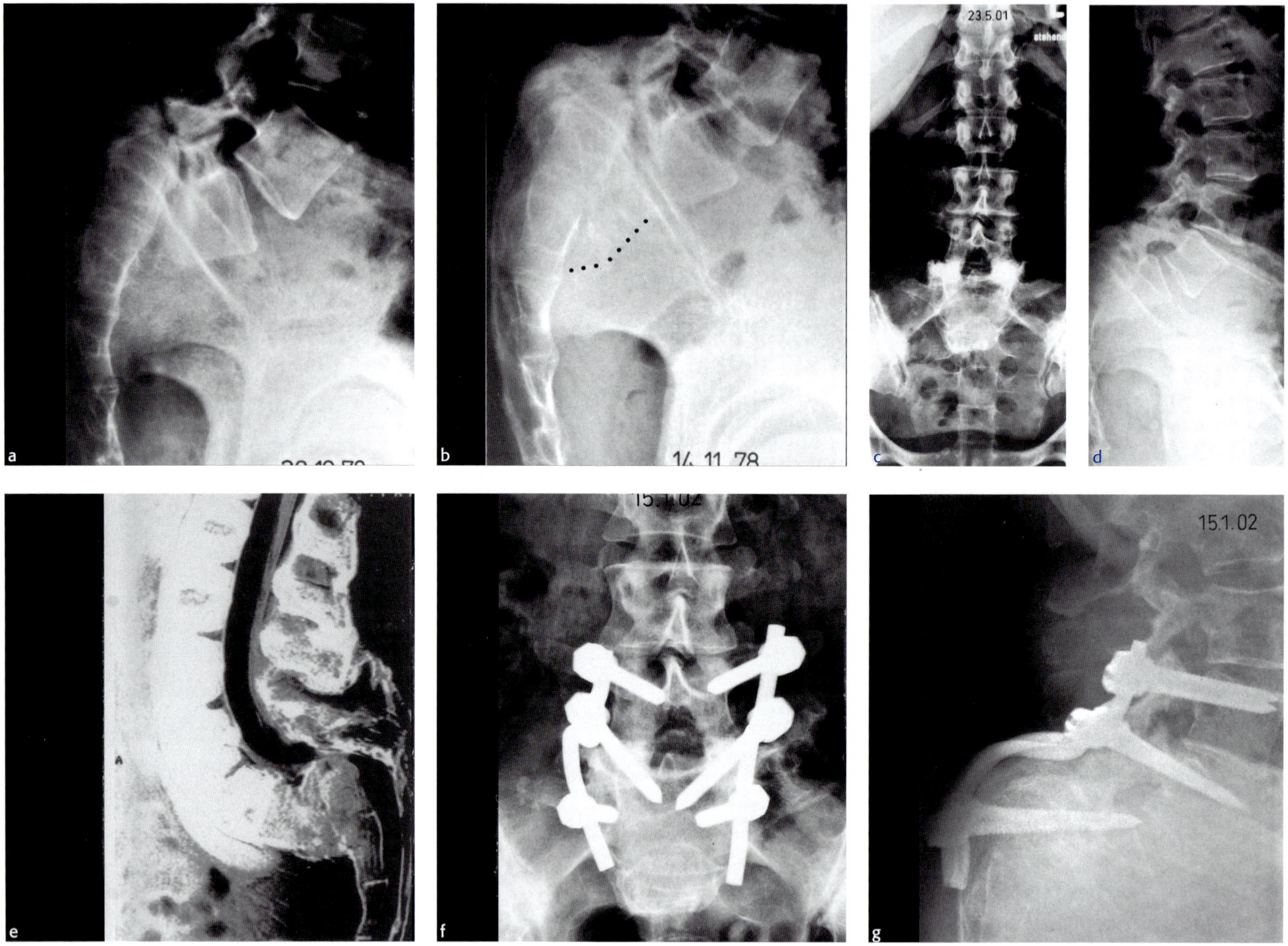

Fig. 7-20a–g Spondylopthosis with in situ presacral fusion.

a Spondylopthosis at age 19.

b Transperitoneal approach, retroperitoneal exposure, application of a large mass of autogenous bone graft (outlined). 2 months' bed rest after surgery.

cd 23 years later: sound in situ fusion of L5 against the front of the sacrum. The current problem is 1 year of low back pain from secondary disk degeneration L3/L4 and L4/L5.

e MRI: ideal fusion L5/sacrum, no diskherniation proximally.

fg 9 months after posterior instrumentation and grafting: fusion has occurred, symptoms have disappeared.

5.2 Humerus and forearm

Autogenous bone grafts are suitable for various pathologies.

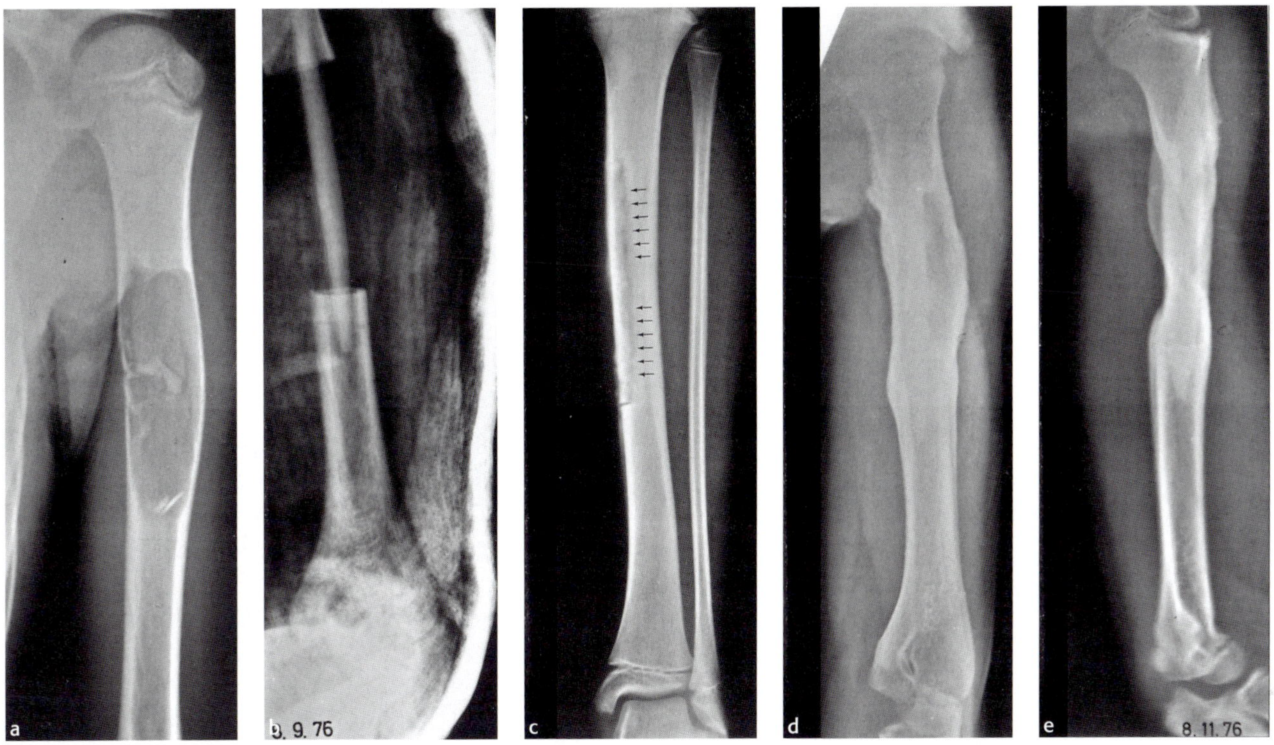

Fig. 7-21a–e Large unicameral bone cyst.

ab The cyst is excised and a tibial corticocancellous graft is inserted to keep limb length.

c The donor site 1 month after surgery (arrows).

de 2 months after surgery: the tibial graft is surrounded by a completely regenerated humeral shaft.

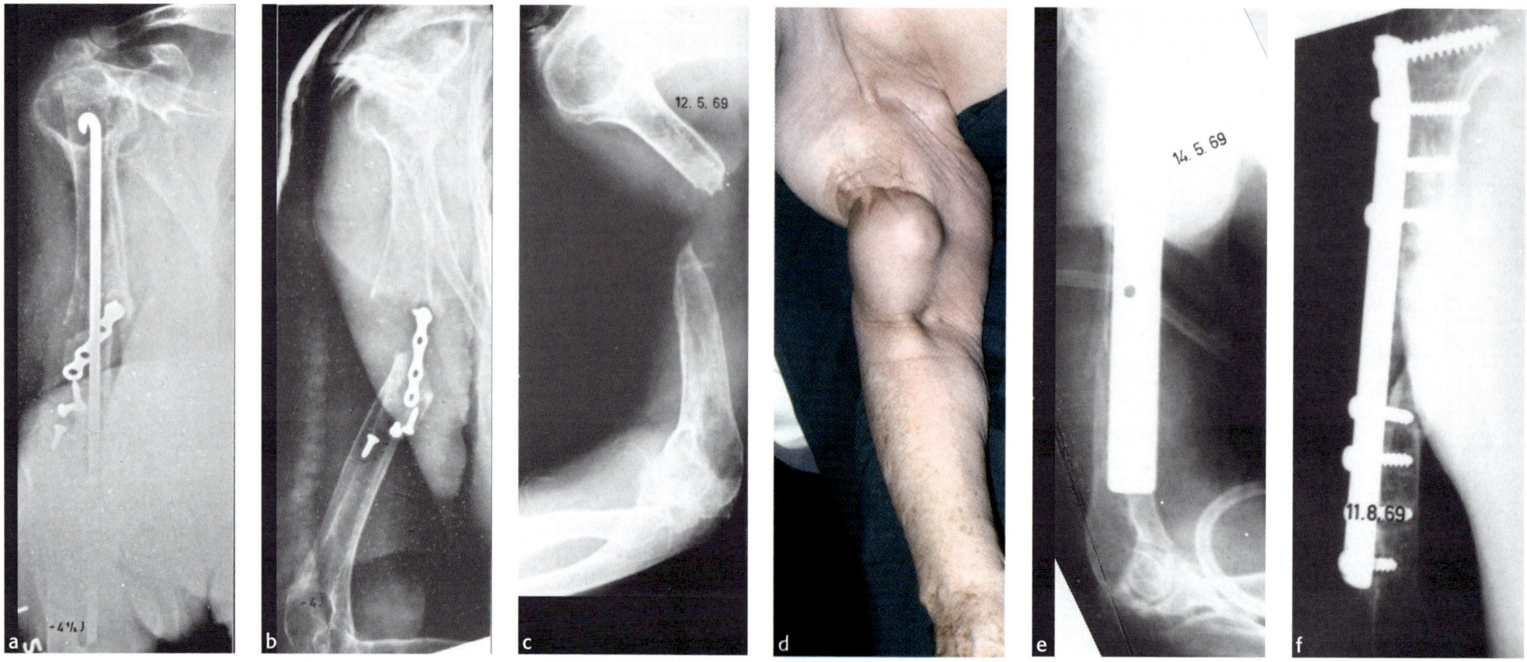

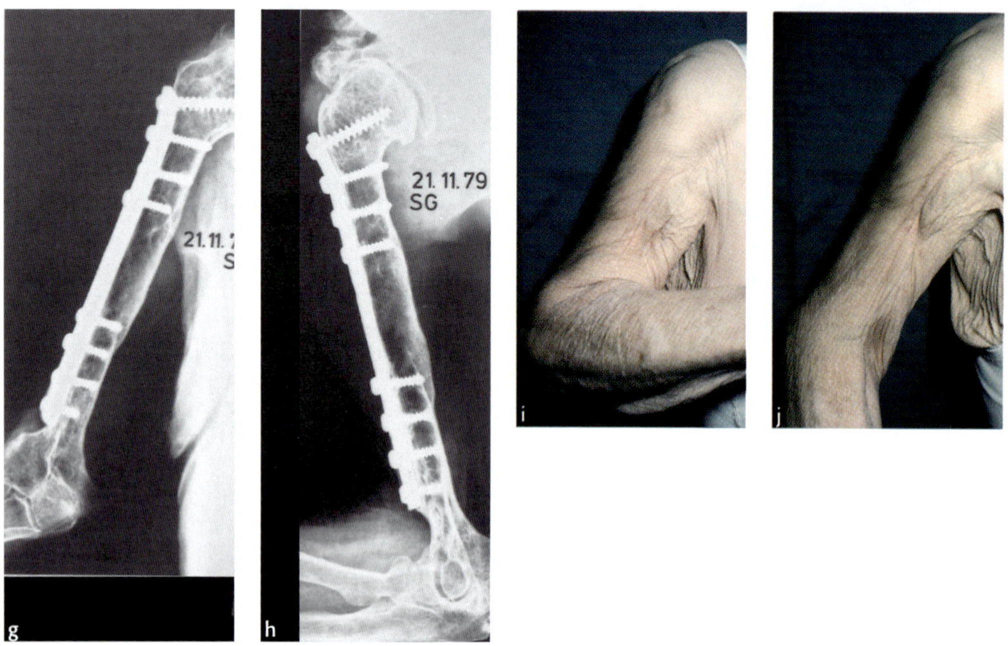

Fig. 7-22a–j Bone loss after fracture of the humerus.

ab The old lady has had 14 operations!

cd At admission 4 years later, 12 years after the original injury: large defect with atrophic fragments. Excellent mobility in the non-union, but frozen shoulder and halfway stiff elbow.

ef 3 months after plating and autogenous bone grafting.

gh 10 years after surgery: the nonunion had healed after 1 year. Useful function of the arm has been regained.

ij Different look and function of the arm 10 years after surgery.

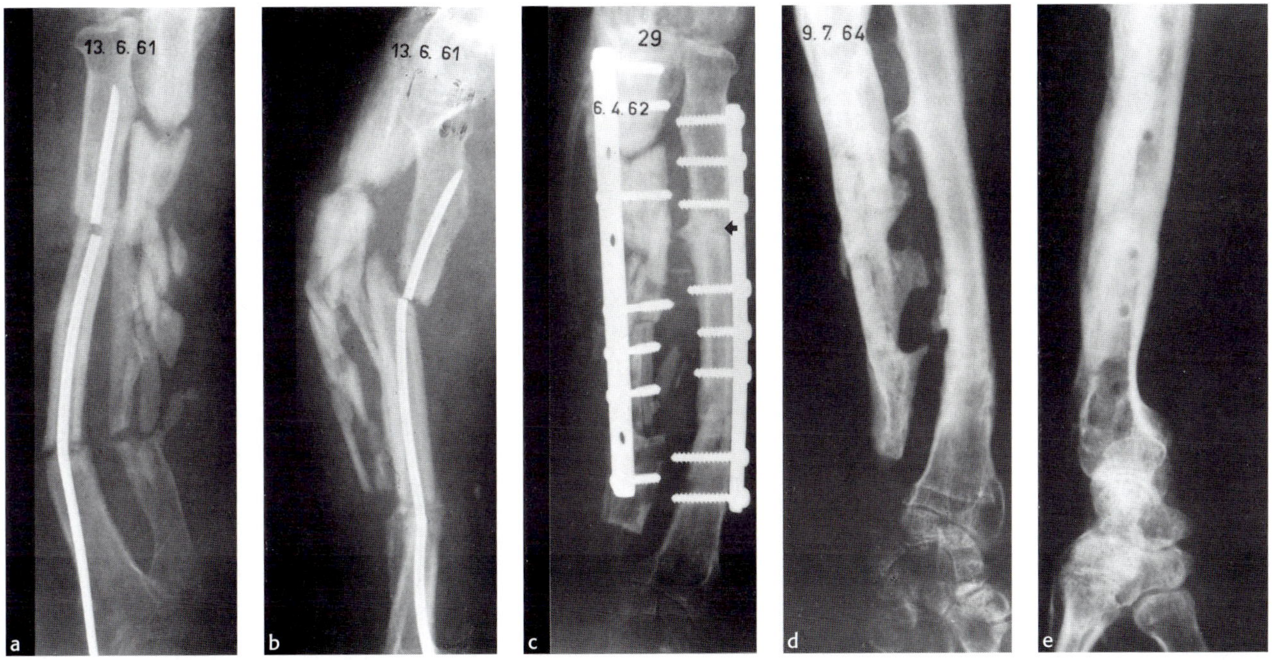

Fig. 7-23a–e Multiple nonunions following high-energy injury of the forearm.

ab 3 years after injury: multiple nonunions, poor function of the lower arm.

c 29 weeks after reconstruction: the capitulum ulnae was used as autogenous graft for lengthening in the nonunion of the radius (arrow).

de Late follow-up at 3 years, 1 year after metal removal: the worker has regained usable function of the arm.

5.3 Proximal femur

Femoral head necrosis and benign tumors are indication for autogenous bone grafting.

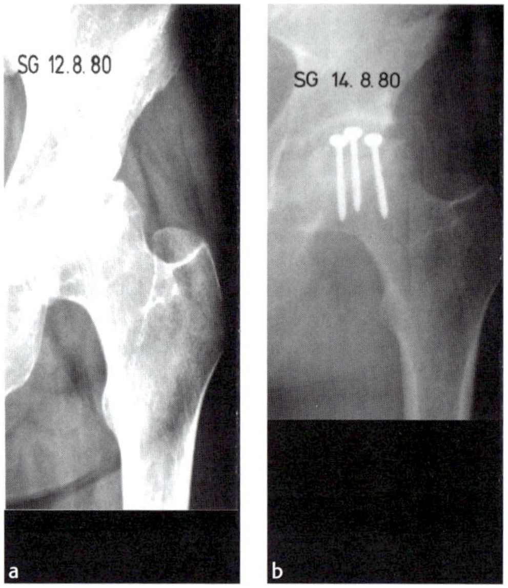

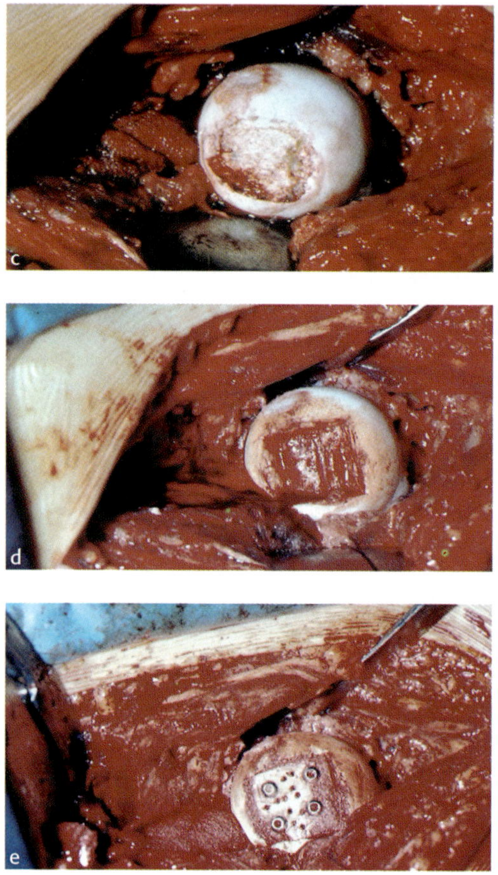

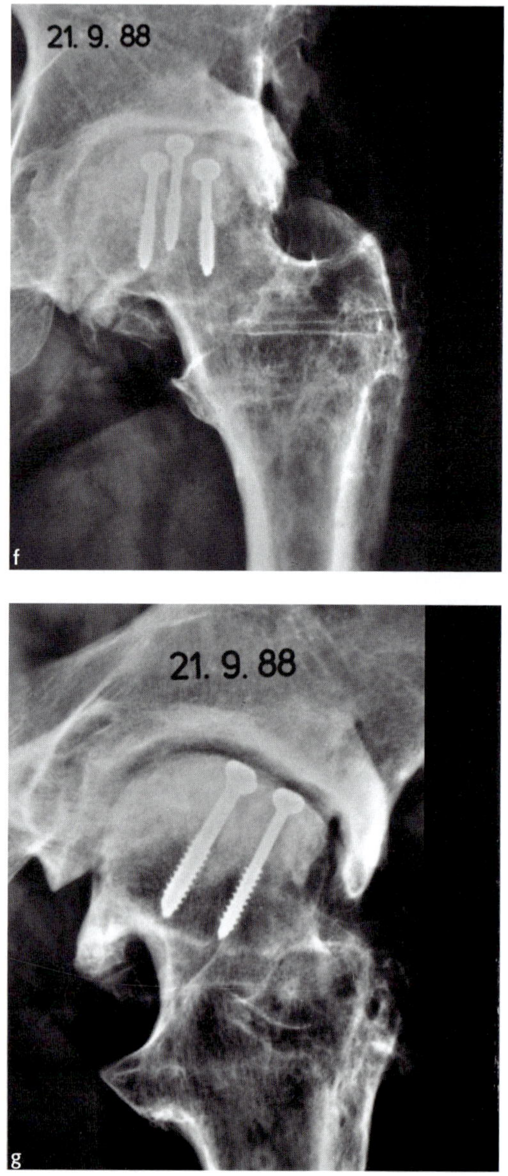

Fig. 7-24a–j Idiopathic head necrosis.
Selected cases of idiopathic and posttraumatic (after neck fracture) necrosis were treated accordingly. The result lasted up to 18 years. Total hip replacement was delayed for more than 10 years in all eleven cases, which is important for younger patients.

ab Large necrotic zone and postoperative x-ray.

cde The operative technique. Excision of the necrosis down to bleeding bone. A pelvic graft is slotted into the defect and fixed with lag screws. The graft is thereafter trimmed to roundness. The remaining cortex is perforated to encourage connective tissue in growth and coverage.

fg At 8 years; at 4 years an intertrochanteric osteotomy was done to correct fixed external rotation of the leg. The hip is free from pain with flexion range of 90°. The man, a foreman in building construction, does manual labor.

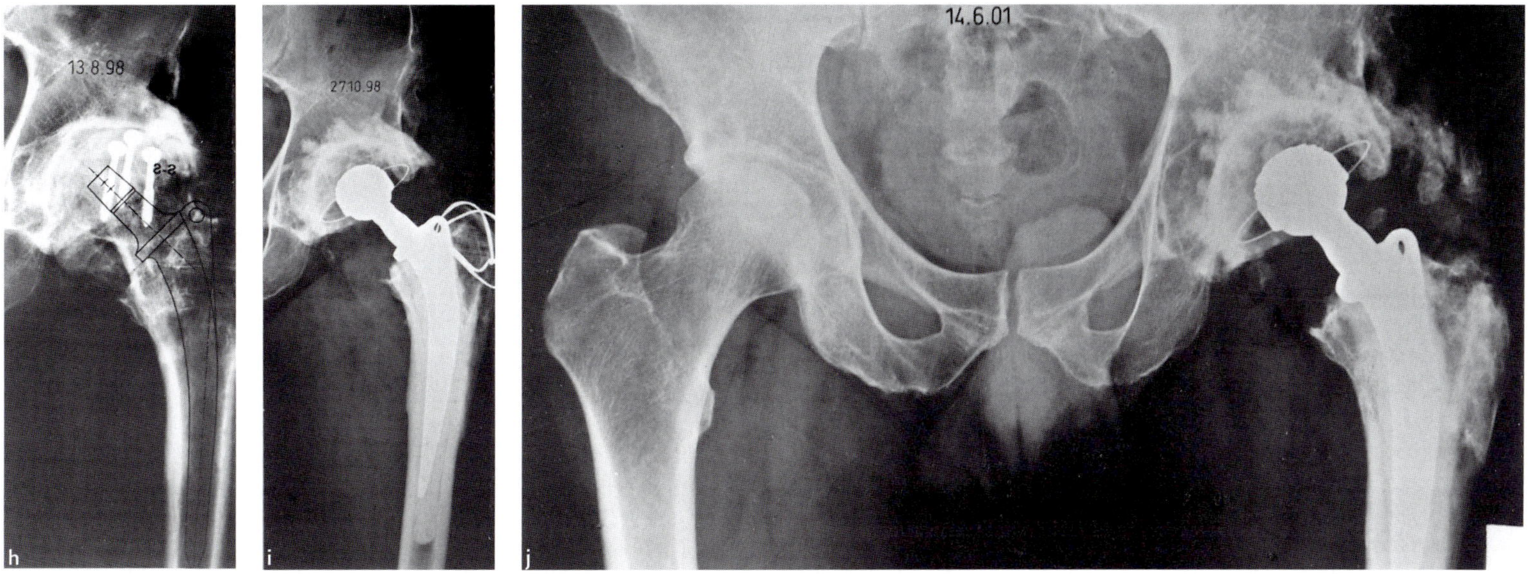

Fig. 7-24a–j cont.

hi 18 years after grafting: only now total hip replacement is indicated.

j 3 years later: the foreman is working 100% with no complaints.

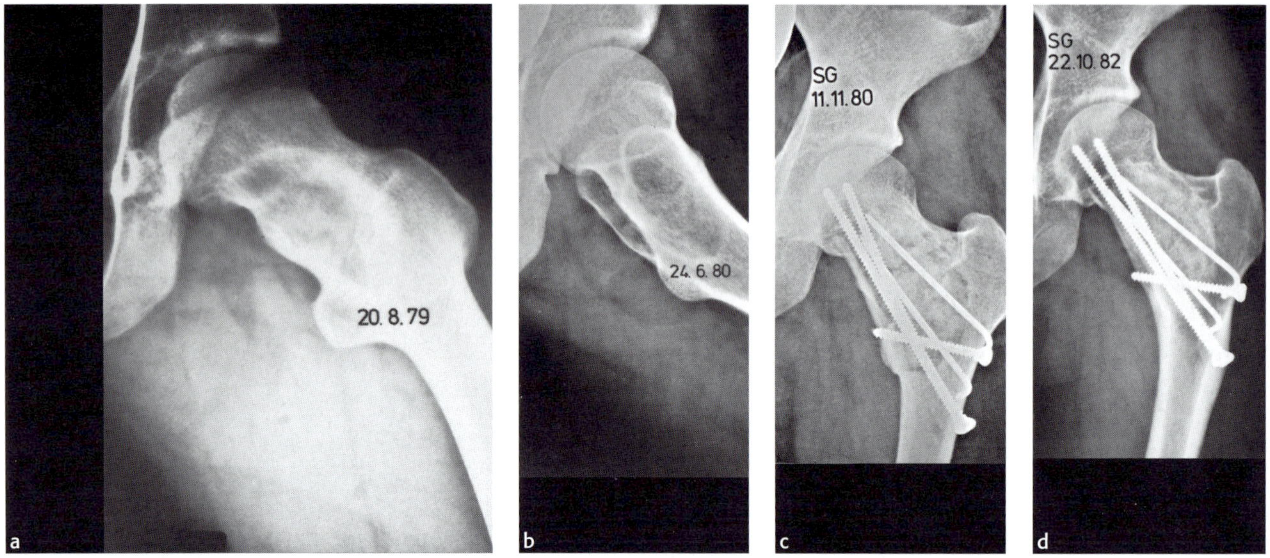

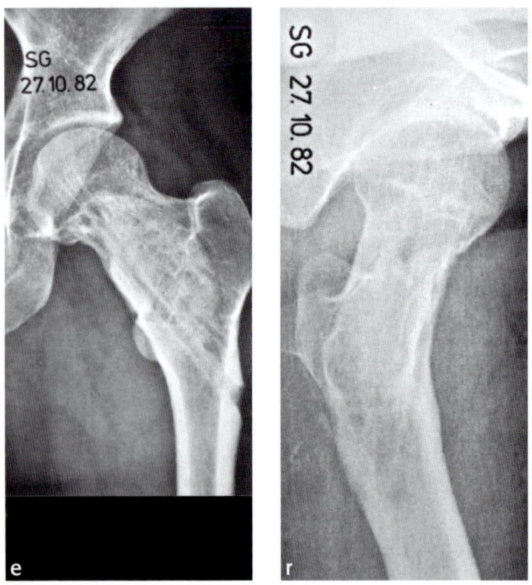

Fig. 7-25a–f Osteofibroma of the femoral neck.

ab Slow growing tumor, risk of spontaneous neck fracture.

c 1 month after surgery: resected calcar femoris is replaced by a tibial cortical graft. The tumor void is packed with pelvic grafts. Reinforcement with three screws and two K-wires

def 2 years after surgery, the metal is removed. The proximal femur shows anatomical and stable reconstruction.

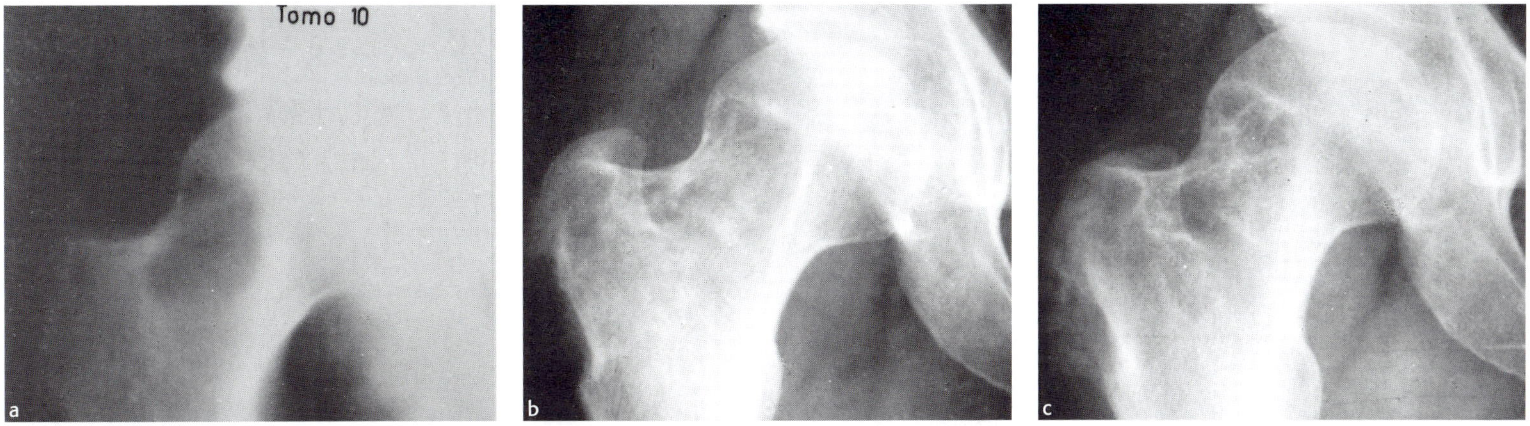

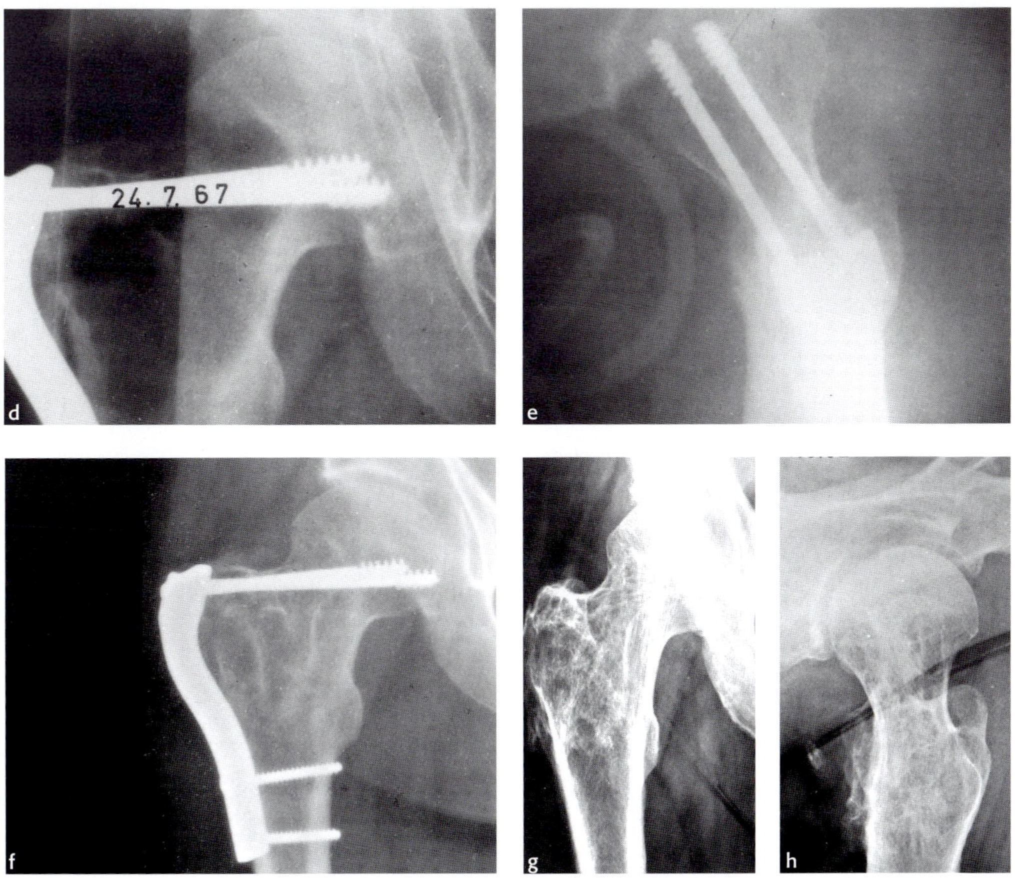

Fig. 7-26a–h Osteoclastoma, giant cell tumor, vanishing bone.

- a The bone defect in the tomogram.
- b 1 month after curettage and packing with autogenous grafts from the lateral side.
- c Recurrence has started.
- de Second radical excision of the tumor from the front of the femoral neck. Packing with autogenous grafts, preventive internal fixation (tension band).
- f 1 year after excision-reconstruction. 1 year later the metal was removed.
- gh 35 years later, no recurrence, sound hip joint.

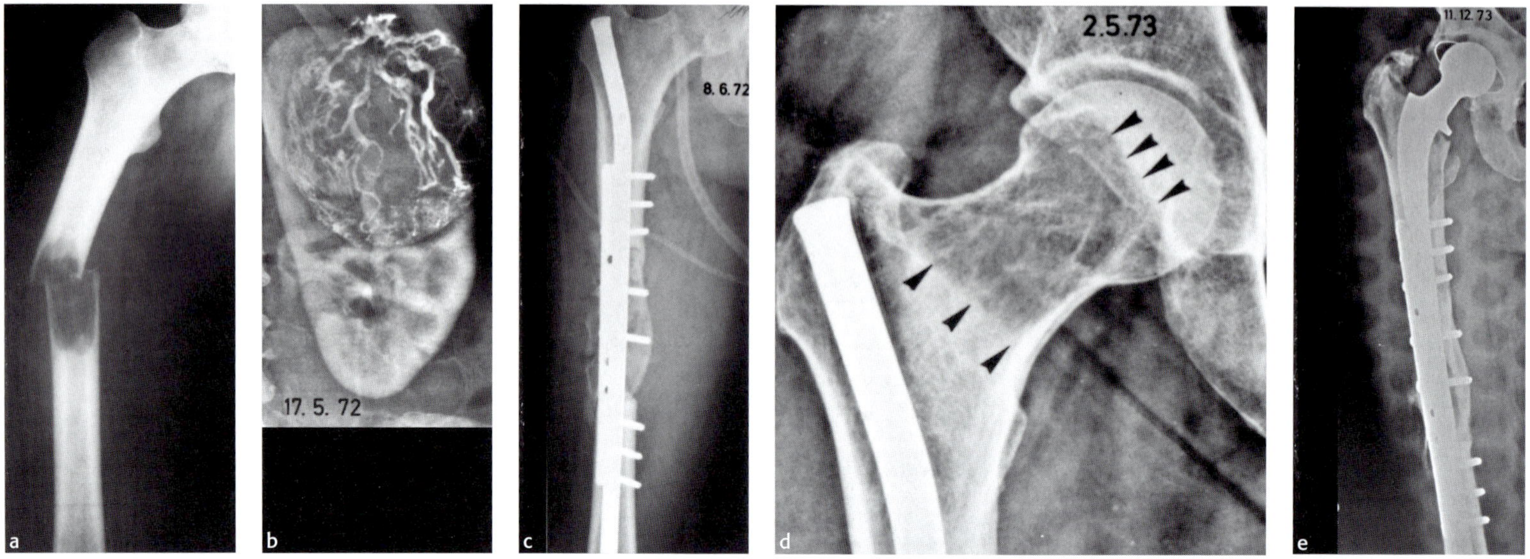

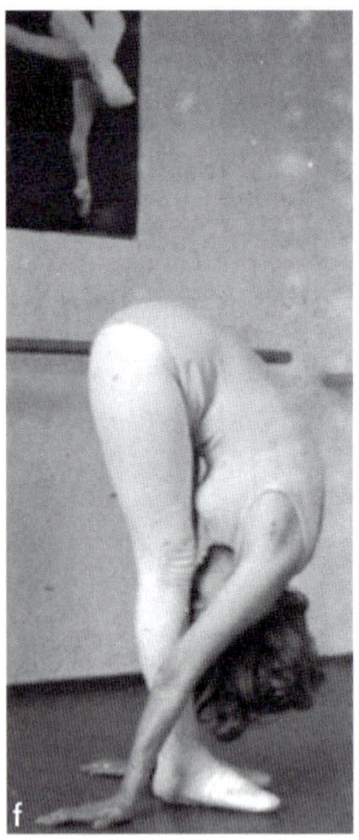

Fig. 7-27a–f Hypernephroma.

a Metastasis with fracture.

b Hypernephroma (angiography).

c The metastasis is resected with a wide margin. The gap is filled with iliac crest and cancellous bone. Internal fixation with a tibial (!) nail and with plate.

d 1 year later: metastasis of the femoral neck (arrows).

e Total hip replacement after tumor resection of the proximal femur. The femoral shaft is free of tumor recurrence.

f The patient, a professional ballet dancer, continued to dance for 3 years until her death from generalized metastatic disease.

5.4 Shaft of the femur

Defects of the femoral shaft are treated differently in the absence or the presence of infection. Also different is the treatment for benign or malignant tumor disease.

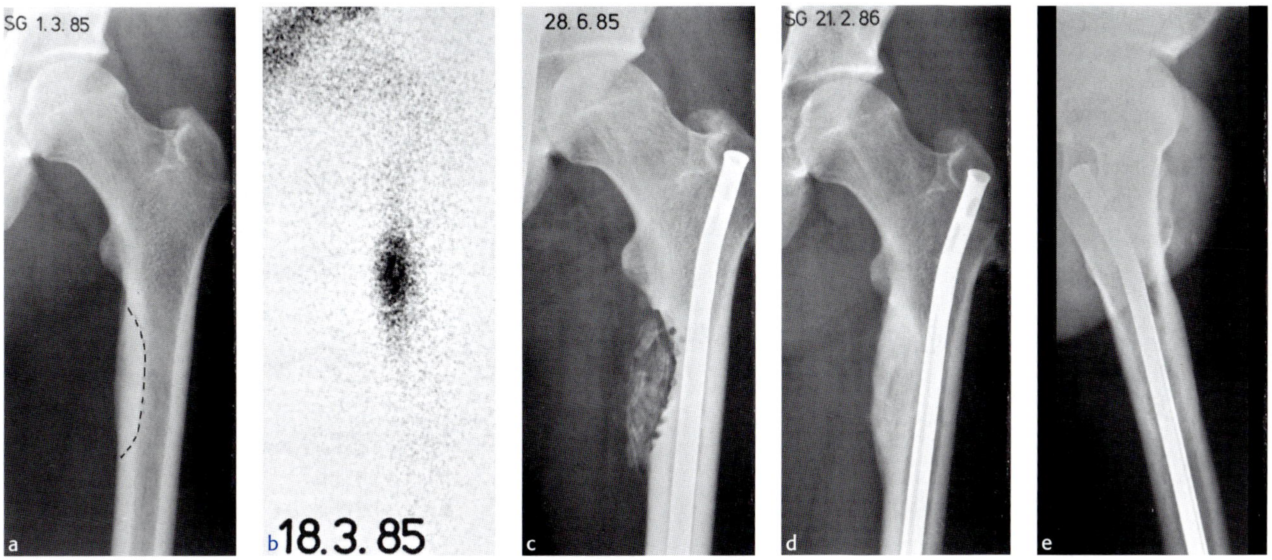

Fig. 7-28a–e Osteoid osteoma, eosinophilic granuloma in the proximal metaphysis.

a The bone area to be removed is outlined.

b Scintigraphy. Hot spot.

c The tumor is removed, the defect is filled with autogenous grafts. Intrinsic stability is present. To prevent spontaneous fracture, stability is increased with a tibial slotted nail.

de 8 months later: incorporated and remodeled grafts. The nail is removed at that stage.

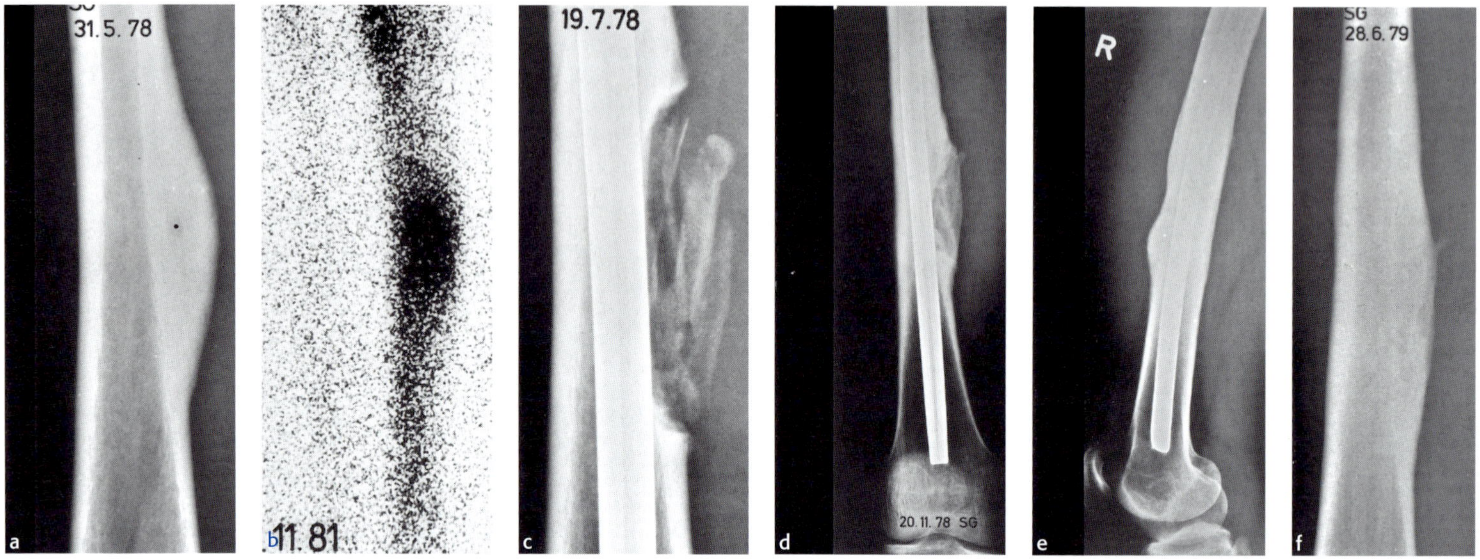

Fig. 7-29a–f Osteoid osteoma, eosinophilic granuloma of the midshaft.

a The tumor with nidus (black dot).

b Scintigraphy: hot spot.

c The tumor is resected, the defect is filled with autogenous cancellous flakes, the femur is reinforced with a medullary slotted nail.

de 4 months after surgery.

f 1 year after surgery, after removal of the nail. The grafts are remodeled to a new cortex.

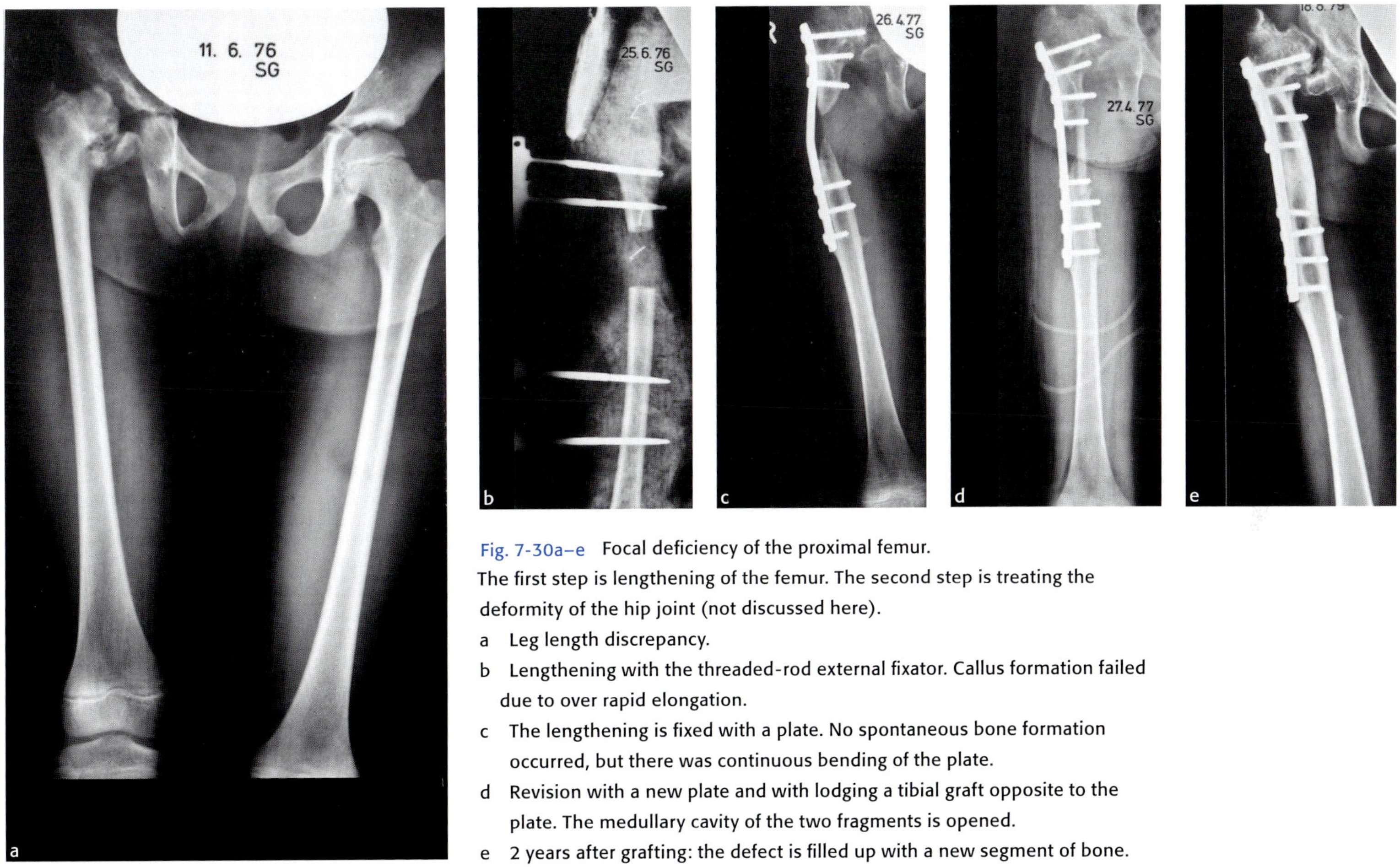

Fig. 7-30a–e Focal deficiency of the proximal femur.
The first step is lengthening of the femur. The second step is treating the deformity of the hip joint (not discussed here).

a Leg length discrepancy.

b Lengthening with the threaded-rod external fixator. Callus formation failed due to over rapid elongation.

c The lengthening is fixed with a plate. No spontaneous bone formation occurred, but there was continuous bending of the plate.

d Revision with a new plate and with lodging a tibial graft opposite to the plate. The medullary cavity of the two fragments is opened.

e 2 years after grafting: the defect is filled up with a new segment of bone.

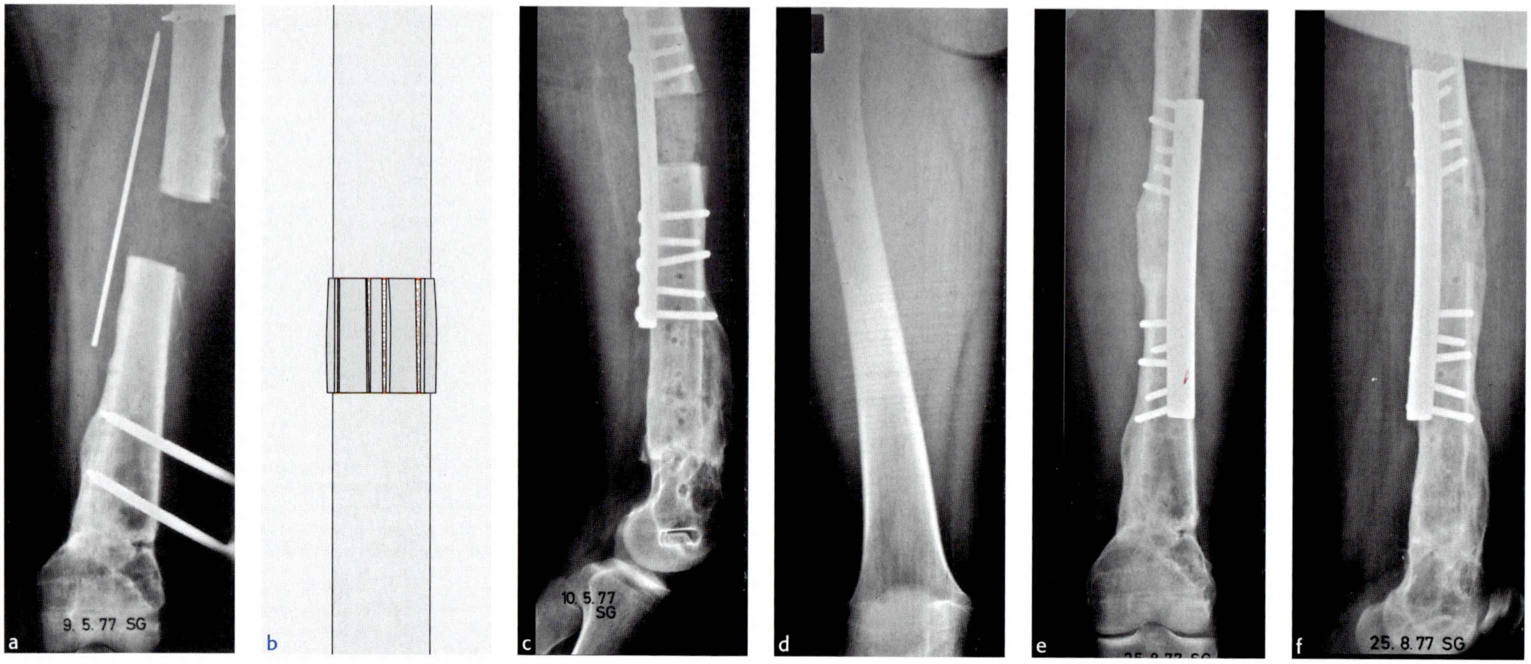

Fig. 7-31a–f Lengthening and primary grafting in the adult.

- a 17-year-old girl, valgus deformity and shortening following peripheric Salter 3 injury of the distal femur 4 years earlier. Valgus deformity has already been corrected with supracondylar osteotomy.
  Lengthening of 5 cm is performed with Wagner apparatus in 2 weeks.
- b The technique of gap filling with corticocancellous pelvic grafts to offer intrinsic stability.
- c Posterolateral plating with the grafts in situ.
- d The sound femur for comparison.
- ef 3 1/2 months later: incorporation, remodeling, mass augmentation of the grafts due to CAF, ie, weightbearing. Plate removal 1 year after surgery.

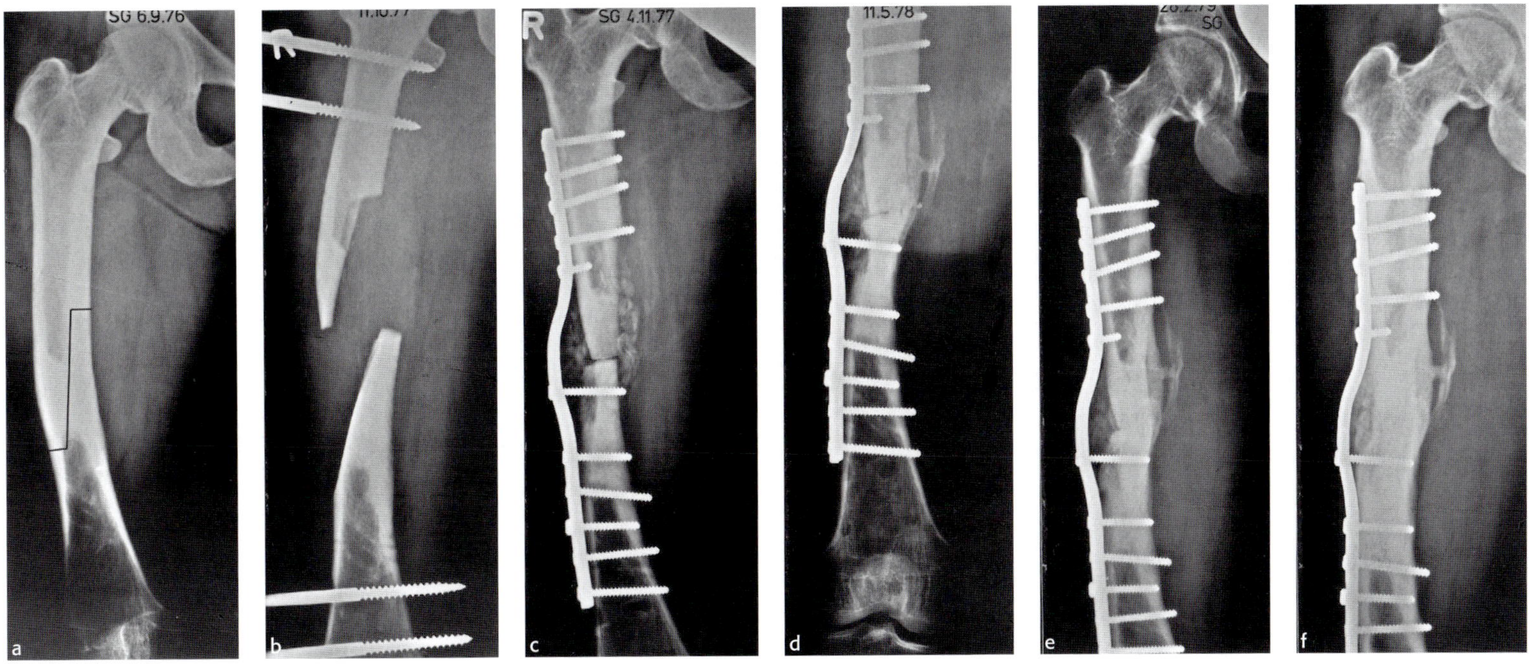

Fig. 7-32a–f Posttraumatic lengthening in the adult.

a The step-cut osteotomy for lengthening is outlined.

b Distraction or lengthening 8.5 cm in 3 weeks, ie, 3 mm per day.

c The fragments are opposed to each other, offering intrinsic stability. A plate is contoured to a waveplate and fixed. Autogenous grafts are added. The biomechanics of the waveplate: tension band opposed to the medial bone contact. Grafts are placed between femur and plate.

d 6 months after grafting.

e 15 months after grafting.

f 3 years three months after grafting and plating: perfect remodeling of the femoral lengthening. The plate is removed at that time.

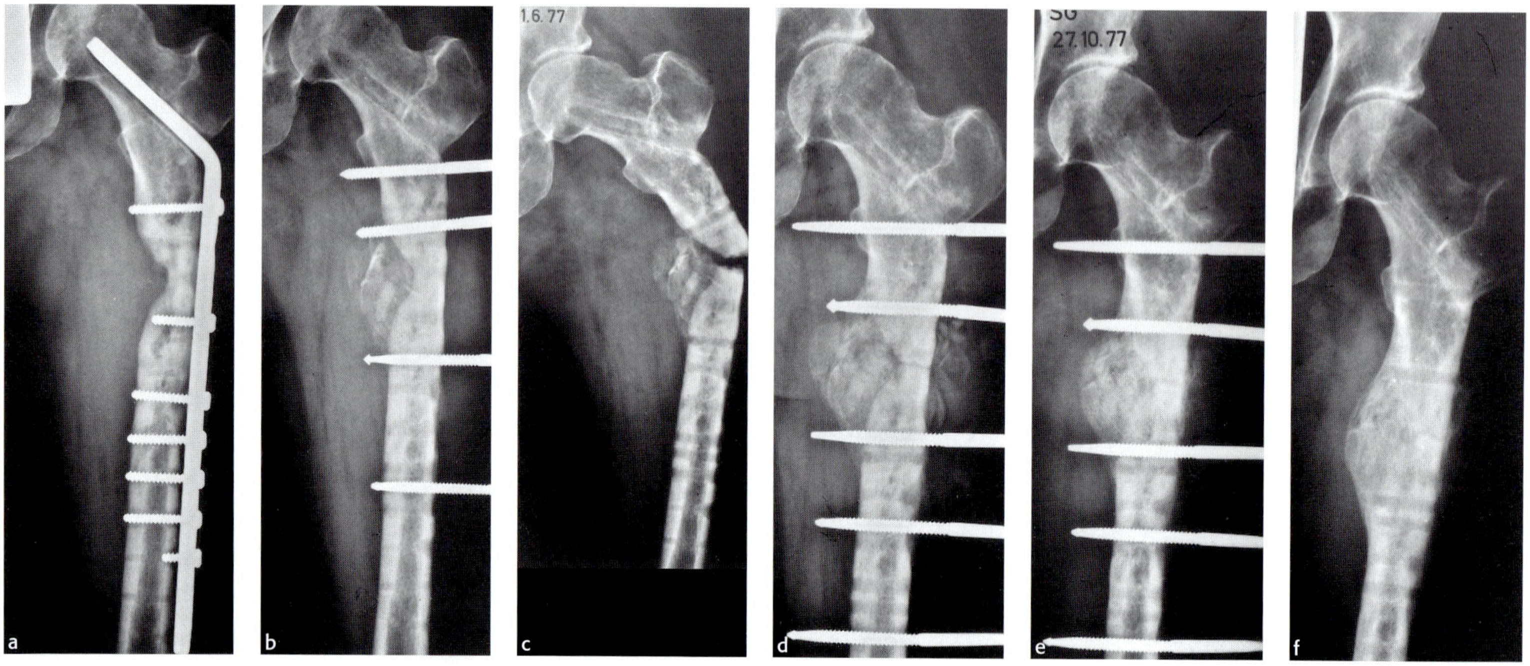

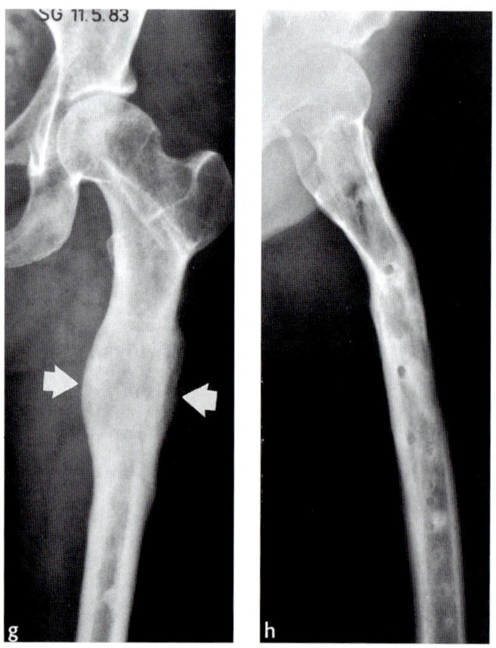

Fig. 7-33a–h Lack of lateral tension resistance of the femur followed by fatigue facture.

- a At admission: subtrochanteric fracture 1 year ago, internal fixation followed by infection. Sequesters were removed. Low-grade infection with Staphylococcus albus, two small sinuses.
- b The plate is removed, an external fixator of tension-band type is inserted and a massive autogenous bone transplant is applied on the medial side of the femur.
- c 3 months after successful grafting, 1 week after removal of the external fixator: spontaneous fracture due to lack of tension resistance of the lateral cortex.
- d Second external fixator now with grafting on the lateral side (arrow) in analogy to the waveplate technique.
- e 4 months later: grafts have remodeled under CAF, ie, weightbearing.
- f Another 3 months later, immediately after removal of the external fixator.
- gh Follow-up 5 years after admission: remarkable remodeling of the graft area, especially on the lateral tension side (arrows).

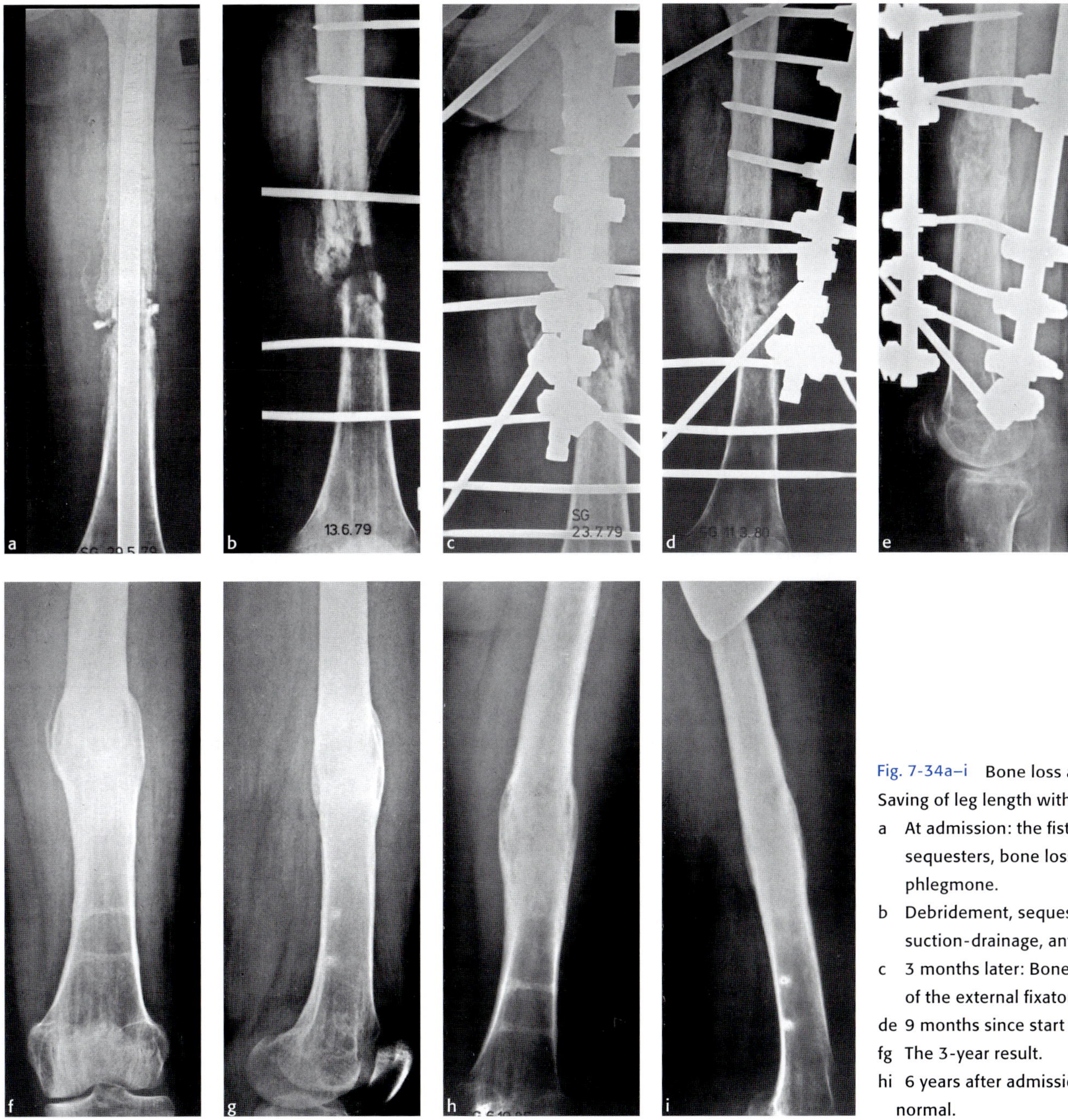

Fig. 7-34a–i Bone loss after infected fracture. Saving of leg length with grafts.

a At admission: the fistulography shows the sinus, sequesters, bone loss, and the local medullary phlegmone.

b Debridement, sequesterectomy, external fixator, suction-drainage, antibiotic treatment.

c 3 months later: Bone grafting and reinforcement of the external fixator.

de 9 months since start of reconstruction.

fg The 3-year result.

hi 6 years after admission and treatment: back to normal.

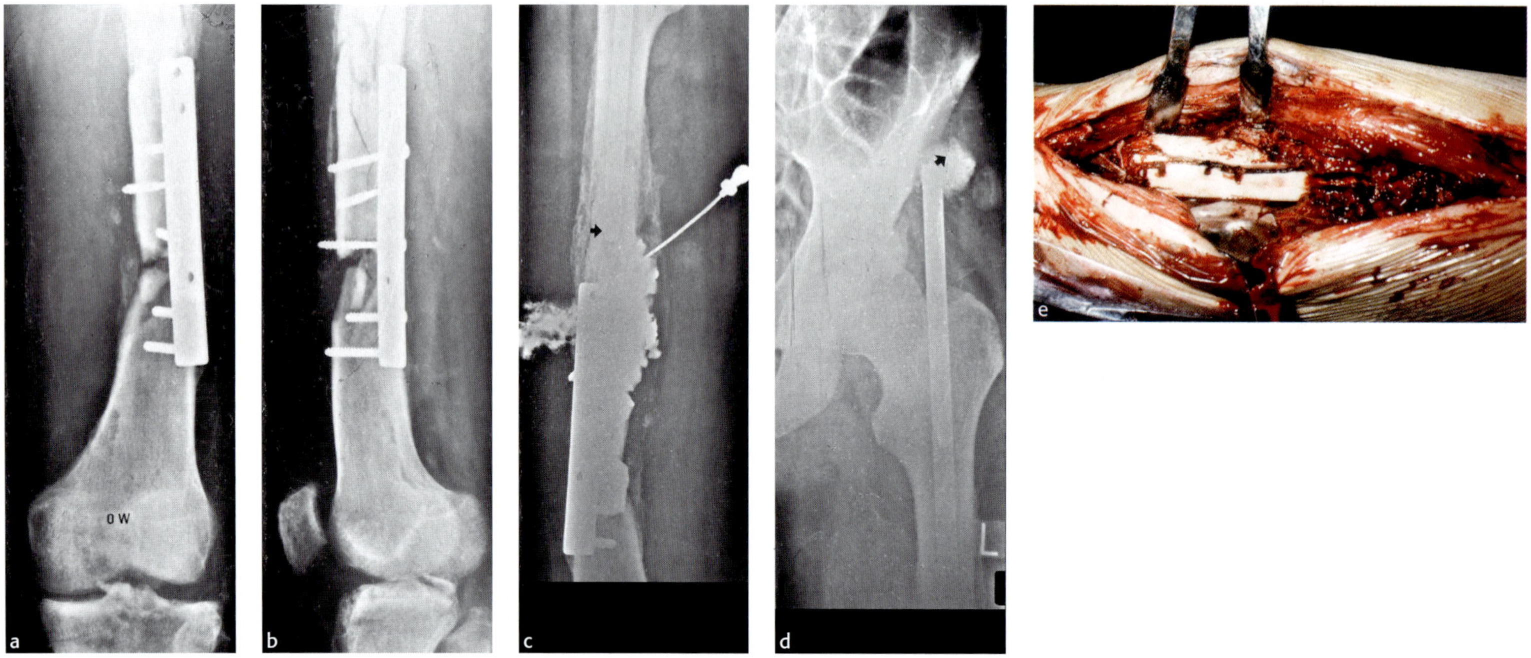

Fig. 7-35a–m Infected fracture with bone loss of the midshaft.

ab At admission: 12 weeks after failed nailing and instant plating, followed by infection.

cd Fistulography: the dye expands from the fracture to the upper end of of the nail (arrows).

e At surgery: sequesters to be removed. Debridement made, external fixator applied. 3 weeks later bone grafting is performed.

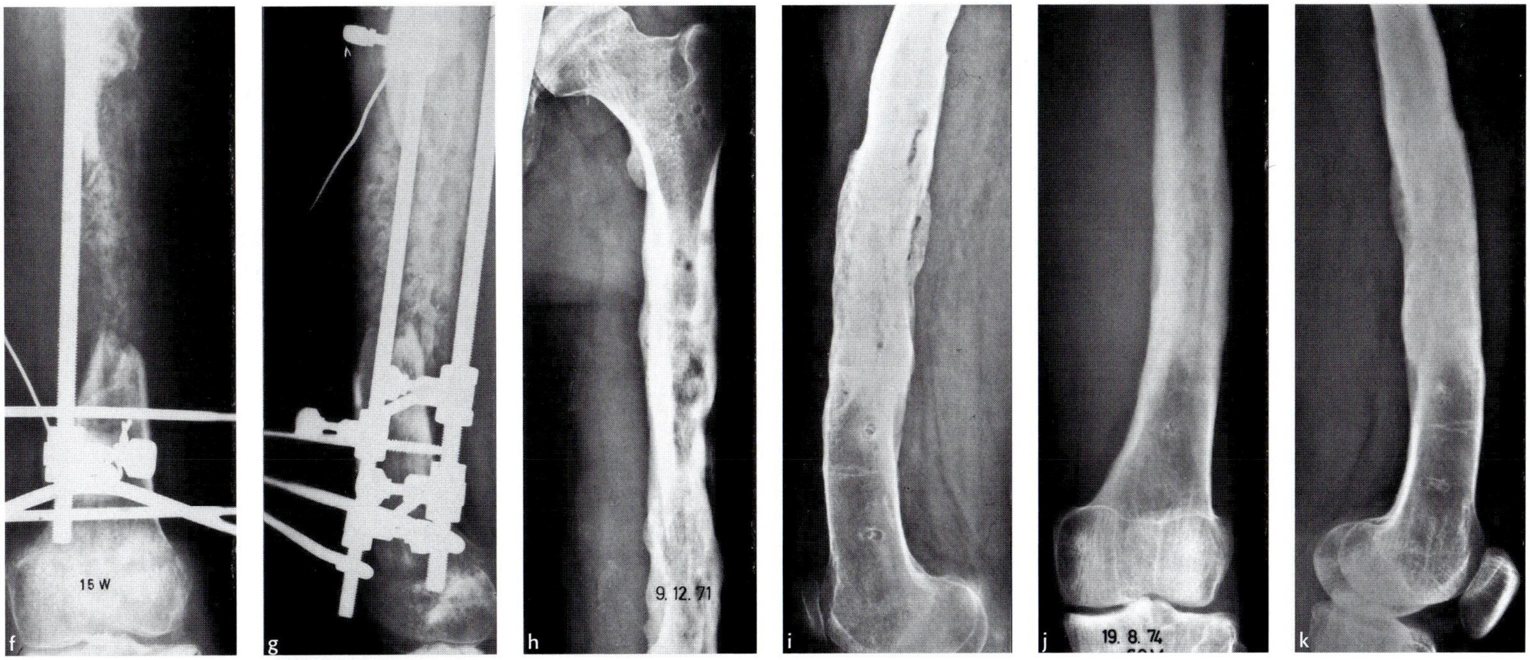

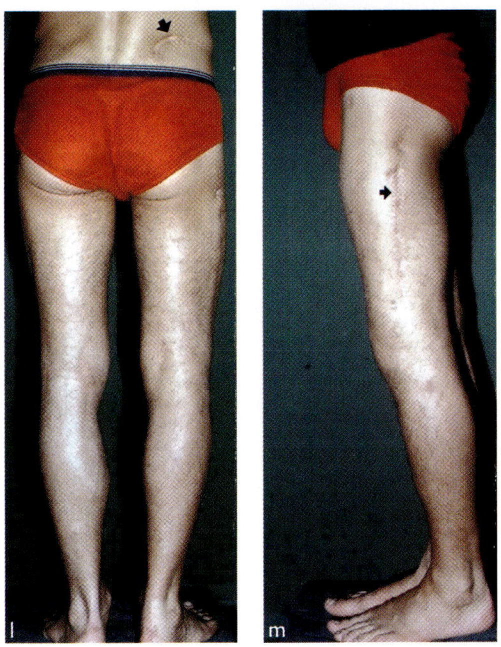

Fig. 7-35a–m cont.

fg 12 weeks after grafting and CAF, ie, partial weightbearing, the grafts have started to remodel.

hi 2 years after surgery, 1 year after removal of the external fixator, reappearance of a medullary cavity.

jk 5-year follow-up: the femur is restored.

lm The patient at that stage: back to normal except for loss of knee flexion of 20°.

Note: scar from graft harvesting and from reconstruction (arrows).

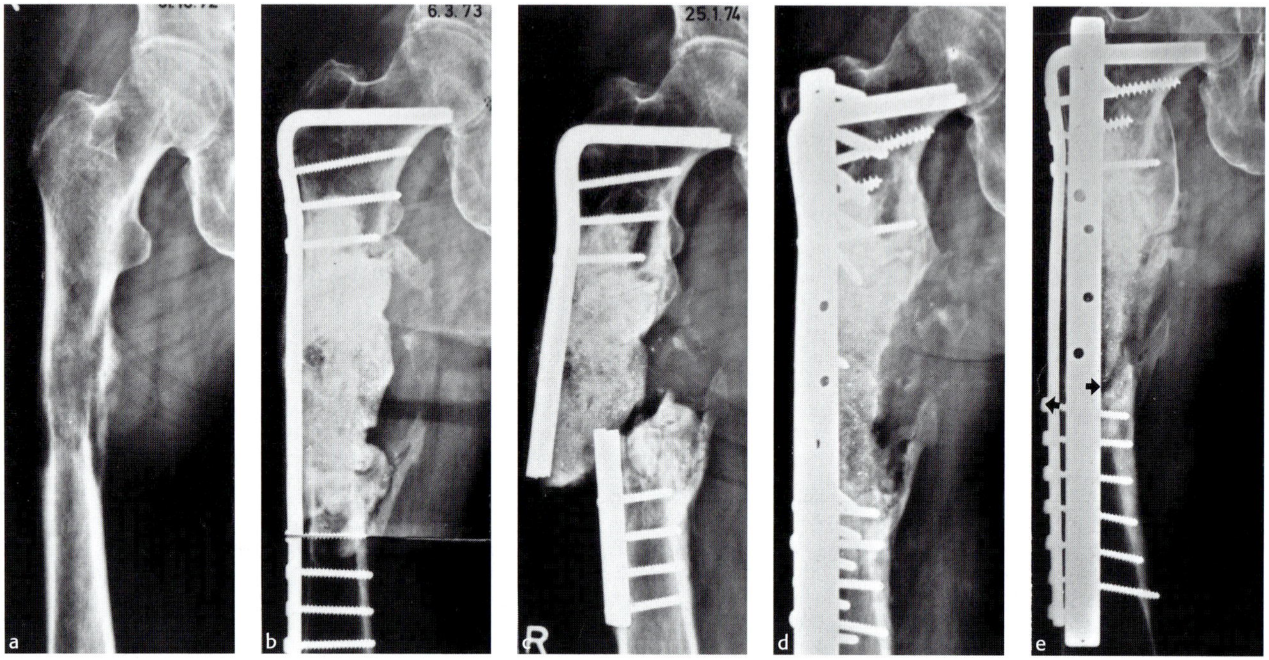

Fig. 7-36a–e Breast cancer metastases. Different policy of treatment.
The grafts are not incorporated into malignant tumor tissue. To offer the patient life quality for the limited life span, pure mechanical stability of the involved bone segment is strived for.

a Tumor metastases in the femur.

b 4 months after tumor mass resection and compound internal fixation with bone cement and tension-band plate.

c 15 months later: fatigue fracture through plate and bone cement.

d 1 month after re-stabilization with double plate.

e 5 1/2 months later: impending second breakdown of the fixation (arrows). The patient died 1 month later of generalized breast cancer metastatic disease.

5.5 Shaft of the tibia

Benign tumors are treated with excision, grafting, and stabilization. Bone loss after fracture and with infection is a much more serious and more frequent problem.

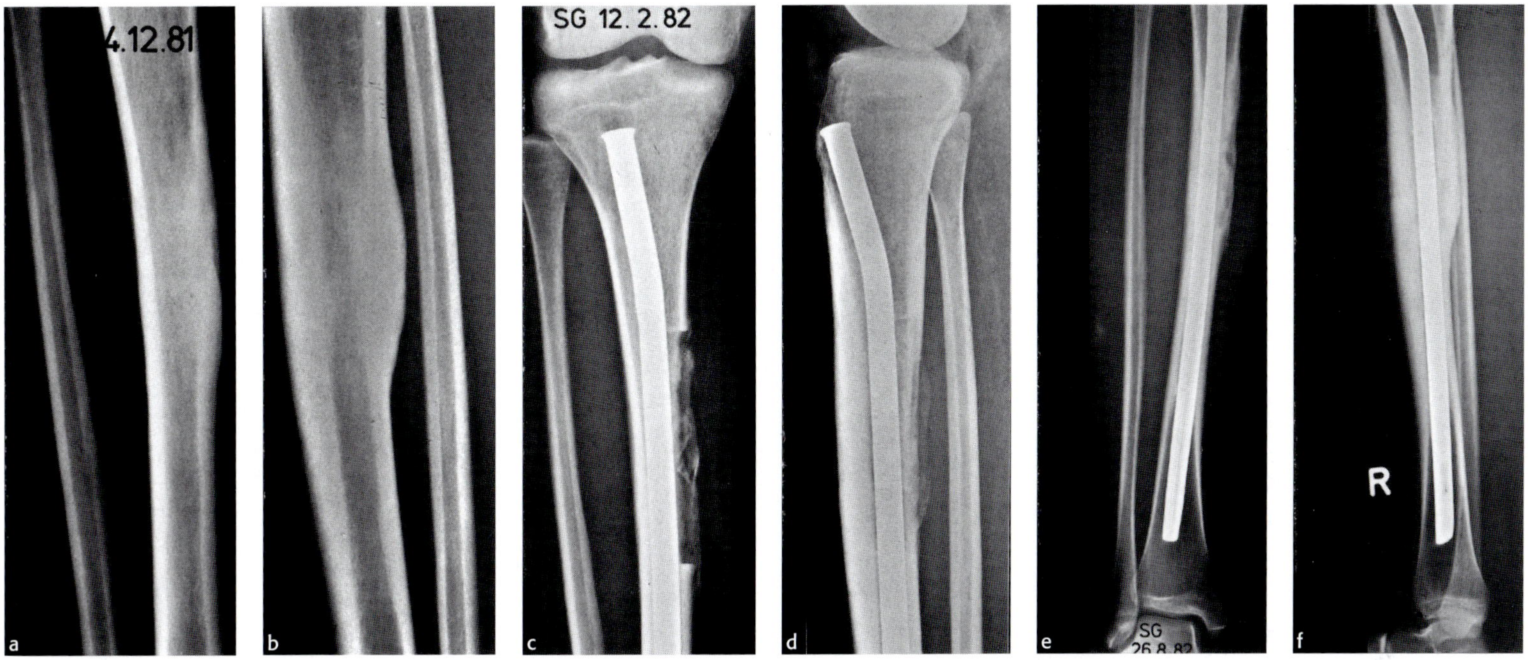

Fig. 7-37a–f Osteoid osteoma, eosinophilic granuloma of the diaphysis.

ab Posteromedial thickening of the tibial midshaft cortex.

cd Resection, grafting, protective nailing with an 8 mm slotted and gently reamed tibial nail.

ef 6 months after surgery and CAF, ie, weightbearing: grafts are solidly incorporated. The nail is now removed.

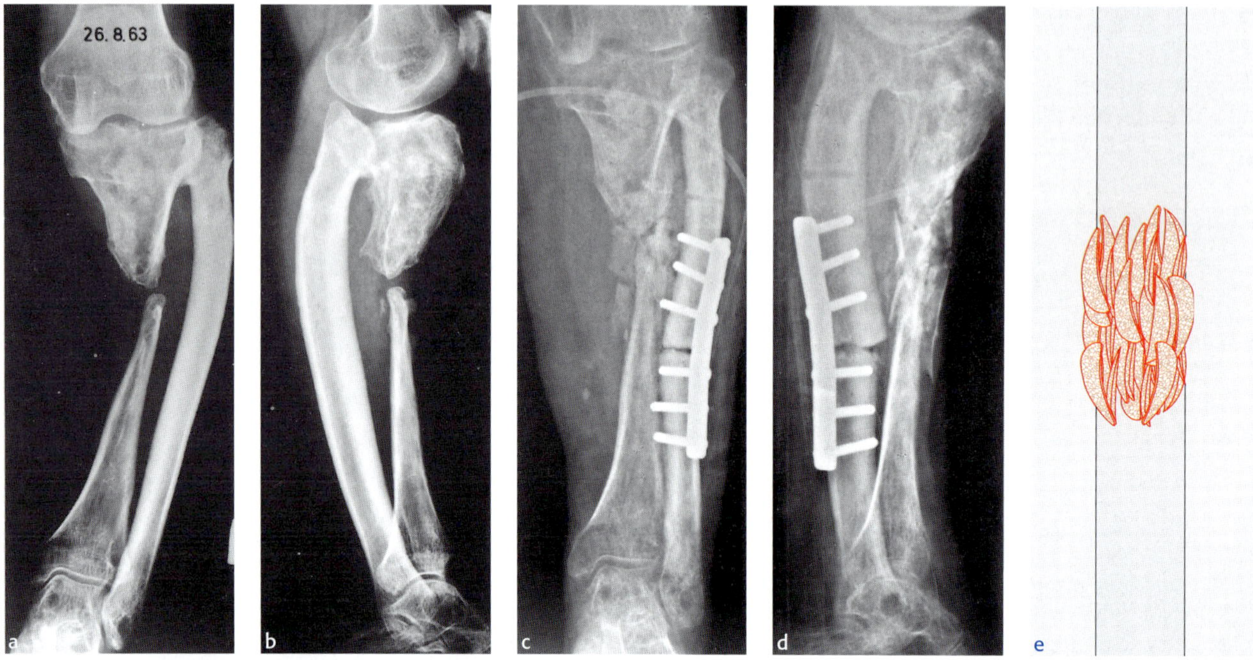

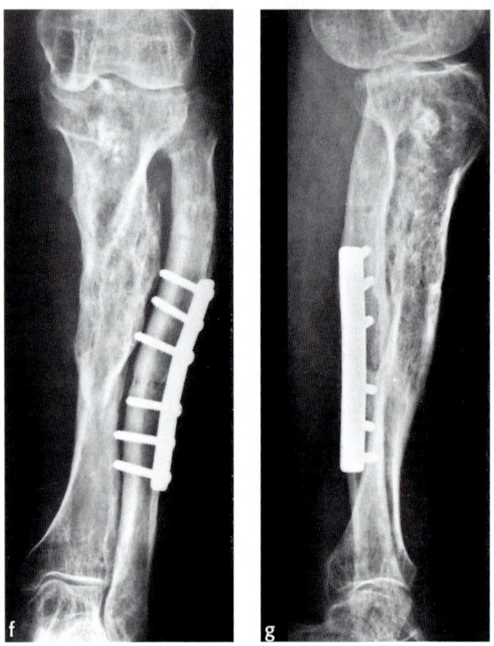

Fig. 7-38a–g Defect of the tibial diaphysis after fracture and infection 20 years ago, no current infection.

ab The starting situation for reconstruction: atrophic defect nonunion of the tibia. Secondary hypertrophy of the fibula with varus bowing for 20 years.

cd Reconstructive surgery: osteotomy of the fibula with correction of deformity. Grafting of the tibial defect.

e Technique of grafting with cancellous bone slivers.

fg 9-year follow-up: nonunion healed in 1 year. The grafts have since been remodeled into a solid tibia.

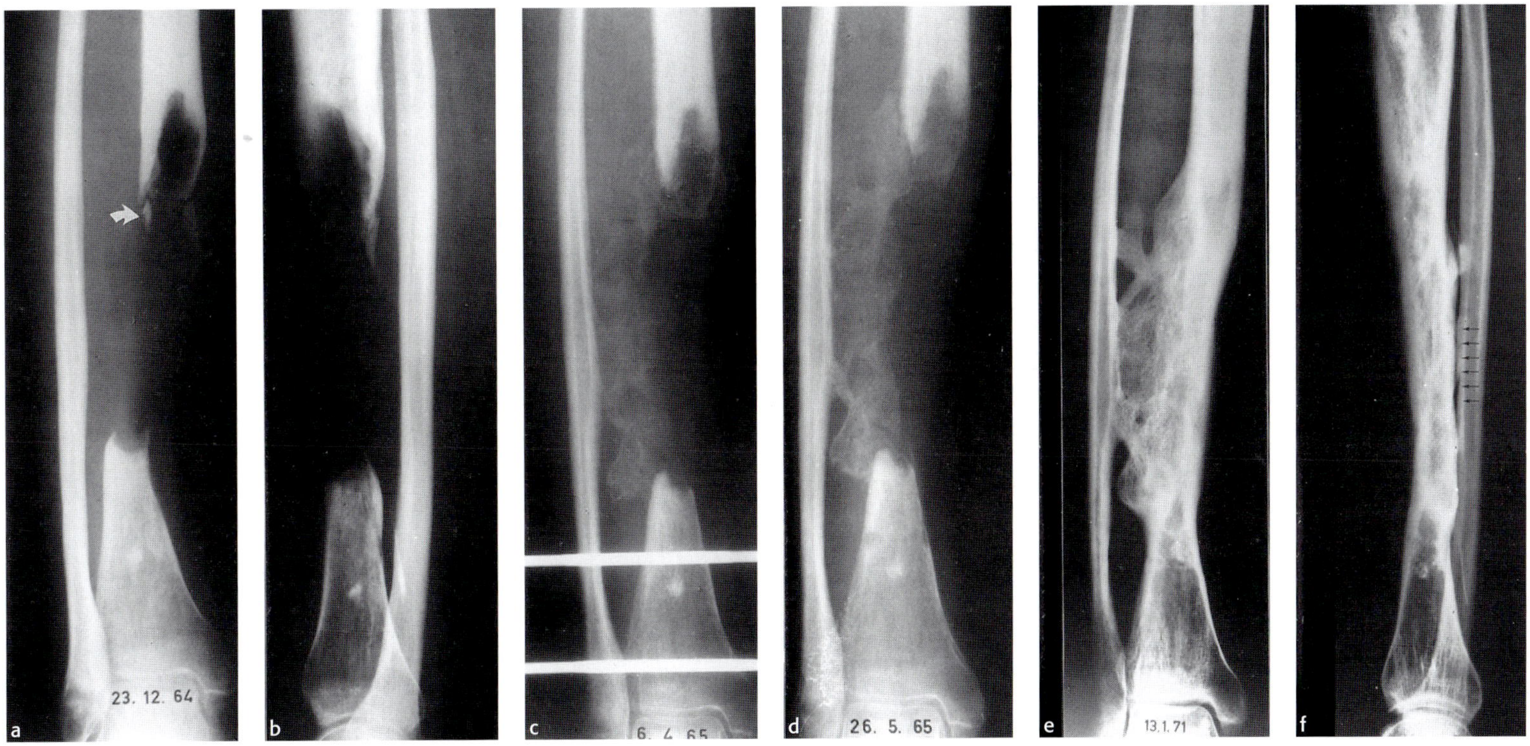

Fig. 7-39a–f Defect of tibial diaphysis after fracture and infection. Injury 5 years earlier.

ab The starting situation for reconstruction: atrophic defect nonunion of tibial shaft. Small sequester proximally, sinus discharging medially (arrow).

c 3 months after sequesterectomy, 2 1/2 months after bone grafting type fibula-pro tibia from Harmon approach (arrows).

d 5 months after surgery, immediately after removal of the external fixator, after CAF, ie, weightbearing: the grafts increase density and improve structure.

ef Late follow-up after 6 years: tibia is ‘remade’, fibula is again spontaneously mobile against the tibia (arrows).

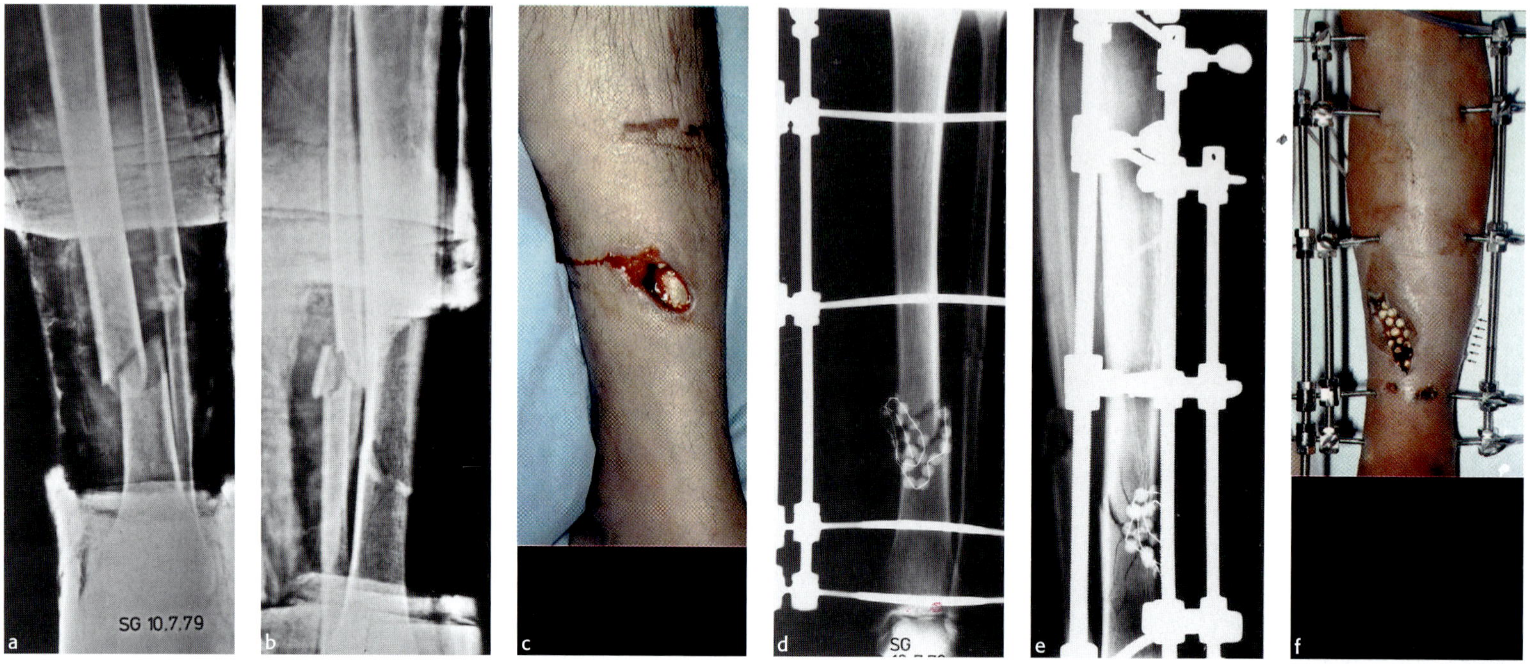

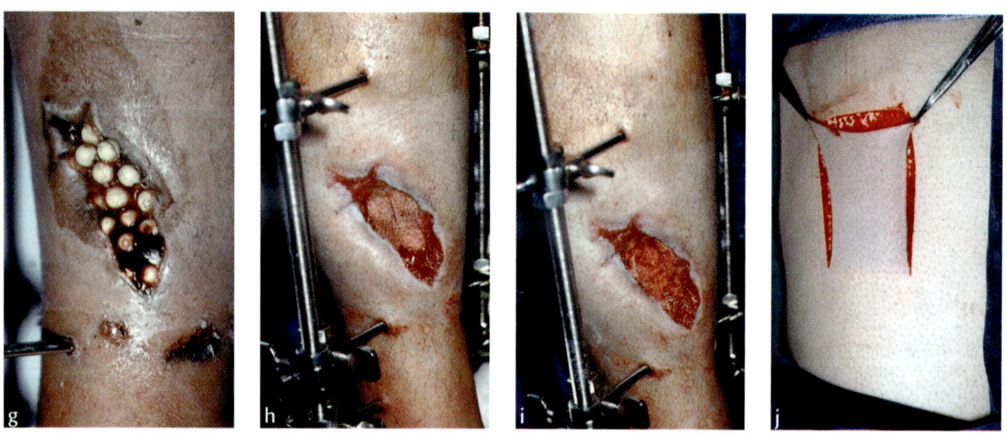

Fig. 7-40a–t Fresh infected open fracture grade 2. Open grafting.

ab The open fracture grade 2, 2 months ago abroad. The patient is now admitted.

c The infected fracture with skin defect.

de Rigid fixation with external fixator frame, debridement, Gentamycin beads.

f The open wound: wound with the beads is sealed with a radiolucent tape (arrow), the vacuum-drain was in situ for 10 days.

g 10 weeks after the debridement. The beads are removed, open cancelleous bone grafting is performed now.

h 1 week after open grafting, the grafts sealed with radiolucent tape.

i 3 weeks after grafting: grafts are vascularized under the radiolucent tape and therefore not infected.

j A split skin graft is taken.

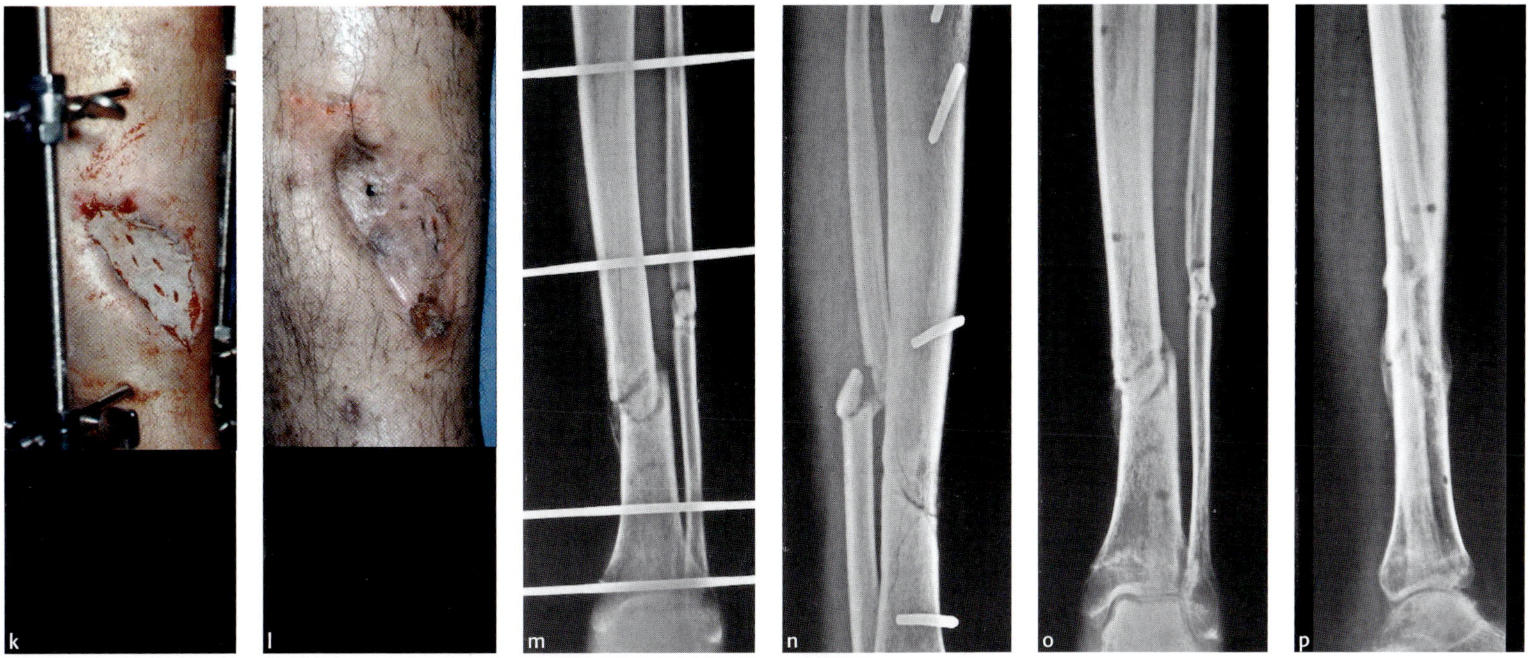

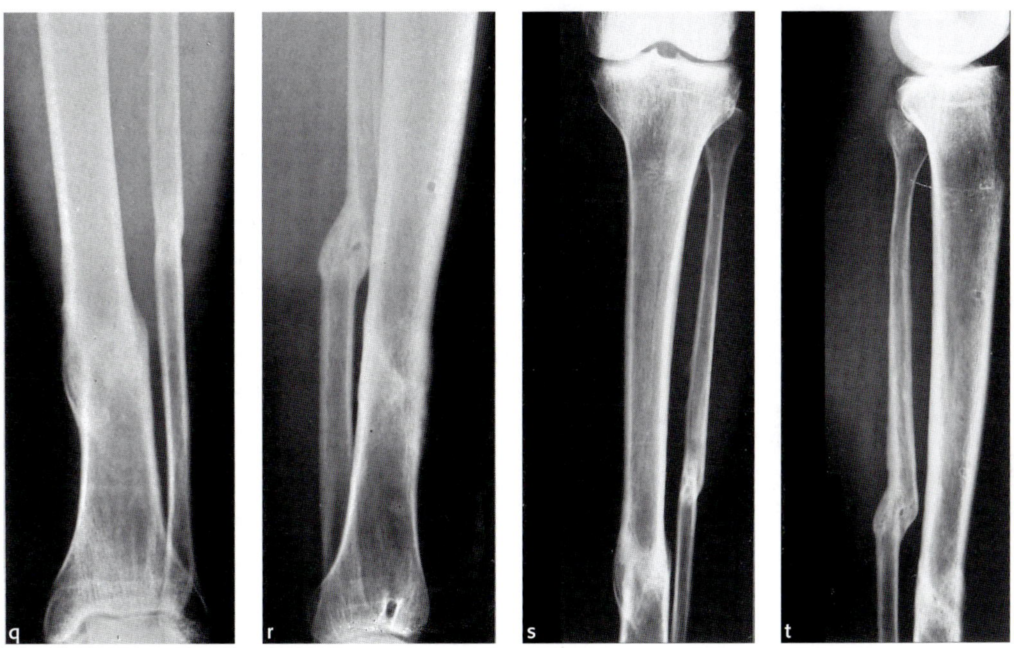

Fig. 7-40a–t cont.

k The graft is sutered into the open wound and covers the vascularized cancellous bone.

l 10 weeks since the beginning of the treatment of the open and infected fracture.

mn 3 months since admission of the patient at the time of removal of the external fixator, the fracture has started to consolidate. CAF, ie, weightbearing continues with a protective lower leg caliper.

op 1 month without external fixator, fracture healing is in progress.

qr 3 1/2 years after admission; fracture shows sound union.

st 18 years after beginning reconstruction; back to normal.

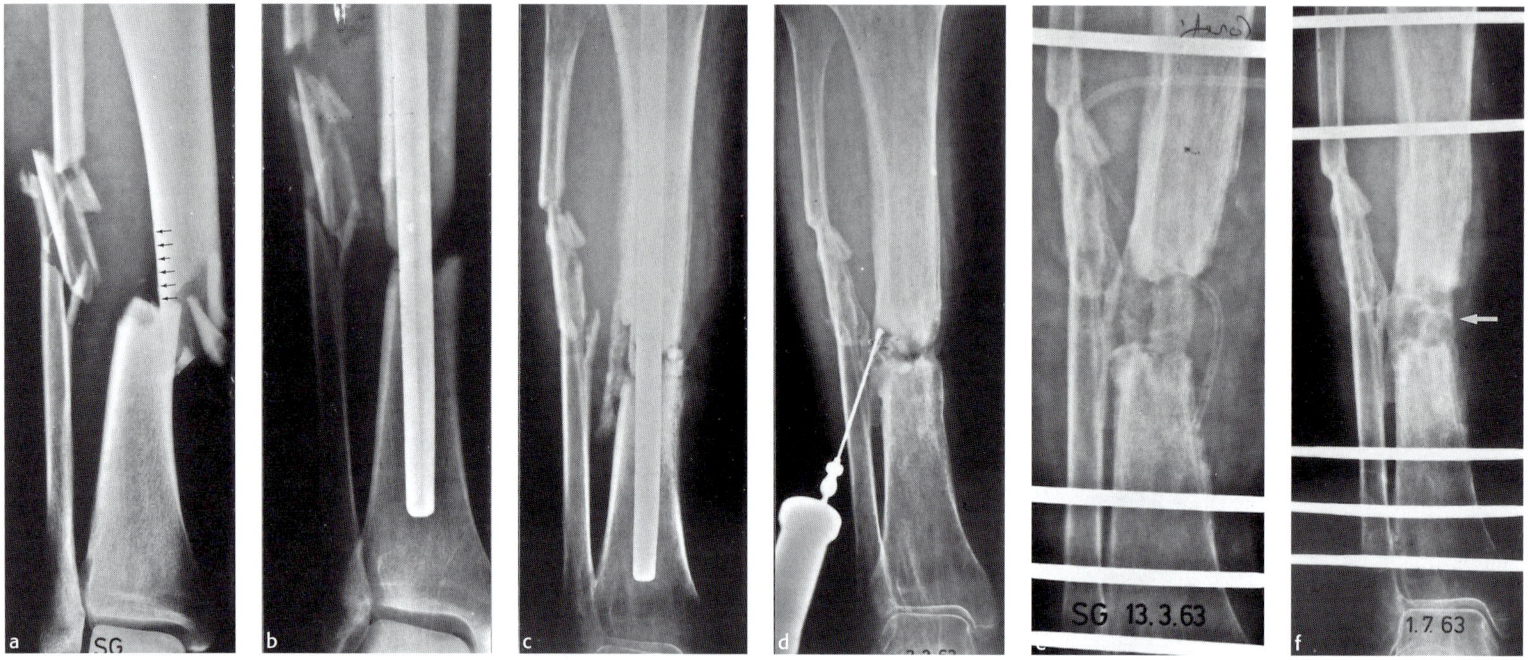

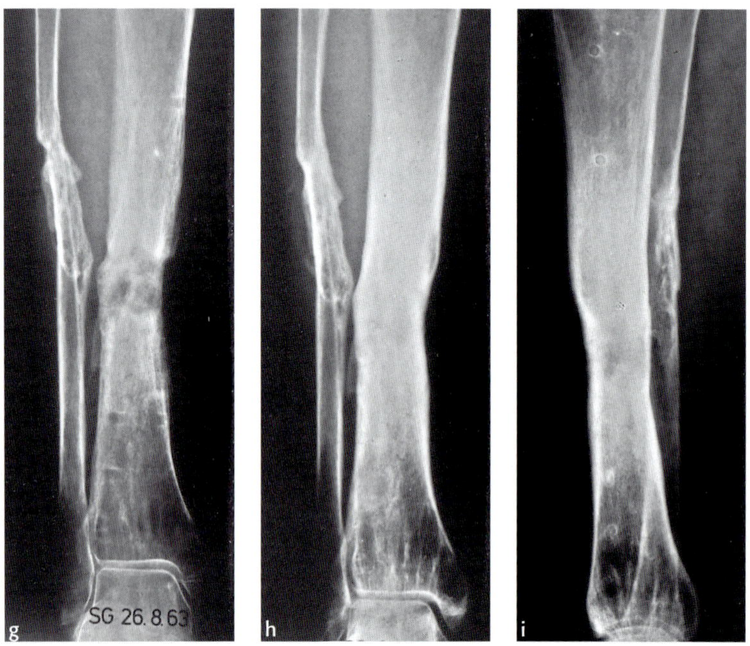

Fig. 7-41a–i Open fracture grade 3 followed by infection.

a The fracture grade 3 would be suitable for an external fixator and secondary bone grafting. The proximal fragment is stripped of periosteum, but the medullary blood supply is still present, as for the distal fragment. Note: periosteal stripping (arrows).

b The surgeon preferred nailing and removing small loose fragments. Distraction of the fragments caused dead space. Infection occurred.

c 7 months after the accident: infected nonunion.

d 18 months after the fracture, at admission: infected nonunion with sinus, with bone defect, with infection.

e A prestrained external fixator is applied, radical debridement is performed, massive corticocancellous iliac bone blocks are locked with compression of the external fixator.

f 3 1/2 months later after CAF, ie, partial progressive weightbearing: grafts are incorporated (arrow), external fixator is removed.

g 5 months since admission: tibia is solid. The patient walks with a protective caliper for another 1/2 year.

hi 3 years since admission and treatment of the infected nonunion: fracture healed, leg almost restored back to normal.

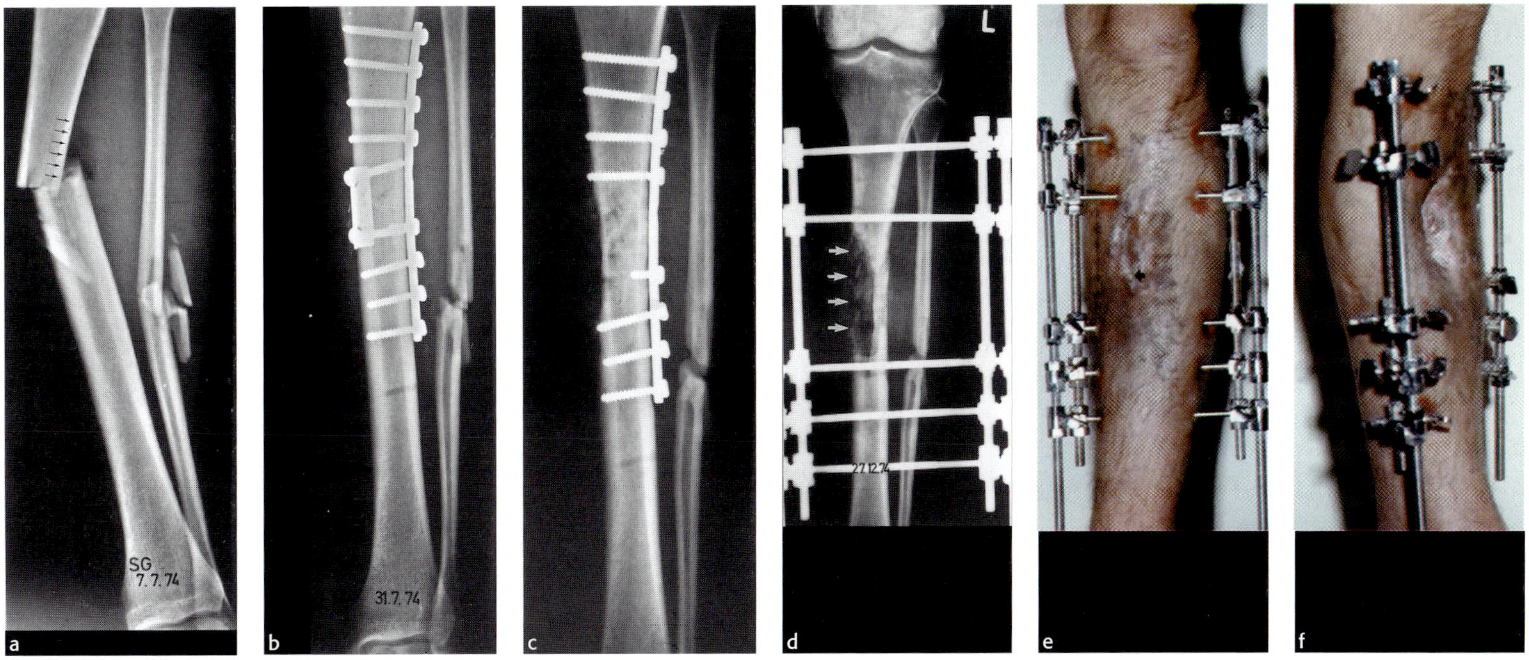

Fig. 7-42a–o Open fracture grade 1 followed by infection.

a The periosteum is extensively stripped from the proximal fragment (arrows), the medullary blood supply, however, is intact. An open reduction and external fixator would be the adequate primary treatment.

b The surgeon, however, prefered to extend periosteal stripping by double plating. Infection followed. The medial plate was removed and then the patient admitted.

c On admission: infected fracture with open wound over the tibia medially.

d The first step of reconstruction: external fixator frame, meticulous debridement, the wound left open. 3 weeks later: grafting (arrows) from a posteromedial approach. The open wound improved with granulations that were covered with small Reverdin patch grafts.

ef 2 months later, the open wound is almost closed (arrow) and finally closed after local sequesterectomy. External fixator in situ with CAF, ie, weightbearing for a total of 1/2 year.

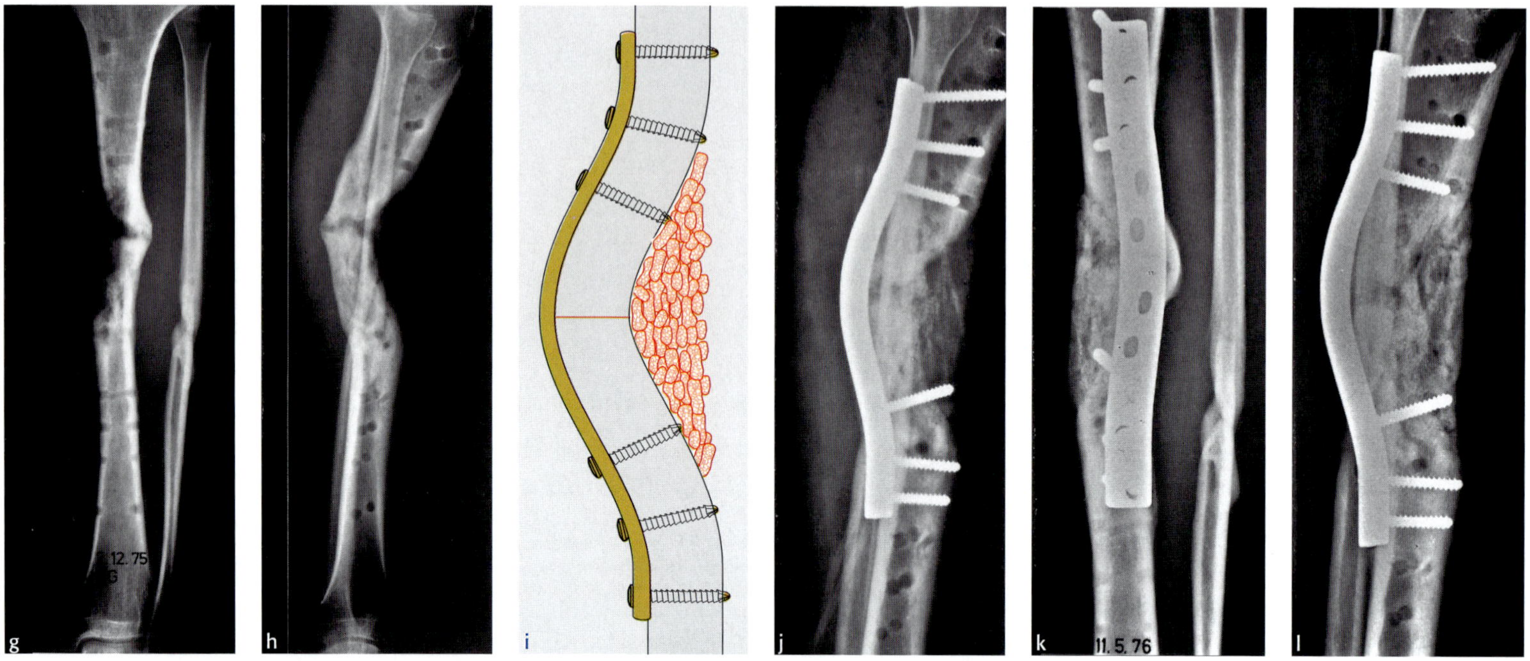

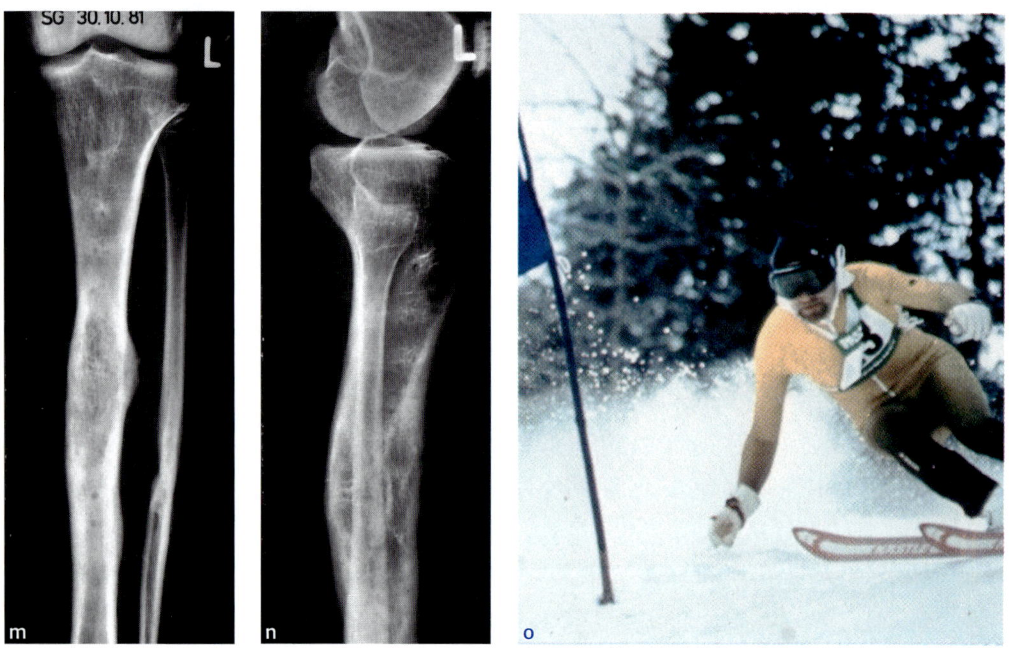

Fig. 7-42a–o cont.

gh 1 year after admission, after external fixator, grafting, caliper, CAF: the autogenous graft has improved regarding mass and structure. A vital eutrophic nonunion remains. No infection present.

i The next step of treatment of the nonunion: defect grafted and bridged with a wave plate.

j The treatment of the uninfected nonunion 1 year after admission.

kl 5 months later: remodeling in process.

mn 7-year follow-up, 4 years after plate removal: back to normal.

o The patient performing competitive downhill skiing again.

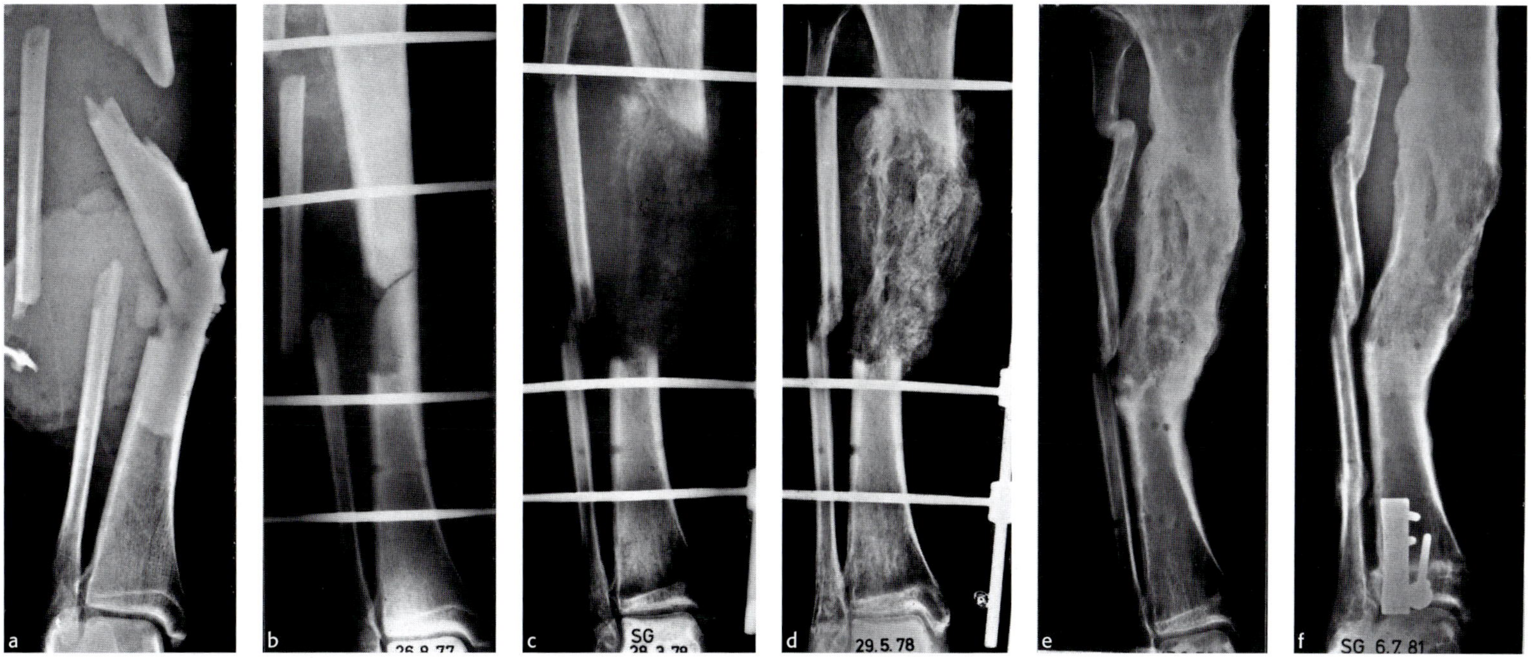

Fig. 7-43a–j Open segmental fracture grade 3 followed by sequestration and infection.

a The midshaft segment is devascularized.

b Deprived of periosteal and medullary blood supply, the necrotic segment suffers infection and is removed 2 months after the injury. With a Picot-flap the skin loss on the front of the lower leg is covered.

c 7 months after injury: successful skin coverage allowed bone grafting from a posteromedial approach 2 months ago.

d 5 months after bone transplant and CAF, ie, weightbearing with a cane: impressive remodeling of the grafts. Removal of external fixator, patient's leg is protected with a caliper for 1/2 year.

e 18 month since grafting: a new tibia has developed.

f Varus deformity is corrected with a supramalleolar closed wedge valgus osteotomy.

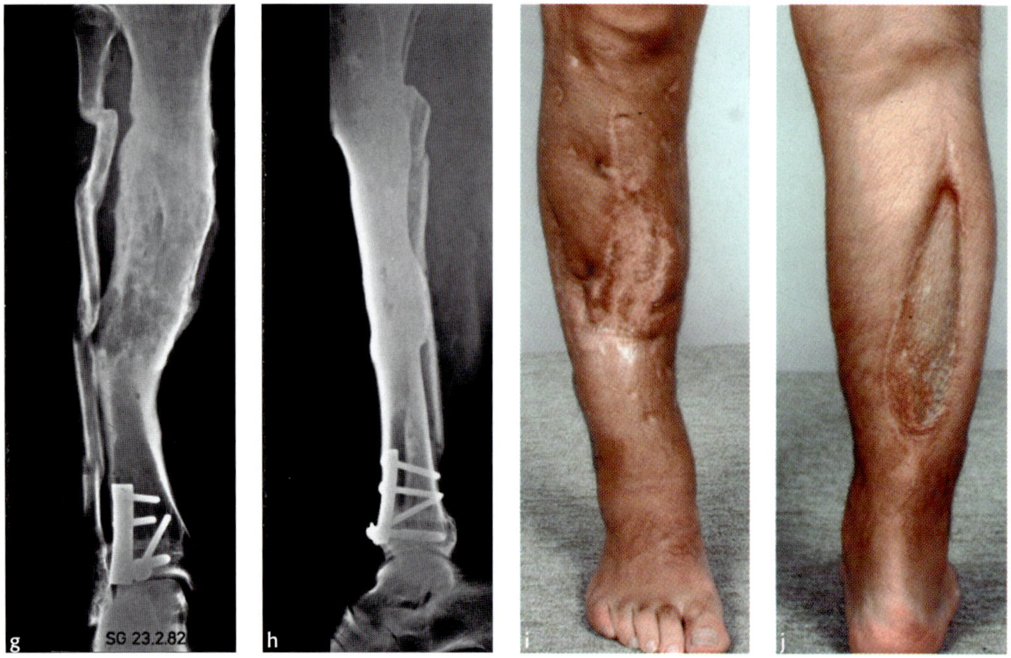

Fig. 7-43a–j cont.

gh 4 years 4 months after the injury: reconstructed tibia.

ij With the Picot-flap, the skin defect on the front of the lower leg was closed, the incision of the calf covered 4 weeks later with a split-skin mesh graft. The unsightly calf was finally corrected with two sequential excisions of the mesh graft area.

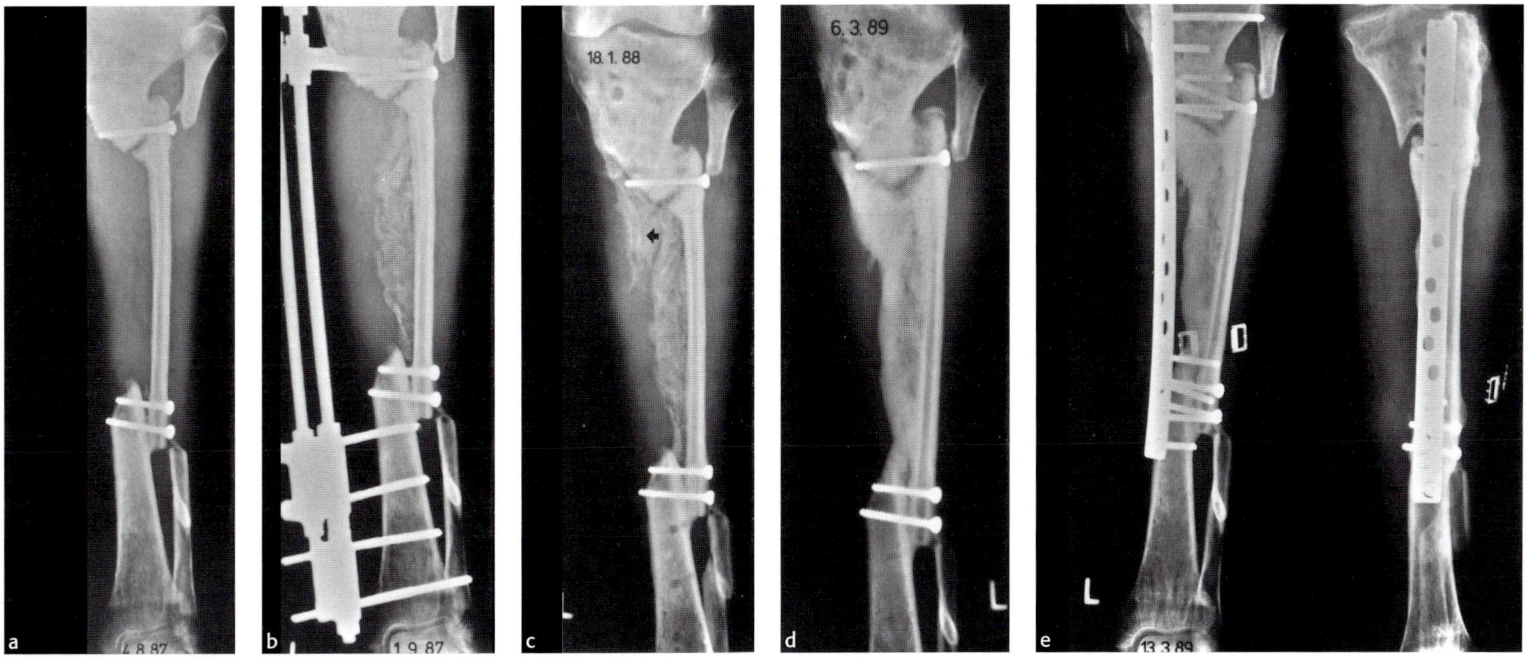

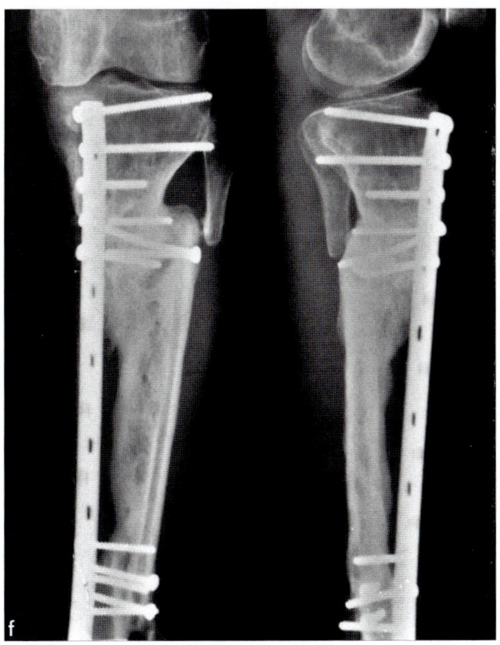

Fig. 7-44a–i Repercussions after open fracture grade 2, followed by infection, by sequestrectomy and by fibula-pro tibia shift. Amputation recommended.

a The starting situation on admission from abroad where the patient had rejected the proposal of amputation.

b First step of reconstruction: unilateral prestrained external fixator. 3 weeks later, first session of bone grafting along Harmon approach.

c 6 weeks later a second bone transplant was performed from a posteromedial approach (arrow). The external fixator was left 3 1/2 months. CAF, ie, weightbearing is continued with a caliper.

d 18 months since beginning of reconstruction: grafts are remodeled, but the nonunion has persisted.

ef A heavy bridging plate is applied subcutaneously. The stabilized nonunion consolidated thereafter.

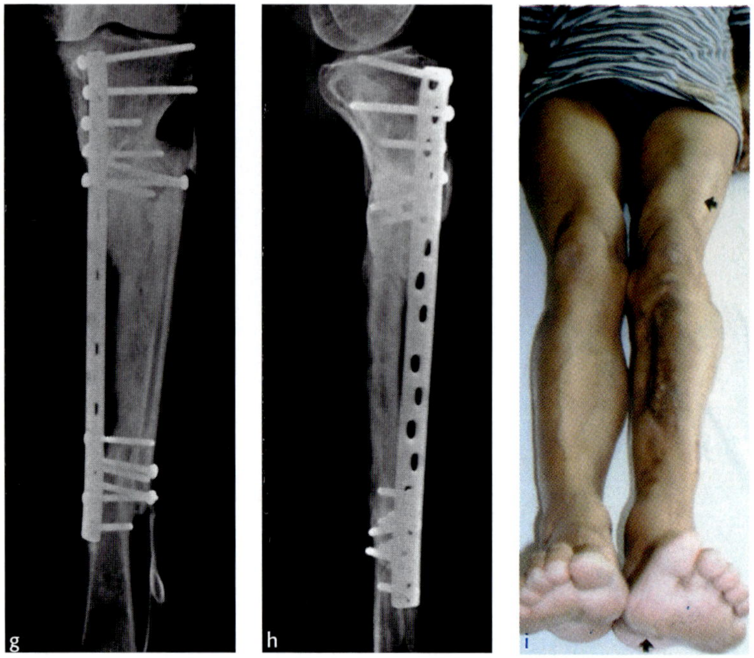

Fig. 7-44a–i cont.

ghi Late follow-up 12 years after admission: The leg is functioning to the patient's satisfaction. Note: normal leg axis, normal horny skin of the foot sole (arrow), and symmetrically developed quadriceps muscles (arrow), which shows the benefit of symmetrical use of the legs.

6 Conclusions and summary

Autogenous bone grafts, transplanted to well-vascularized surroundings are integrated under strain and stress of function in an amazingly short time. Uninfected defects, without malignancy, restore faster and better, the better the stability with internal or external fixation. Infected defects first need debridement and mechanical stability, as a rule with an external fixator. Grafting is safest when performed along a sound route, typically in the lower leg, where skin coverage is often deficient. In certain situations, open cancelleous bone grafting in the medial defect is possible. Otherwise skin coverage precedes defect compensation.

On the femur or other sites, grafts are accepted in the presence of mild infection under the condition of local stability and blood perfusion of the surrounding tissues (muscle).

Bone transplant is mostly single, or occasionally—when needed—sequentially staged.

The healing times with autogenous grafting are short—in my opinion, shorter than with other techniques.

Morbidity at the graft donor site is minimal when the described rules are observed.

Local infections are avoided when the entire reconstruction of bone defects is performed under sterile enclosure conditions or at least under otherwise maximal aseptic precautions (see chapter Asepsis).

Epilogue

Since its foundation, the AO has developed in size and structure from a small group to a worldwide global organisation. However, the AO's basic principles of anatomical reduction, rigid fixation, care for blood supply, and functional after treatment, are not followed generally.

In 43 years of the AO, two tendencies have been observed:

1. The school of St. Gallen: Rigid fixation is asked for all joint fractures and for many shaft fractures. Operative spine fracture treatment with open reduction and internal fixation (ORIF) was an early activity. Plate fixations were refined, as were those with external fixators. Since 1967, the highest attention has been paid to the blood supply of bone and all other tissues, which has required more slender fixation than was originally done for 'biological' as well as bridging fixation with plates or external fixators.
   The St. Gallen method of fracture care has taken advantage of the sterile enclosure facility from 1970 until now. Sir John Charnley, whom I had the good fortune to meet in 1960 in England and thereafter repeatedly in Whrightington, with the International Hip Society and on many other professional occasions, deserves highest esteem for his work on:
   - Closed treatment of common fractures
   - Compression arthrodesis
   - Total hip reconstruction
   - Sterile enclosure, greenhouse technology

   The safety from wound contamination and infection is why we, in St. Gallen, had no motive to refrain from open reduction and internal fixation. Open reduction and internal fixation became ORI(E)F, where E stood for economic.

   The MINIMAX principle grew together with the original AO principles in mind and with the goal of restoring the status 'back to normal'.

   This book focuses on important aspects of the St. Gallen method of fracture care. This way of solving problems is not forgotten by all those who were trained in our institution. Some of them have encouraged me to write 'The book' that documents one branch of the developing AO.

2. The official AO, mastered by more and more Unfall-Chirurgen, ie, accident surgeons, developed fracture care with their non-orthopedic understanding. They 'bridge' not only complex, but also banal fractures with 'sophisticated' nails and plates. Anatomical reconstruction is not striven for—only bone healing—which is what the bone could do without any surgery at all.

I end this book with an expression of thanks to the AO Founders and to my teachers M.E. Müller, M. Allgöwer, H. Willenegger, R. Schneider. They accepted me not only as a junior colleague in AO teaching, in the AO Technical Commission, but also as co-author of all the AO Manuals under their leadership.

Bernhard G. Weber
Fall 2002

Index

Page numbers in italics refer to figures

C

D

E

F

G

H

Q

R

S

T

U

V

W

X

YZ